Praise for *Asking for a Pregnant Friend*

"*Asking for a Pregnant Friend* is so brave, essential, and thorough. Bailey Gaddis's writing is conversational yet poignant, revealing yet compassionate, and bold and feminine. To have answers to these sensitive and vulnerable questions — given with such care, intelligence, humor, and practicality — is absolutely crucial for all mothers, whether it's their first pregnancy or fourth. As a mother to two children, I wish I'd had this book as my ally earlier! It's going to become my go-to gift for every expecting family."

— **Rachel Kolar McCord**, writer and artist

"Guilt and horror, be gone! Nothing you are feeling or experiencing on this wildly life-altering journey is wrong, weird, or shameful. Bailey Gaddis sets it *all* on the table and unpacks it with thoughtful care, honesty, kindness, and a rich (and comedic) personal experience. *Asking for a Pregnant Friend* is a treasure trove of information on pregnancy, childbirth, and early motherhood, delivered in the most modern, supportive, and encouraging format. Bailey's pitch-perfect, sage, and sure-footed advice feels like it's coming from the best friend you wish you had."

— **Kristen Vadas**, writer and producer

"*Asking for a Pregnant Friend* is a fun, relatable book that will resonate with moms and moms-to-be around the world."

— **Nita Landry, MD, OB-GYN**, cohost of *The Doctors*

"*Asking for a Pregnant Friend* fills a void as the wise, funny, witty, and commonsense mama mentor that we all need during pregnancy but is so difficult to find in our society. This book is laugh-out-loud funny and relatable for anyone who has found themselves pregnant and questioning what on earth is going on with their body and emotions."

— **Brittany Sanders**, artist (and mama)

"Bailey Gaddis isn't just an engaging writer; she brings a wealth of experience in pregnancy, birthing, and motherhood to this book. She dares to go to the places that every woman wonders about. Let her hold your hand and lead you there. You will feel more at peace after you have navigated your own wilderness."

— **Meghan Rudd Van Alstine, PhD**, psychologist

"*Asking for a Pregnant Friend* is the book mamas-to-be have been waiting for! Bailey Gaddis's candid, loving, and no-BS voice will soothe and calm you before, during, and after your pregnancy. This is the book I wish I'd had for each of my three pregnancies. Reading it now lets the thrice-pregnant me feel relieved, informed, and taken care of by my dear friend Bailey. A must-read for any person considering having a child."

— **Carrie Ruscheinsky**, actor and producer

"Bailey Gaddis has an instinctual, profound talent in making you feel empowered with her words of wisdom. This is a must-read that will give you the confidence and the insight you need as a first-time mother-to-be."

— **Alanna Ubach**, actor in *Coco*, *Legally Blonde*, and *Girlfriends' Guide to Divorce*

"In *Asking for a Pregnant Friend*, Bailey Gaddis has the best way of speaking the unspeakable and connecting us to the psychological aspects of pregnancy, which is vital for all mothers and moms-to-be to better prepare for and endure this monumental experience. I highly recommend reading this book!"

— **Jennifer Ollestad**, psychotherapist

"Bailey Gaddis has written the book every woman of childbearing age wants to curl up with and devour. This is the book that answers the juiciest questions, concerns, and what-the-hecks, and it's written with the warmth of a knowing, open, hilarious friend. This book will liberate so many mothers."

— **Sophie Ward**, author of *Heart of Bold* and founder of Milk + Seed

"*Asking for a Pregnant Friend* tackles the most pressing (and sometimes embarrassing) questions about pregnancy and birth with striking thoughtfulness and honesty. Bailey Gaddis is a bright and refreshing voice in a sea of predictable pregnancy resources. I will be pointing my expecting friends in Bailey's direction!"

— **Marisa Belger**, coauthor of *The First Forty Days: The Essential Art of Nourishing the New Mother*

Asking for
a Pregnant Friend

Also by Bailey Gaddis

*Feng Shui Mommy: Creating Balance and Harmony
for Blissful Pregnancy, Childbirth, and Motherhood*

Asking for a Pregnant Friend

101 Answers to Questions
Women Are Too Embarrassed to Ask
about Pregnancy, Childbirth, and Motherhood

Bailey Gaddis

New World Library
Novato, California

New World Library
14 Pamaron Way
Novato, California 94949

Illustrations by Amanda Sandoval
Text design by Tona Pearce Myers

Library of Congress Cataloging-in-Publication Data

Names: Gaddis, Bailey, author.
Title: Asking for a pregnant friend : 101 answers to questions women are too embarrassed
    to ask about pregnancy, childbirth, and motherhood / Bailey Gaddis.
Description: Novato, California : New World Library, [2021] | Includes bibliographical
    references and index. | Summary: "Frank girlfriend talk and expert advice about
    everything women experience in pregnancy, childbirth, and early motherhood,
    including postpartum concerns"-- Provided by publisher.
Identifiers: LCCN 2021005124 (print) | LCCN 2021005125 (ebook) | ISBN 9781608687176
    (paperback) | ISBN 9781608687183 (epub)
Subjects: LCSH: Pregnancy--Miscellanea. | Childbirth--Miscellanea. | Motherhood--
    Miscellanea.
Classification: LCC RG551 .G34 2021 (print) | LCC RG551 (ebook) | DDC 618.2--dc23
LC record available at https://lccn.loc.gov/2021005124
LC ebook record available at https://lccn.loc.gov/2021005125

First printing, June 2021
ISBN 978-1-60868-717-6
Ebook ISBN 978-1-60868-718-3
Printed in Canada on 100% postconsumer-waste recycled paper

New World Library is proud to be a Gold Certified Environmentally Responsi-ble Publisher. Publisher certification awarded by Green Press Initiative.

10   9   8   7   6   5   4   3   2   1

*To Eric and Hudson — thank you for loving the whole me,
weird bits and all.*

Whenever I see a taboo, I just think that's something we need to drag screaming out into the light and discuss. Because taboos are where our fears live, and taboos are the things that keep us tiny. Particularly for women.

— CAITLIN MORAN

Contents

Mothering 181

Introduction

Hey, mama. I see you. I see the questions you push away in embarrassment at your prenatal appointments. I see the wariness you feel over the bombardment of emotions you've been navigating as your belly blooms. I see the dark thoughts you have about motherhood. I see you doing everything you can to lead a healthy, happy, and informed pregnancy but still feeling confused, like there's a big chunk of information and support missing from the sea of guidance on pregnancy, childbirth, and early motherhood. I see you wondering if you're the only one who feels this way.

I see you because I am you. When I was pregnant with my son Hudson, there were so many deep, murky layers of the baby-making journey I found perplexing and, in many ways, shame-inducing. This confusion and shame stuck because I didn't think I could talk to anyone about what I was experiencing. I felt like I was hiding. Hiding my insatiable lust. Hiding my kinky dreams. Hiding my swollen labia (you're welcome, world). Hiding my "Should I have gotten an abortion?" question. On the outside I looked like a bloated, fairly content, baby-grower with shiny hair. On the inside, I had pulled out all that shiny hair and was cowering in a corner while judgy fingers pointed at me.

To soothe my fried nerves and scrambled brain, I tried to secretly find candid answers to my questions, especially those society has labeled taboo.

(I also developed a "Clear Browsing History" obsession.) I thought that if I could just find an online resource or book that named what I was feeling and told me it was normal, I might stop feeling like I was broken. But I didn't find it. I found only watered-down answers to the G-rated cousins of my questions, and lots of books that told me how to glow during pregnancy, not die during childbirth, and breastfeed during motherhood. Sure, they were helpful, but they weren't what I was looking for. And so my pregnant brain logically assumed everyone else just magically knows about the super strange physical changes of pregnancy, that no one else has morbid, scary thoughts about childbirth, and that all the other ladies have the whole postpartum sex thing figured out.

I didn't discover how wrong I was until I started teaching childbirth preparation classes and my clients pulled me aside to ask questions. Their questions were my questions, and I was thrilled. I wasn't alone! I wasn't broken. Hearing other women name many of the unspeakable queries I had on my journey into motherhood emboldened me to start asking physicians and mental health specialists these questions. The answers I received were fascinating and liberating. Turns out there were totally legit reasons for every thought, physical phenomenon, and emotion that had made me feel different or unfit for motherhood. I started adding this information to my classes, and the response has been awesome. When I talk about how orgasms during pregnancy won't hurt the baby, or what all the weird smells from all the places mean, women light up (and men often blush and shuffle off to the bathroom). They're getting answers to the questions they were praying someone else would ask. But the coolest part is, my bringing up these topics often gives them the confidence to share their experiences with said topics. We get into some really interesting conversations.

These moments of sharing and connection in my classes caused me to become That Lady at dinner parties, conferences, back-to-school nights — and heck, pretty much every other social situation — asking unsuspecting women about all the stuff they never thought they could talk about during pregnancy and beyond. Sometimes people slowly back away, but most of the time they open up.

I've learned that we're part of a massive secret society. There are thousands of us slipping away from prying eyes to scan chat rooms and forums, flip through books, and make our fingers numb with Google searches as we look for answers to the same things you came to this book wondering about — maps to the same paths you're wandering. But I don't want you to feel like tracking down answers is a full-time job. I want you to have all the answers in one place, from a friendly, accurate source. I also want those answers to come from a friend who would never judge or make you feel like a weirdo for asking that "TMI" question.

So…can we be friends? Can I be the person who never judges you and is always up for talking about sex, smells, scary thoughts, feeling like you want to lock your partner out of the house, and all the other stuff we deal with as we make, birth, and nurture babies?

It's my hope that during this friendship you will be freed from many of the barriers to a joy-filled journey into motherhood. I also hope that this friendship will bolster your confidence so that you can begin speaking more freely about the "underbelly" of your motherhood experiences IRL. And I hope you start finding women you trust and talking with them about the things they're also worrying about or confused by. But hey, even if you just talk to this book, I hope the experience fills you with relief, and compassion for your amazing self, who is doing the best she can.

Where Did These Questions Come From?

These questions have been sourced from women just like you over the past five years. Even when I wasn't aware that I was collecting these questions, I was collecting these questions. They've come in whispers after childbirth classes, from girlfriends who look over their shoulder at the café to make sure no one is listening, or from my YouTube viewers and social media buddies who email their questions because they don't want them seen on public forums. And when the idea for the book was sparked, I began asking everyone who would talk to me what their hidden questions were during the wild entry into motherhood. People talked, fascinating discussions were had, and juicy questions emerged.

Why Are These Questions So Embarrassing?

The questions are embarrassing because they require that we come to terms with the fact that we don't have it all together, they force us to develop a new relationship with our bodies and sexuality, and they often uncover emotional or mental challenges. This is big stuff. It's stuff we innately shy away from because it's usually really uncomfortable to take an honest look at who we are and how pregnancy and motherhood are changing us. Sometimes we shy away from these questions so fiercely we don't even know they're our questions until we see or hear them.

But the beauty of shared questions and experiences is that they often wipe away the grime of embarrassment. Think about it: If you're walking down the street and you trip in front of a group of people, you're probably going to feel embarrassed. But if another person trips just as you're getting up, much of that embarrassment will dissolve because, hey look, you're not the only one who trips! It's all good! That's what this book is, all us ladies tripping through pregnancy, childbirth, and early motherhood together, then helping one another up.

Who Is Answering These Questions?

Mostly me: Bailey Gaddis. I'm a mother, the author of *Feng Shui Mommy: Creating Balance and Harmony for Blissful Pregnancy, Childbirth, and Motherhood*, a childbirth preparation educator, birth and postpartum doula, and certified hypnotherapist. As I answered the 101 questions in this book, I also drew on the experience of midwives, OB-GYNs, and doulas I've worked with over the years, and my lady buddy, Meghan Rudd Van Alstine, PhD, who is a licensed psychologist. Insights from peer-reviewed studies were also a big piece of the puzzle. I bundled all this wisdom together into a book of science, intuition, and experience-based guidance for ladies who are ready to be liberated from those taboo curiosities and crippling fears that keep them up at night.

So here they are, the juicy and totally legit things a woman would only ask that treasured friend who never, ever judges. The questions some women get brave enough to ask online but are then flayed by trolls about and never ask again. Welcome to the first step in leading a shame-free and super empowered journey into motherhood.

Pregnancy

It's happened. The miracle of life has been sparked, and it now spawns surprise flatulence, sore boobs, all the feels, all the time, and questions... lots of questions.

This is an intense time. You're facing massive physical and emotional changes, and people are dropping endless opinions on you. These opinions can be annoying, helpful, or completely terrifying, but no matter what they trigger, they're often lacking a key element: information that answers your deeper questions — the questions you might be too embarrassed to even think.

During pregnancy I got so bummed when people would share stories and opinions and none of them addressed the stuff that was waking me up at three in the morning. No one shared their crippling fears of stillbirth, strange sexual urges, or concerns that emotions toward a partner weren't just hormones but a sign of impending divorce. No one brought that stuff up, so I assumed I was a weirdo.

I've since discovered that while I am a weirdo in many ways, those thoughts and physical reactions to pregnancy didn't make me "other"; they made me part of a sisterhood also consumed with thoughts, fears, and physical idiosyncrasies they rarely or never talk about. The questions and answers in this book were crafted to give that pregnant sisterhood a voice, and a starting point for discussing these topics.

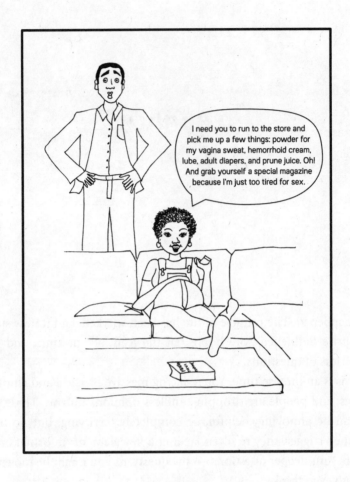

Relationships

1. I'm really sick of everyone talking to me only about pregnancy, childbirth, and babies. How can I still have conversations about other aspects of my life and be seen as more than a pregnant woman?

Talk about an identity shift, right?! One day you're viewed as a woman unique for her special sauce of personality traits, talents, and interests, then the next day your belly is blooming and most people lump you into the pregnancy/mommy crew, assuming you just want to talk about labor positions and the merits of cloth diapers over disposables. It's frustrating. And sometimes it's identity crisis–inducing. Most women already have that little voice, constantly worrying about how they'll change as they wander into motherhood, so it's understandable that they freak when folks seem to stop perceiving them as dynamic individuals and see only the generic "mom." (I don't care who you are, you're not a generic mom — you're a badass individual.)

But before we start ragging on those nameless folks, it's important to note that most people don't actually think of you as a generic mom; they are simply latching on to something about you they can relate to. More than almost anything, humans want to connect and feel understood, so when we see someone showing visible signs of something we have experience with, we want to talk about that thing. I'll bet that if people find out you're an architect (for example), and they have a passion for design, they'll happily shift the conversation.

It's also common for women to feel guilty about not wanting to always talk about pregnancy, birth, and the mamahood when they're in the thick of those experiences. Some feel like it's a betrayal of the baby to be irked when someone asks yet again whether you're planning on having a vaginal birth. But let it really sink in: you have every right to feel like you're more than a vessel for new life — because you absolutely are. You are a well-rounded woman who will be a better mother because you are committed to holding on to the things that make you feel like you. A dedication to the nourishment of your whole self will teach your child that they also deserve a life in which their personal interests and needs matter.

What to do

When someone starts chatting you up about everything your belly makes them think of and you're not feeling the mommy-talk, try one of the following:

- **Come up with a go-to question or response for changing the subject.** For example, you can describe how pregnancy is impacting your career, or how you're concerned motherhood will change your interests. This will hopefully inspire the other person to start talking about similar experiences, allowing you to learn what their interests are and giving you golden material for a new topic of conversation. "Oh wow, so you worked in the circus before you became a parent? Did you know the bearded lady?"
- **Straight-up tell them you don't feel like talking about birth or babies.** "You know what? I'm usually so down to talk baby stuff, but I feel like that's all I've been going on about lately. Can we talk about something else? Maybe some Bachelor Nation gossip?"

Besides navigating tricky conversations, it's also good to remind *yourself* that you have many fascinating layers. So add the following to your to-do list:

- **Commit to putting yourself in situations that stimulate your favorite parts of who you are.** For example, taking a class or joining a club that's devoted to one of your interests will allow you to hang with people who are probably more interested in the activity or topic you're there to explore than in what's going on in your uterus. And spending time with colleagues can help you connect to the side of you that's passionate about your career, as it's easy to find not-baby-related common ground with these people.
- **Nurture your dynamic layers after birth.** When baby is born, you can hold on to parts of your pre-pregnancy identity by making a plan with your support team for engaging in the activities you love. For example, maybe you'll schedule your mom to watch baby for an hour every other day so you can work on a passion project.

Something I found so amazing about motherhood was that after I got through the first few months of postpartum chaos, I was filled with inspiration. I started writing the book proposal for *Feng Shui Mommy*, crafting and pitching a TV show I'm now so grateful never graced the small screen, and volunteering for a cancer resource center. It was like my newfound purpose as a mother awakened all these other sources of purpose. And I'm not unique. Most moms I know began their most exciting endeavors soon after having a baby. I'm not telling you this to make you feel like you need to change the world while you're still trying to figure out how to get your boobs to stop leaking. I just want you to feel hopeful that your best self and life might be yet to come.

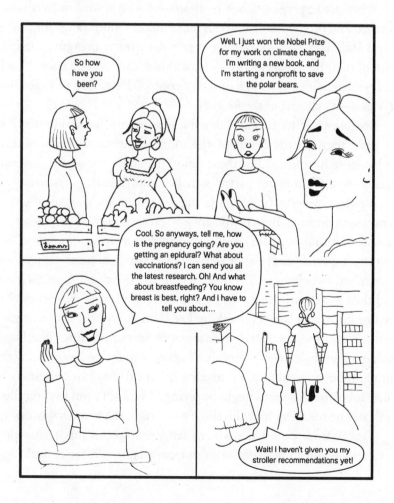

2. Why do I think my partner is the most irritating person in the world? How can I start liking them again?

Don't tell my husband, but I was pissed he didn't have to live off saltines for three months, didn't have an always-aching groin, and didn't have to do the whole push-a-baby-out thing. Pissed. I felt enraged by the injustice of his simply having to contribute sperm. Beyond that, just about everything else he did irritated me. Left a drop of pee on the toilet seat...Aargh! Didn't shut the silverware drawer all the way...Why, I oughta! Didn't get the right kind of ice cream...I won't even go there. There was a lot of rage. But I never talked about it. I didn't want to be seen as the irrational pregnant woman who stirred up conflict for no reason. But it turns out there *was* a reason.

When we're pregnant, our bodies flood with a confused cocktail of estrogen and progesterone that can make our emotions range from crying over a Hallmark card to wanting to pop the tires of that guy who cut in front of us at the grocery store — all within a sixty-second span. It's a lot. And we shouldn't feel wrong, or out of control, for having this cacophony of feels — it's all part of the journey.

Because your partner is likely the person you feel emotionally safest with, they get the brunt of the more unpleasant emotions stirred up by those hormones. But those emotions aren't always the hormones talking — sometimes our partners are just really freaking irritating.

A potential cause for this irritating behavior is the changes your partner is going through. Both of you are navigating a massive shift — a rite of passage our culture doesn't appropriately acknowledge or support. Men are often especially inept at processing this change because most of them were raised to believe they should manage their emotions on their own. And then society tells them they shouldn't complain because they're not the one growing a baby (something I've been guilty of saying to my husband). Sometimes men aren't even aware of how impending fatherhood is molding their behavior — they don't see how their fears over losing their autonomy or masculinity are making them extra selfish and annoying. Their subconscious mind might be saying, "I will not bend to parenthood. I will still be me. Here look, I'll show you!" (Cue the annoying behavior.)

I speak from experience when I tell you that this mix of hormones in us and aggravating behavior in our partners can make us feel rage...

and fear...and sadness...and more rage. While you have every right to feel these feelings, I'll also take a wild guess and bet it doesn't feel great to always feel like you and your significant other are on opposing teams. During this time, more than any other phase of life, we crave companionship and harmony. So it can be frustrating when our emotions offer up the recipe for the total opposite.

What to do

First off, let yourself feel the emotions. When irritation pops up, resist the urge to talk yourself out of it or ignore it. Go to a private space where you won't be tempted to unleash that irritation on your partner, then let yourself go. Talk smack about them in the mirror, stomp your feet, do a silent scream. Then count to ninety. People much smarter than me have found it takes any emotion ninety seconds to pass through the mind and body... if we do nothing to shut it down. So let it flow. Then...

- **Take a few moments to examine what just happened.** Look at what triggered you. In the case of your partner pissing you off, determine whether the offending action is something they do repeatedly that you would really like them to stop doing — like if they said something that was offensive and that warrants an apology — or is something that really wasn't a big deal and can be let go of. Because you've released the emotions around the event, you're able to make a more logical, objective decision about how to move forward. The gist: give yourself alone time when your partner makes you steam.
- **Check in with your partner once a week.** When you're both well rested, not distracted, and in a good headspace, sit down for a talk about how you're both feeling. Before you begin, lay some communication ground rules — for example, avoid name-calling, don't cut off the other midsentence, and be dedicated to finding solutions and common ground instead of trying to prove that you're right. Airing your feelings on a regular basis can keep you from feeling like a powder keg, and it will help you feel more heard and connected — all things that will make your partner seem way less irritating.
- **Assign parenting tasks.** During one of those weekly check-ins, break down the impending parenting responsibilities and decide who will

tackle what. Because a hunk of the stress you and your partner are feeling probably stems from all the unknowns of parenthood, this planning session can be a surprisingly effective salve, helping you get clear on what to expect from parent-life.

To start, make a list of everything that needs to be done when you have a baby (e.g., diaper changes, feeding, cooking meals, taking out the trash, washing dishes, doing laundry, setting up health insurance for baby, paying the bills, researching childcare, etc.).

Then, go through each item and discuss who will take responsibility for it. If you decide to share responsibility for a certain task, break down what that will look like. Make sure to write down your decisions so there's no confusion when your brains are eventually possessed by parenthood and no sleep.

In addition, make sure your name isn't next to 75 percent of the tasks. Women often have to put in double the work to be seen as an equal contributor. That's a BS social dynamic we need to change. Split the tasks evenly because you deserve equality in your home just as much as you deserve it at work...and everywhere.

3. My partner and I are fighting all the time. Can the baby hear us? Are we emotionally scarring them?

When I was pregnant, I wrapped a blanket around my stomach when Eric and I argued, figuring this would protect Hudson from our un-perfect relationship. I soon discovered I didn't need to be as worried about what our son heard in utero as about the stress hormones he was exposed to. And before we all get stressed about being stressed, know that it's impossible to have a completely stress-free pregnancy, where only rainbows and unicorn smiles pass through the placenta — stressor hormones are a normal part of life. But regularly elevated levels of said hormones don't have to be.

So why do so many women experience elevated stress during pregnancy? As this Q&A implies, tension with a partner can be a big factor. As your body and many aspects of your life (and your partner's) change — or prepare for change — it's common to argue about finances, shifting priorities, intimacy, wet towels on the floor (oh wait, that's always), and so much more. For many, our partner is our rock — our numero uno for emotional and physical support. So when it feels like they're our adversary, we can crack.

When I was in my second trimester and Eric was in the throes of graduate school, he had a meltdown one evening while I was partaking in a joyful perineal tissue massage. He started sighing really loudly, which is usually my cue to say, "What's wrong?" But I didn't — I was focused on stretching out my vagina so a head could fit through it. His sighs turned to grunts, and I snapped. "Just say what's bothering you!" I barked from the bathroom. And then it happened. He erupted in tears, complaints, and infuriating raised eyebrows. The pressure of school, working full-time, and having parenthood looming in his near future was too much. He didn't think he could do it, and he was terrified.

Usually, I would see this as a cry for help and let him vent as I furrowed my own brows and nodded. But not this time. I was pregnant, and he wasn't. In that moment I believed he was just trying to make my life harder — that he was implying pregnancy was more difficult for him. I went off. We yelled, cried, and blamed…then he left. It was the worst fight we'd ever had, and I was a puddle. I convinced myself that he was never coming back, and that Hudson and I would have to forge ahead alone. I was shaking, and Hudson was going crazy in my uterus.

Something had to change. While Eric and I would obviously argue again, I had to make a plan for keeping things civil. My body and baby were giving me clear signals that what had just happened was toxic for all.

After Eric and I reconciled, I made a list of how to avoid that toxicity in the future — you'll find it in the "What to do" section. I also researched the effects of high levels of stress on a fetus. It's not great. When a pregnant woman is regularly in "fight-or-flight" mode, cortisol, adrenaline, epinephrine, and other stressor hormones flood the body. According to a study published in *Frontiers in Human Neuroscience*, a fetus's exposure to these hormones could potentially cause symptoms of anxiety, depression, and increased stress reactivity later in life. In addition, a study published in *Women & Birth* found that maternal stress could increase the risk for preterm birth. The final study I'll drop, published in *Obstetric Medicine*, reported that prenatal stress could result in low birth weight and impact the child's learning and memory. For mama, high levels of stress can lead to anxiety or depression, headaches, nausea, cramping, digestive issues, and sleep issues.

When I read about these risks I was overcome with guilt, certain that my blowout with Eric had led to irreparable baby-damage. But hold up. While studies like this can be frightening, they're not saying our babies are doomed to a challenging life just because we're occasionally stressed. After I chilled, I saw the potential risks as encouragement to do everything I could to limit my stress, work that list I made, and remember that while prenatal stress isn't dire, it should be avoided as much as possible. So how do we do that? We do that by empowering ourselves to take back some control over our stress levels and creating a more harmonious relationship with our partners.

Note: If the fighting you're experiencing contains even a thread of emotional or physical abuse, seek support. The National Domestic Violence Hotline (thehotline.org) offers guidance and referrals for women who are experiencing domestic abuse or wondering whether certain aspects of their relationship are unhealthy. It's best to seek help now. As much as we want the birth of a baby to heal a deeply fractured relationship, it often does the opposite. You and your baby deserve an environment of emotional and physical safety and support.

What to do

Make a list of everything that stresses you out. When you get to how your partner stresses you out, be really specific about the topics you often argue about and the triggers you both have. This exercise takes the mystery out of your relationship stress and gives you a jumping-off point for resolution and eventual maintenance. With your list in hand, try out the following argument- and stress-reduction tools.

- **Pause.** When you feel your anger sparked, resist the urge to vent. Instead, take a pause. Go to a private space, take ten deep breaths, and look at what's going on. Is your partner being a total jerk, or are you just reading into what they're saying? Are they doing something that requires a talk, or can you let it go because your reaction's coming from something else that's going on with you? Take a hot second before you pounce on the opportunity to argue. (I used to be so bad at this.) This feels super awkward the first few times you do it, and if your partner's not used to it, they may respond by trying to get you to react immediately. But if you stick with it, you can likely keep those stress levels in check and avoid unneeded disputes.

- **Fill your partner in on what it's like to be pregnant.** So many of the fights I had with Eric revolved around him not getting what I was going through. I thought he should just know what it's like to have cankles that feel like they've been injected with Play-Doh, to feel bullied by the constant shifts of the hormones responsible for regulating my emotions, to be freaked by the idea of pushing a human out of my vagina. But he didn't just know. So finally I told him. Do the same with your person. Tell them the nitty-gritty of what you're experiencing, and then get specific about how they can help. Remind them that this is an incredibly tender time for you, and you're going to need a lot of slack to be cut.

- **Give compliment sandwiches.** Partners can be irritating and sometimes incredibly hurtful, which means there will be times when you need to speak up. And because all humans have sensitive egos (even those who swear otherwise) you can avoid critique-backlash by using the trusty compliment sandwich. Here's one I remember recycling often when Hudson was a baby: "Hey babe. I love your dedication to surfing — it's awesome to see how happy you are afterward. While I definitely want you to keep having time to do that, it would be great if you could shorten the surf sessions. Maybe you could try to be back in two hours instead of three? Hudson and I really love having you around and it would be amazing to see more of you on your days off." Kind of cheesy, but it usually worked. The times I forgot about this sandwiching technique and threw out, "It's selfish and ridiculous how long you spend surfing!" he would usually peace out for even longer, and then we would fight. #SayYesToTheSandwich

- **Practice gratitude maintenance.** The longer we're paired with another human, the easier it is to see their annoying qualities and the harder it is to see their lovely ones. This natural phenomenon breeds contempt.

   One of the quickest ways to replace contempt with appreciation is for you and your partner to make a list of ten things you appreciate about one another. It can be really specific, like, "I love the way you make a smoothie" or "You're really skilled with your tongue" (never hurts to throw in some kinky gratitude!). When you have your lists, read them to each other. Don't follow this up with lists of the things you *don't* appreciate — just sit in the space of gratitude for a few minutes. Whenever you feel the contempt creeping back in, repeat the exercise.

- **Give hugs.** It's really hard to hold on to stress and be mad at someone you love when you're engaging in a long, warm hug. While it's beautiful to embrace after you've resolved a conflict, you can also do something wild and initiate the hug midargument. If you feel yourself spinning out or notice an argument is becoming unproductive, step forward, ask your partner if you can hug them, and then do it. Make it a long one. Hold the embrace until you feel them soften. This can be one of the simplest and most effective ways to hit the reset button.

Regarding the other life-stuff that stresses you out, try the following when the going gets gruff:

- **Sing.** Music helps control cortisol levels. So when you feel stress escalating, turn on your favorite jam and belt it out.
- **Decompress.** Even when all seems merry and bright, pregnancy hormones can dump a load of stress on you. When this happens, wind down from the tension by meditating, taking a warm bath, getting a prenatal massage or acupuncture, listening to good ole Enya, or doing anything else that helps your mind and body release.

And finally, ask your partner to do any or all of the above. As much as we try to shield ourselves from our partner's moods, they still impact us. So getting your person to utilize some of the same argument-soothers and stress-relievers you're trying can help you both land in emotional equilibrium.

4. I feel certain my partner is going to stray while I'm pregnant. They've never shown warning signs, but I'm still terrified it will happen. Should I talk to them about it? Should I just ignore the fear?

There's bad news and good news. The bad news is that 10 percent of males cheat when their partner is pregnant, according to the book *What's Your*

Pregnant Man Thinking? by psychologist Robert Rodriguez. Many other studies have mirrored these findings. While there's not much research on infidelity in same-sex female relationships during pregnancy, studies done on general infidelity have found little difference between same-sex female and heterosexual couples.

So what's the deal with prenatal cheating? Some suspect two primary factors at play in this unfortunate statistic. First, some women have a big drop in their libido during pregnancy, or are so physically ill that the only thing they want to slip under the sheets for is sleep. It's also believed that this cheating might stem from the partner's unmet emotional desires, as many women are navigating so many changes during pregnancy they don't have room for their partner's emotional needs. Of course, neither is an excuse for cheating. But these factors do provide a good jumping-off point for the conversation we'll get to in the "What to do" section.

The good news is, you're not a statistic! You and your partner are individuals who make autonomous decisions. It's not a foregone conclusion that infidelity will play a part in your pregnancy. Your partner might even be one of the folks who's incredibly turned on by your pregnant body and can't get enough of you. Or because of a drop in testosterone (something that commonly happens to males during their partner's pregnancy), they might have a diminished sex drive. Remember that your relationship is unique, and that there's so much you can do to bypass infidelity.

What to do

Talk to your partner ASAP. In many situations, so much grief can be avoided if partners summon the courage to be candid with one another. Here's how to navigate the conversation:

- **Kick off the conversation.** When you're in a good headspace — for example, after you're well rested, well fed, and not distracted by to-dos — ask your partner for a sit-down. Preface the convo with a reminder that you're not accusing them of cheating. You can even blame me: "This book I'm reading was talking about infidelity rates during pregnancy, and I just thought a chat would calm my fears."

    Then, you can share some of the catalysts for cheating I listed: lack of sex or need for emotional nurturing. Ask your partner straight-up how they feel about those aspects of your relationship. If they try to shrug it off, remind them that opening up is one of the best ways they can help you have a more relaxed pregnancy.

- **Navigate challenges.** As you get deeper into the conversation, some challenges might come up. For example, your partner might say they feel like you're not attracted to them. Or maybe it comes out that both of you feel emotionally detached from the relationship. Whatever it is, resist the urge to blame, and instead commit to making a plan. If sexual connection is the issue, discuss ways to reignite the spark (covered in this book!). If the emotional glue is dissolving, brainstorm ways to fortify it. As you wrap up the conversation, I encourage you to commit to re-engaging in this honest sharing anytime either of you feel your lust or emotional intimacy slipping.

- **Consider counseling.** If this talk makes you realize how much you don't trust your partner, it could be a sign that you need to seek additional support to discover how to move forward. I recommend reaching out to a therapist in a private practice, or utilizing complimentary counseling services through a local pregnancy support organization. This mental health professional can help you determine where your concerns are coming from, and if further action is required.

Even if you're not questioning your relationship, seeking some form of counseling can seriously nourish your pregnancy journey. This healthy outlet allows you to explore all the layers of your experience that pregnancy is exposing and to receive the emotional support you might not be getting enough of at home (which is so normal, even in the healthiest relationships). This release in a counselor's office might also give you more patience and desire for nurturing your partner's emotional needs, thus sidestepping that second aforementioned infidelity trigger. And while it's hard to encourage someone who isn't asking for help to see a counselor, it could be a good gentle suggestion to make if you see your partner struggling with emotions you don't feel equipped to handle.

When I was pregnant, I had a lot of therapy — for many reasons. But a big one was the fear of infidelity. Eric couldn't get enough of me, but I was still terrified he would stray. We became pregnant early in our relationship, and he had an ex who reached out more than I liked. That was enough to totally freak me out. Even though he showed no signs of straying, "What if?" kept scrolling through my mind. Even though my therapist urged me to talk with him, I hid my thoughts, thinking I would seem "hysterical" if I gave them a voice. I didn't realize holding them in was what made me hysterical.

It all bubbled out the day before our baby shower. We were making a Costco list, and suddenly fat teardrops distorted the words "brownie mix" and "Metamucil." A three-hour conversation, with lots of hugs, commenced. The results: a promise to encourage said-ex to cool it on the communication and a commitment to share our fears and concerns, no matter how out of place they seemed. While we still have plenty of issues, we've become obsessed with communication, piping up when anything feels off in our relationship. And I still frequent therapy.

5. I don't like the idea of my partner watching naked women in birth videos. Should I ask them to not watch the videos with me?

When I first watched a birth video with Eric I immediately wondered if he was lusting after the woman's bare breasts. They were full and round and probably four cup sizes larger than mine. However, the only part of the video that seemed to faze him was the liquid pouring out of the vagina as the head popped out. I asked him about the boobs, and he said he didn't notice them. Whether or not he was fibbing doesn't matter. What matters is that I was forgetting why we watched the birth video. We didn't watch so I could compare myself to other women, or fall down the rabbit hole of doubt about whether my partner thought I was attractive — we were watching to expand our knowledge of birth and prepare for our journey as parents.

That's my long way of saying I relate to this question. It's normal to have a slew of insecurities during pregnancy, when our bodies are undergoing rapid-fire changes. And naturally, these insecurities can bleed into our romantic relationship. It can come to a head when we're watching a video of a beautiful naked woman handling birth — a process we might not think we can get through — like a pro, all while our partner looks on. So. Many. Triggers.

While it's absolutely okay to avoid watching birth videos with your partner, I also think it's a missed opportunity. Watching birth videos that depict an empowered, peaceful birth can help you and your partner realize that such a birth is possible for you. As a childbirth educator, I can talk for hours about how wonderful birth can be, but few parents really get it until I show the videos. This visual depiction of birth allows all the information I've shared to really sink in.

Of course, it's most important for *you* to watch these videos, but getting your partner in on the action helps them develop a more positive perspective on birth. This shift in perspective will support them in bringing an enhanced, trusting, serene energy to your pregnancy and birth experience. And let me tell you, the energy coming off your partner makes a big difference, whether you're aware of it or not.

What to do

First, figure out what it is about watching birth videos with your partner that makes you uncomfortable. Is it just the idea of your partner looking at naked women? Or is it more than that? For example, I was afraid Eric would be thinking, "There's no way Bailey is strong enough to birth like that lady." (A thought that was my own, not his.) Write out your particular triggers, then follow one of my all-time favorite recommendations — talk with your partner.

Sharing your concerns gives your partner the chance to assuage many of them — because in most cases, the partner is not at all thinking about the naked woman; they're just worried they'll pass out when they see the blood. So this conversation allows you both to get out your questions and concerns so you can move into the exciting process of watching birth videos with confidence and a fortified sense of partnership.

How to find the right birth videos: Because all birth videos are not created equal, I recommend an internet search for "calm birth videos," "gentle birth videos," or "HypnoBirthing birth videos" to help ensure you discover encouraging videos that won't strike fear in your uterus.

6. I'm no longer with my baby's father and am so nervous about all the questions and judgments that will be coming my way. How should I handle this?

First off, if you left your partner because you were in an unhealthy relationship, you are my hero. It takes Wonder Woman strength to stand up for your well-being and get out of a relationship that isn't good for you, especially when faced with impending parenthood — a journey that makes many yearn for a partner. But as you probably know, being partner-free can be better than having a toxic relationship.

If you broke romantic ties with your partner because you realized the two of you are better friends than lovers, kudos to you, too. It's really easy to convince ourselves to stay with someone we don't want to be romantically involved with if they're a good person and friend. By beginning to create a new structure for your relationship now, the two of you can hope to have a solid system and healthy dynamic by the time baby arrives.

And now for one of the trickiest types of separations: If you were left by someone you still want to be with, this split might be one of the most painful things you've ever experienced. Being abandoned by the person you probably thought would stay by your side no matter what can feel like an insurmountable betrayal. And if cheating was a factor, you can heap another pile of pain into the mix.

Regardless of the nature of the separation, you're likely navigating a maelstrom of confusion, loss, and maybe anger and fear. The last thing you need to worry about is how others will react to the news. But whether we like it or not, reactions will come. Hopefully, your people will understand and do nothing but offer comfort and support. But some might have a hard time accepting your situation, making your life even harder.

Oh, mama. You're dealing with so much. I wish I could wrap you in my arms and make sure you get all the love and support you deserve. I hope I will have the privilege of doing that someday, but for now, here's a strategy for moving through this super tricky time in a way that nourishes your mental and emotional health.

What to do

Build your support system. Think of the people who will understand your situation and won't do that thing where their face gets really judgy when you tell them about your new relationship status. Find these people, and ask them straight-up if they'd be willing to be one of your rocks. If they agree, make a plan together for how they can support you during pregnancy and early motherhood. Be really specific with your needs, so they can be really specific about how they can help.

During this vulnerable period I also recommend scheduling regular times to connect with these support people. When we're struggling and in pain, it's all too easy to hide and not reach out. So it's important to prepare for this by scheduling regular check-ins. If you and your sister, for example, plan for her to come over every Wednesday evening to talk, and for her to call you every morning to boost your morale, it's going to be a lot harder to resist support.

Once you've set up this solid support network, you'll likely feel braver and more assured in your decision to leave your partner, or more secure in the single status that was thrust on you. Now, with confidence and enhanced calm fueling your creativity, write a loose script for what you'll say to acquaintances when they ask about your baby's father. Then, think about what you'll tell close friends and family members — likely you'll offer them a more extensive breakdown of what happened. If you fear they'll urge you to question your decision, or to try to get your partner to take you back, add an addendum to your script where you lovingly tell them you'll request their advice if you want it. To fortify your nerves for the family-and-close-friends conversations, bring along someone from your support system who can back you up, or get you out if anyone is hurtful.

7. I have a friend who is devastated because she can't get pregnant. I'm afraid to tell her I'm pregnant. How should I handle this?

A friendship can get tricky when one friend's pain intersects with another's joy. The emotions experienced by someone facing infertility, miscarriage, or stillbirth can be truly understood only by those who have navigated the same sorrow — it cuts deep and can feel like a cruel joke. I speak from experience, as I've had a miscarriage.

While every woman who experiences this painful journey will do so in her own way, a common thread is feeling frustration, desolation, and even resentment when they see babies and pregnant bellies, or hear about the healthy pregnancies of their loved ones. Being around pregnancy can be so triggering. Because of this, it's fair to feel nervous about sharing your amazing news with someone who will understandably see it as a reminder of what they don't have. It's not a fun conversation. But it has to happen.

While it's normal to want to hide this information because you don't want to cause pain, you'll actually cause more by hiding it. I have a close friend (we'll call her Megan) who experienced a late-term stillbirth that rocked her world. I was devastated when I heard about her loss — so I can't even begin to piece together how she felt — and still feels. Then one of Megan's friends (we'll call her Anna) became pregnant, and had a get-together where she shared the news with all their mutual friends. Anna did not invite Megan. Sharing the news with Megan was left to her husband, who heard about the pregnancy secondhand, and this made Megan feel that a secret was being kept, like Anna would rather hide than face Megan's pain. She felt betrayed. If Anna could have pushed past her discomfort, they would have had a potent opportunity to connect, as one of the main things Megan wanted was for people to be willing to talk to her about her child who had passed. To be willing to hear about her pain. She wanted people to not be scared of her story and her grief.

So in some ways, the situation you're in with your friend is a gift. It's an opening, an opportunity to let her know you're there for her no matter how uncomfortable her emotions and life circumstances make you feel. While initially uncomfortable, this conversation could be one of the most unifying and transformational encounters you'll ever have. It will force you to summon your strength and compassion, and connect with another human in a raw, deeply authentic way.

What to do

To start, don't post anything on social media or have a big pregnancy announcement party until you've spoken to your friend. News travels fast in the age of instant information, so hold it close. Then consider the following:

- **Make a plan for when and where you'll tell her.** First, think of a day and time that will give both of you plenty of time to talk and allow room for decompression before either of you step into another activity. Next, figure out a private, safe space for her to freely express whatever emotions might arise. (Her house might be a good choice.)
- **Figure out how you'll tell her.** To get started, write down some ideas about how to deliver the news. For example, you can preface the news by telling her you're fine with any reaction she has, as this can make

her feel safe to express sadness or frustration if that comes up. In addition, knowing that you didn't come into the conversation with expectations about how she should respond will likely make her feel emotionally held.

You can also write a reminder to remain neutral when you tell her you're pregnant. While it's natural to want to gush about how happy you are and share all the details, know that such a reaction might exaggerate her pain.

Below is an opener I helped a client write. You obviously don't have to say this verbatim, but it can provide a starting-off point. You also don't have to walk into the convo with the script, but it's helpful to review it beforehand to ensure you don't forget the most important points.

If you feel your friend would rather receive the news via email, compose a letter along the lines of what's written below, and end with an invitation to talk whenever she feels ready.

Sample Script for Informing a Sensitive Friend

"I want to start by saying how much I love you and appreciate our friendship. Before I jump into my news I also want you to know I have no expectations about your reaction — you should feel safe to express whatever comes up. With that said, I want you to be one of the first people to know that I'm pregnant. [Pause for reaction.] I can't even begin to understand what you must be going through, but I want you to know I'm always here for you. I promise we absolutely do not have to talk about my pregnancy when we hang out. You are an amazing woman, and it's an honor to know you."

- **Determine how to manage your emotions.** An important aspect of preparing for this talk is recording ideas (see the invisible shield exercise on the following page) about how you'll manage your own emotions or triggers if she doesn't seem happy for you. She's moving through a challenging experience, and it's natural for her to not be excited about your news. Her reaction is not personal — it does not mean she doesn't love you or thinks you don't deserve to become a mother.

- **Actively listen.** After you've said your piece, allow her to lead the conversation, and practice active listening. Avoid going into details about your pregnancy, like due date and birth plans, unless she asks, and for the love of uteruses, do not offer any advice on conceiving or drop fertility platitudes. "Everything happens for a reason," "It will happen for you when the time is right," and other such sayings are not helpful.

- **Protect yourself.** Something else to consider as you plan for this conversation is that *your* fears could be triggered. For example, if your friend experienced a miscarriage or stillbirth and wants to talk about it, you could begin wondering if the same will happen to you.

  To protect yourself, create an invisible shield before you meet by closing your eyes and envisioning a golden light around you. Allow this light to represent energetic protection from whatever your friend says. Remind yourself that this conversation is for her, and that all you need to do is be there for her — you don't need to absorb her pain or fear. When I went through this exercise with a client she asked if it was selfish, saying, "Shouldn't I be willing to feel her pain and really go there with her?" The thing is, "going there" with her sucks energy away from your ability to support her. If you spiral into the what-ifs of your own journey, you'll have little concentration, or even willingness, left for nurturing her. In addition, gifting yourself this energetic protection can prevent you from becoming defensive or angry if her response is hurtful.

- **Keep reaching out.** After you have the talk, avoid the temptation to ghost her. It's normal to want to hang only with people who lift your mood and are cool talking about baby stuff 24/7, but continuing to give friendship-TLC to her can be good for both of you — she feels supported, and you're reminded of what a solid friend you are. (Just don't talk baby unless she's the one bringing it up.) With that said, she might request space from you. She might find it's just too hard being around you during your pregnancy and that she needs to take a step back. While you want to honor her choice, it doesn't hurt to continue checking in on her occasionally, letting her know you're thinking of her and are there if she ever needs anything.

8. I used an egg (or sperm) donor to conceive and still haven't told anyone. Do I have to share this information?

Nope. That decision is super personal, and you can do whatever you like with it. In the age of oversharing, some people feel it's their right to know all your business, which can make you feel pressure to share it all — even the aspects of yourself you want to hold close. This can even result in you feeling like you're lying or inauthentic if you're not completely open about your journey to conception. I don't want that for you. I want you to feel free to choose who you do and do not share this intimate information with, and to know that you're not less-than if you don't feel like shouting it from the rooftops.

You might also still be processing how you feel about using a donor. Maybe you're exploring what it's like to be pregnant with a child who is not biologically related to you. Or maybe you're supporting your partner through that journey. It can muddy the emotional waters to share information you're still unpacking.

On the other hand, you might also be yearning for a few special people to talk with about your donor decision — a few people who won't judge or ask insensitive questions. Creating this carefully curated group can give you a pillow of support when you do tell people who might not be as understanding as they should (for example, uptight parents or in-laws) and your child, when they're old enough to understand.

What to do

Think long and hard about the people you trust implicitly. The people who never raise their eyebrows when you tell them something deeply personal. The people who have your back no matter what. Make a list of names. If you have a partner, make this list with them. Then do the following:

- **Tell those people.** I recommend having a private meetup with each of the individuals on your list, where you share your exciting news. You can also request that they don't share this information with others until you give the go-ahead.
- **Request support.** If you're struggling with emotions around your genetic connection to the child or are nervous about telling certain people, ask your core group if they'd be willing to support you through this process. They'll likely appreciate you being up-front with your needs and will probably jump into action to make you feel held.

  With this team of ride-or-die confidants in place, move on to phase three…telling the family members you're not excited to tell.
- **Having the tricky talks.** Before we dive into this, I want to note that it's not absolutely necessary to tell anyone — even family members. I cover how to share this information with family because many women feel it's easier to tell them than to try and preserve the secret. But of course, whatever choice intuitively feels right for your unique situation is the right one.

  If you choose to share your decision to use a donor with the family, make a loose script for what you will say, writing down any information you're willing to provide and what you're keeping to yourself. You can also create a script for what to say if they ask questions you don't want to answer or are judgmental. For example, if they start hammering you about why you used a donor instead of doing X, Y, or Z, clearly tell them that you're not there to discuss your reasoning and have no obligation to do so. Express that you're telling them out of courtesy and do not need them to agree with your decision. State that you've shared everything you're willing to share, and request that they find a way to support you. This might seem harsh, but I want you to remember that you don't need their approval. You're an adult who is following the path to parenthood that is right for you and, if applicable, your partner.

  If you're really nervous about having these conversations, ask someone from your support group to accompany you so they can back you up, or pull you out if the situation gets toxic.

You are a champion for moving through the intense journey of conceiving with the support of a donor. It's a long road, and you deserve to be honored for your commitment to bring a new life into this world. Don't let anyone dim your light.

9. Pregnancy has made me so irritable I can barely stand being around people. Will I always feel like this? How can I stop being so mean?

"I hate all of them," my client Shelly said. "First it was just all the people that aren't pregnant and can bend over, and poop, and eat more than crackers. And then I started hating all the pregnant women too. They all glow more than me, yet sweat less. There's no way they're as scared, or angry, or tired as me. And then there's my husband — he really sucks. I hate that! I hate all of them, but I can't stop it. And…and…and…" Shelly went on for a while. I felt for her. She was taking my childbirth prep class and had stayed behind to talk.

Shelly said the moments of excessive annoyance began almost as soon as she peed on the stick. But the rage didn't fully blossom until the beginning of her third trimester. She couldn't tolerate being in public because she couldn't hold her tongue — she couldn't stop her eyes from giving away how dumb she thought everyone was. "I got a foot massage last week and asked the woman if she was *trying* to do a bad job. I could barely feel her hands, but still, I was such a bitch. She teared up. I'm not usually like this. Before I became pregnant I was that person who struck up conversations with strangers in the checkout line. I would leave waiters big tips even if they did a horrible job. I think I'm possessed," she said. She was possessed. But not by the Spawn of Satan, just by the Hormones from Hell — and a few other pregnancy demons.

What Shelly experienced was an extreme version of the mood shifts many women have during pregnancy. The changes in estrogen and progesterone throw your neurotransmitters — the chemicals in the brain that help regulate your mood — for a loop. Like a giant, nauseating roller coaster loop. In addition to the hormones, the fatigue, the stress of preparing for a new baby, and the changes to your metabolism contribute to the whole "other people are insufferable" thing. While this is all normal, it doesn't feel great, and each time you see red it can cause a surge of the stress hormones epinephrine, cortisol, and adrenaline, in addition to a constriction of blood vessels.

A study published in the *Journal of Obstetrics and Gynaecology* found that pregnant women with chronic high levels of anger had high levels of cortisol and adrenaline, in addition to low dopamine and serotonin levels, and that these women tended to have babies with high cortisol and low dopamine levels. These babies also had issues with sleep, orientation, and motor maturity after birth. The good news is there's a lot you can do to minimize the spike in these rage hormones, as well as the dips in your happy hormones.

What to do

Avoid other people. Seriously. While I'll get to ways to manage your irritation when you *have to* be around other humans, I want to stress your right to honor your needs — even if those needs include being a hermit for a few weeks. Maybe your irritable mood is a much-needed invitation to step out of the social scene and spend more time connecting with your baby — a person who, at the moment, cannot talk back and demands nothing of you (beyond most of your nutrients).

If you've *always* felt like you'd rather stare at a blank wall than interact with other humans, this may be a sign of social anxiety, chronic depression, or other common conditions, which might be something you can explore with the support of a mental health specialist. But if this is a state of being that popped up with pregnancy, it'll likely subside after baby comes and the hormones chill. So instead of stressing about other people stressing you out, give yourself permission to avoid people as much as possible. Give yourself permission to retreat in ways like these:

- Pop on your headphones when you're at work (or anywhere) so people aren't tempted to talk to you.
- Tell your partner you need alone time and slip into bed with a good book or the remote.
- Pull the pregnancy card when friends ask you to go out, or an invite to a family gathering arrives.

If any of your people are offended, be straight-up. Tell them pregnancy hormones are making you exceedingly irritable, so you'd rather avoid people than be mean to them. You can also remind them (and yourself) that you'll be back to your more social self after your hormones regain equilibrium. Until then, just send your regrets. #SorryNotSorry

However, there will be times when you just can't avoid interacting with fellow earthlings. To make those situations less infuriating, try the following:

- **Discover what relaxes you, then do it.** Analyze all the activities you engage in, or want to engage in, and pinpoint what makes you the most relaxed. For example, maybe a walk every morning, a nap in the afternoon, or a massage once a week pushes your reset button. Or maybe your thing is bingeing on *Dr. Pimple Popper* or knitting baby booties. Or whatever. Just do what soothes you at least once a day, as this will fill you with a greater capacity to deal with irritants when you have to leave your bubble.

- **Follow the healthy norms.** I know eating nutritious food and not being a total couch potato is talked about ad nauseam, but it's for good reason. These activities help combat the factors that can make you susceptible to anger and irritation, like fatigue, headaches, and bloating, while also pumping you full of endorphins.

- **Walk away.** When someone triggers you and you feel a red-hot response on the tip of your tongue, swallow it and walk away. Go somewhere private (the bathroom or car are my favorite choices), and let your rage spill out there. Say everything you wanted to say to that person. Bang your fists. Let it out. This helps avoid the escalation of interactions that don't need to escalate, and prevents you from saying something you'll later regret. If you need to return to that person, wait until your anger has subsided so you can engage from a calm space.

- **Pull the pregnancy card.** If those red-hot words spill from your mouth and you wish you could shove them back in, blame it on the baby. "I am so sorry I said that. These hormones are out of control." However, if that person deserved those red-hot words, skip the excuse, and as the singer Lizzo would say, do a hair toss and walk your fine self out the door.

- **Intentionally rage.** Release your inner pressure cooker on *your* terms by finding activities that allow you to express your anger without hurting anyone. For example, I've been known to scream into pillows, pound said pillows, or write a scathing letter to someone I'm mad at, then burn it. Find your thing, then do it as often as needed.
- **Practice nostril breathing.** Most people hold their breath when they get mad. Pull yourself out of this state by practicing the very strange, yet effective, technique of nostril breathing, also called the "subtle energy clearing breathing technique." To do this, close your right nostril with your thumb, then take a deep inhale through your left nostril. Next, close your left nostril with your finger, then exhale through your right nostril, and then inhale through your right nostril. Now close the right nostril, and exhale through your left nostril. That's one cycle. For optimal results, do it for five minutes. It may sound confusing, but it gets easier with practice.

   Safety Note: Stop this breathing technique if you begin feeling light-headed.
- **Practice muscle release.** In addition to holding their breath, people tense their muscles when they're mad. So when you feel anger coursing through your muscles, counteract it by envisioning a warm, euphoria-inducing liquid being poured into the top of your head and flowing down through every muscle, nerve, and cell in your body until it reaches your toes. Track this liquid as it slowly moves through you, feeling your muscles relax as the euphoria moves through them. Keep repeating this visualization until you feel the anger subside.

Medical Care Providers

10. I can't stand my medical care provider, but I'm just weeks from my due date. What should I do?

This is one of the most frequent questions I receive. As our culture sets doctors up to be authority figures (something that can be comforting in many cases), we often feel like we're stuck with the first person we receive treatment from after we pee on the stick. Most of the time, that person is the OB we started going to because our insurance covered it or a few friends recommended them. But then we start learning about pregnancy and childbirth and might find we're feeling less aligned with that OB — feeling less comfortable asking questions or expressing how we want to navigate pregnancy and childbirth. Under normal circumstances, we would find a new care provider, but discomfort at the thought of firing the person who's been administering those lovely Paps for so long can seem more than our pregnant emotions can handle, especially when we're nearing the end of pregnancy. But the alternative is often a birth experience that is a far cry from what we actually want.

In addition, most of us feel incredibly vulnerable during pregnancy, so when we have a care provider talking with great authority on what we should do, we wonder if we'll be doing ourselves or our baby a disservice if we change care providers. So we stick with them. But this decision is often based on fear rather than on a genuine desire to receive care from the person in question. It's also important to note that some care providers present opinions as fact. They state their views on induction, for example, as gospel, making some women feel silly for having a differing opinion. If you conduct the care provider interviews recommended in the following pages, you'll find that almost every candidate will have a slight (or significant) difference of opinion on almost all pregnancy and childbirth topics. In many cases, a lot of what they say is based on their personal experiences, not on science-based research.

I have a birth story packed with disappointing moments because I didn't feel comfortable being open with my care provider. At the time, I didn't have the courage to find a new one. When I discovered a fertilized egg had landed in my uterus, I went straight to the lady who had given me a painful endometrial biopsy the year before. She was an authoritative grandma type and a high-risk OB. I knew nothing about pregnancy and childbirth and figured it would be good to have a doctor who was well trained in everything that could go wrong. What I soon learned was that she seemed to always be looking for something to go wrong.

I started feeling unsure of my body and my ability to make decisions, and I rarely shared my thoughts on what I wanted my birth to look like. The one time I summoned some courage and told her I didn't want to be induced and didn't want an epidural, she just stared at me. Fast-forward to labor. I had not developed any special circumstances that warranted the watchful eye of a high-risk doctor, so I was primarily left under the care of the L&D nurses, who were happy to let me birth without intervention. Things were moving along fine when my doctor came in and decided to break my water. There was no medical indication for this — she just wanted to speed things up. And of course, I didn't talk back. So that happened…and soon after I was ready to push. I began trying out positions I learned in my birthing class and did a combination of deep breathing and pushing to avoid the burst-a-blood-vessel, high-octane pushing commonly recommended in hospitals. My doctor stood in the corner and watched skeptically for about ten minutes before telling me to put my feet in the metal stirrups and push the way she wanted me to push. Three exhausting hours later Hudson was born. We were healthy, and I had my unmedicated birth, but I didn't feel empowered. I felt like I had been railroaded.

Looking back, I recognize my doctor wasn't "bad," she just wasn't the right fit for me. I wish someone had told me what I'm about to tell you…

What to do

If you're not jiving with your current care provider, find a new one. I can guarantee you won't be the first person to move on from them, and you won't be the last. I can also (almost) guarantee they won't be offended. They have plenty of patients and likely prefer those who happily follow their suggestions, not someone who seems hesitant about their care. So really, you're doing both of you a favor. To find a care provider you gel with, consider the following:

- **Conduct interviews.** These interviews can be done fairly quickly, and sometimes over the phone. You can usually find good suggestions for candidates by asking friends or family members who had the type of birth you're hoping for, or your childbirth preparation educator.
- **Meet with your top choices.** After the initial interviews, have consults with three or four of your favorites, sharing the type of birth you want and paying attention to how they respond. If they seem like they could maybe, possibly support what you want, they might not be a good fit. If they're enthusiastic about your birth preferences and talk about things you can do to set yourself up for your ideal birth — if they make you feel like they'll be your champion — they might be a really great fit.
- **Check in with your gut.** The most important indicator that someone is the right care provider for you is feeling instinctually comfortable with them and excited at the prospect of receiving support and guidance from them. They should be someone you feel you could trust, ask anything of, and tell anything to.

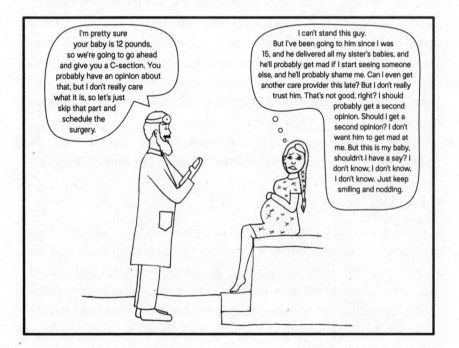

This process can be done at any point during your pregnancy, even a few weeks before your due date. I know a midwife who started caring for a mother the day she went into labor. I also know a woman who had a breech baby and one week before her due date decided to switch from a doctor who was insisting she have a cesarean birth to a care provider who performed breech deliveries.

Above all, you deserve to have a care provider who makes you feel empowered, safe, and capable. And you have every right to hire and fire as many care providers as you need until you find that golden match.

11. I have an STD (sexually transmitted disease). I don't think it's one that impacts pregnancy, so do I have to tell my care provider?

You do. But while the thought of that conversation probably makes you cringe, you have every right to feel *no shame* about sharing this information. According to the Centers for Disease Control (CDC), there were 2,457,118 reported cases of STDs in the United States in 2018 — and many go unreported. That's a lot of people. And I can guarantee all those folks aren't irresponsible miscreants. People contract STDs. It happens. It's something that should obviously be avoided as much as possible through safe sex practices, but despite our best efforts they still occur all the time. This is especially true when we're teens and more prone to in-the-moment "I can't find a condom, but whatever" behavior. And if we contract something like herpes — an STD that can never be erased from the body — we have to deal with those super normal, yet unfortunate, teen decisions forever.

Note: Most care providers recommend testing for human immunodeficiency virus (HIV), hepatitis B, chlamydia, and syphilis during the first prenatal visit.

Although your care provider will provide the most up-to-date information on how your STD could impact pregnancy and what the best course of action will be, here's the lowdown on STD risk factors and the STDs that pose the greatest threat during pregnancy:

- **Can pass to the fetus during delivery:** Without certain medications, chlamydia, gonorrhea, genital herpes, and cytomegalovirus (CMV) can be passed from mother to infant as baby moves through the birth canal.

- **Can infect the fetus during pregnancy:** Syphilis, HIV, and CMV can pass to the fetus.
- **Pregnancy loss:** Syphilis, gonorrhea, HIV, and herpes can all increase the chance of pregnancy loss if left untreated.
- **Chlamydia:** This STD can increase the risk of preterm labor, as well as eye infections or pneumonia in the baby.
- **Gonorrhea:** Eye infections, pneumonia, or infections of the joints or blood in the baby can be caused by gonorrhea.
- **Syphilis:** Syphilis can cause a slew of serious issues for mother and baby, which is why it's often treated with antibiotics during pregnancy.
- **Genital herpes:** Herpes exposure during delivery could lead to problems in baby, like brain damage. Women who have been diagnosed with herpes but don't have active sores will be given medication to prevent an outbreak during delivery. Those with active sores will receive a C-section.
- **Hepatitis B:** As hepatitis can cause serious liver complications, the baby of a woman with this disease will receive the hepatitis B vaccine within twelve hours of birth, in addition to a treatment, called immunoglobulin, that helps prevent a chronic hepatitis infection. Some women might also receive antiviral therapy during the third trimester.
- **CMV:** Cytomegalovirus is a common virus (related to herpes) that often goes undetected. Serious illness could occur if it's passed on to the baby. It's usually managed by giving the mother antiviral medications.
- **HIV/AIDS:** This disease is often managed by giving the baby the medication zidovudine for four to six weeks after birth. In addition, the mother will likely be advised to continue her standard medication regime during pregnancy. A C-section is often recommended if there's an elevated amount of HIV present in the body in the third trimester.

While these risks sound scary, many can be prevented if your care provider knows about your STD as soon as possible and gets you the necessary care.

What to do

Remind yourself that you're not the first pregnant woman to tell her care provider she has an STD. Many women have come before you. Then remind yourself that your care provider is legally obligated to zip it when it comes to everything you tell them — no one else (beyond members of their staff with the clearance to see your chart) will find out, unless you tell them. And because preparation often does wonders for minimizing nerves, think through how you'll tell them the news. As you do this, your head might be filled with visions of your care provider looking at you in horror, or shaking their head in disappointment while making that annoying "tsk tsk" sound. I can almost guarantee they'll do none of the above.

Something else to consider is that you might have omitted this information in numerous prior visits. For example, I've worked with women who have seen their OB-GYN for years, and because of (undeserved!) shame, never told them about their STD. In all cases, the women received treatment for their STDs at a Planned Parenthood. Fast-forward to their pregnancies — now they not only had to tell a person they saw as an authority figure that they had an STD, but also had to let it slip that they had been holding back key medical info for quite some time.

If you're in the same predicament, you might feel the amplified anxiety and embarrassment these women all reported. However, it's important to know that — just like the millions of people who also have STDs — there are likely also hundreds of thousands of other humans who have felt too embarrassed to share this info with their primary care physician. In addition to knowing that you're not alone, know that if your care provider is worth their salt, they won't bring up the fact that you've been keeping this from them. They'll simply mark the info in your chart and discuss how it will be managed. Just another special circumstance. No biggie.

Fears and Worries

12. I just found out my baby's sex and am so disappointed. I desperately wanted a [boy or girl] and don't feel like I can raise the opposite. These feelings are making me feel like I'm betraying my baby. How can I move past them?

Let me tell you a story. I had already picked out outfits for her first Christmas, beach day, and birthday in my head. We had made a long list of girl names, and no boy names because we didn't have to — we were sure we were having a girl. But no. At the twenty-week ultrasound the tech smiled and pointed, "Oh look, there's his little turtle head!" No joke. There was a penis inside of me. I bit down on the inside of my cheek, but the tears still came. Eric was shocked. I immediately felt detached from my baby. I had been connecting to the idea of a girl. I had been thinking about how I would parent a girl. I had been wanting a girl.

Eric had to go to work, so I was left alone to sob in bed. To mourn the baby girl I wasn't having. Waves of disbelief washed over me. And then it happened. The guilt struck. I still had a healthy baby inside me. A sweet little boy whose parents were devastated he was not a she. I started crying again, apologizing over and over again to my boy.

When the tears stopped and rational thinking returned, I realized the sex of my child wouldn't change the way I connect to them. It wouldn't change the way I parent them. It wouldn't change the fact that I was going to put them in ridiculous outfits. And heck, I didn't know how I would connect with or parent them, regardless of their sex, because I hadn't met them. I didn't even know what the baby's gender would actually be. If it had been a girl, maybe she would have identified as a boy, or as neither. Same for my boy. I just didn't know. The only thing I did know was that I would love them completely. Whatever the sex, whatever the gender, whatever the personality, they were my child and I was beyond blessed they had chosen me.

But even after my realizations, it took a few days before we were ready to share the news. I didn't want there to be even a tinge of disappointment in our voices when we said, "We're having a boy!" (We practiced saying it at the same time but could never get in sync.)

So I feel you, mama. It throws us for a loop when we find out we're having a baby who doesn't have the sex we'd hoped for. And I don't buy it when people say, "I don't care what the sex is, I just want a healthy baby." I believe every person expecting a baby has a sex they're rooting for, even if it's just a tiny bit and at a subconscious level. And there's nothing wrong with that. Maybe you have two boys and desperately want a girl. Or maybe you grew up in a household of only women and want the experience of raising a boy. Whatever your reasoning, it's totally understandable. You get to wish for a certain sex. And when it doesn't come true, you get to mourn. You get to freak out. You get to wish the ultrasound tech got it wrong. And then you get to move past the regret and find peace.

What to do

Be upset. Get to a private place and cry. Or scream, "What the [bleep]!" Don't hold back; let your honest emotions and thoughts flow. Write a letter about how friggin' upset you are and rip it up. Then, begin stepping toward acceptance, and even joy, by trying the following:

- **Remember that you're growing a unique human.** As I mentioned before, no mother has any idea who her baby will be, or what gender they'll identify as. Even if the sex had been the one you hoped for, your baby probably wouldn't have perfectly fit into the visions you had of raising a boy or girl.

  Begin connecting to baby as the wholly unique person they'll become by listening to the meditation at this link: yourserenelife.word press.com/babys-gender/.
- **Explore the reasons you wanted a certain sex.** As you envisioned your life with a boy or girl pre-ultrasound, you likely had fantasies of going on certain outings with your girl or boy, maybe guiding them through milestones or connecting over a shared love of literature, pop culture, or whatever your thing is. Write it all down. Then look over those dreams with a new lens — a lens that will help you realize that just because you're having a child that isn't the sex you had hoped for, doesn't mean you can't do the same things with them. The only exceptions I can think of are teaching a boy to not get urine everywhere and to put the seat down, and guiding a girl through her first menstrual

cycles. Beyond that, there's really no bonding experience you can have only with a boy, or a girl.

- **Write a letter to the baby.** If guilt over your disappointment hits, write a letter to your baby explaining how much you love them. Gush over how excited you are. Do whatever you need to do to fill your womb with love as you explore your feelings on the page.

- **Know that your disappointment will fade, but it may take a while.** For many, the disappointment after That Ultrasound will dissolve in a few days, after you get used to your new reality. However, some mothers may feel lingering regret until they deliver their baby. But when you're finally holding your baby in your arms, you'll be shocked you ever wanted anyone who wasn't that exact child.

13. I'm pregnant with my rainbow baby and am so terrified I'll lose this pregnancy that I barely leave the house. What are the chances I'll have another miscarriage/stillbirth? What can I do to avoid it? And how can I calm down and enjoy my pregnancy?

I can't imagine a tragedy greater than the loss of a child. From the incredibly brave women I've worked with who have navigated this heartbreak and from experiencing it myself, I have learned how common it is for fear to encase the heart after loss. Although the conception of a rainbow baby, a baby conceived after a pregnancy loss, is a joyous discovery for many women, it also marks the beginning of a fraught experience. An experience that's a swirl of guilt, hope, anxiety, healing, and fear that the cruelty of loss will strike again. And then there's the stress of being stressed: you know stress isn't good for pregnancy, but you just can't shake the stress that stems from your trauma. It can feel like an impossible situation.

But here's a stat that can hopefully soothe some of those nerves. According to a study published in the *Journal of Human Reproductive Sciences*, only about 2 percent of women will have a repeat miscarriage (pregnancy loss before twenty weeks' gestation) — most go on to have a healthy pregnancy after the initial loss. In regard to stillbirth (pregnancy loss after twenty weeks' gestation), a study published in the *British Medical Journal* found that while women who have had a stillbirth have a higher chance of experiencing another one, the likelihood of this occurrence is rare.

And now for the murkier component of this question, the emotions. Some women feel like they're turning their back on the child they lost by allowing themselves to be happy and hopeful about the new baby they're carrying. But you have every right to let joy bubble to the top of your swirl of emotions. And when you keep making the choice, over and over again, to allow yourself to feel positive emotions — even if it's just glimmers of those emotions — you begin teaching your brain (and heart) that it's able and allowed to move forward, and you begin to realize that moving forward doesn't mean leaving your angel baby behind. Throughout it all, keep reminding yourself that your angel baby will always be in your heart, even on days when you don't think about the loss.

What to do

Find a care provider who is vigilant about helping you understand (as much as possible) what happened in your last pregnancy and is confident about how to support you through this one. This type of care can help you relax a bit more into pregnancy. If you had a stillbirth, consider hiring a maternal-fetal medicine (MFM) specialist.

In addition, ask for more prenatal visits if you feel anxious something will happen in the interim. A family member of mine who experienced a stillbirth requested a prenatal visit every two weeks during the first two trimesters of her next pregnancy, and a visit every week in the third trimester. And don't be afraid to check in if you feel like something is off. Soothing your fears is more important than not calling your care provider too often.

Is there anything else that can help prevent a subsequent pregnancy loss? Maybe. According to the aforementioned study published in the *Journal of Human Reproductive Sciences*, there are various factors that could potentially help you avoid another pregnancy loss, if your initial loss was unexplained. And a study published in *Australian and New Zealand Journal of Obstetrics and Gynaecology* found that 50 percent of miscarriages are unexplained. But many of those are caused by genetic abnormalities, which can't be avoided unless preimplantation genetic testing (PGT) is utilized during an in vitro fertilization (IVF) cycle.

Because there's some debate about the most effective strategies for preventing pregnancy loss, talk with your care provider about whether the following interventions could be useful for your unique situation. Keep in mind that because research is ongoing with many of these treatments, your care provider might not be comfortable recommending them.

- **Folic acid:** Stay on top of taking your 400 mg of folic acid daily, as it helps prevent major birth defects in the baby's brain and spine.
- **Emotional support:** Seeking support from a therapist can help you move through the unique fears attached to your pregnancy. In addition, utilizing alternative support (after your care provider gives you the go-ahead) like acupuncture or hypnotherapy could alleviate stress. You can also use the following link to access a guided meditation I made for women wanting to experience more joy in their rainbow baby pregnancy: yourserenelife.wordpress.com/rainbow-baby/.
- **The norms:** Promote a healthy pregnancy by eating a nutrient-rich diet, exercising regularly, taking your prenatal vitamin, and staying away from no-nos like alcohol, cigarettes, and illicit drugs.
- **Environmental factors:** Limit exposure to harmful products like mercury, solvents, paint thinners, pesticides, and heavy metals. Talk with your care provider about other hazards to avoid.
- **Chronic conditions:** If you have chronic health circumstances such as diabetes, high blood pressure, or other ailments, make a plan with your care provider about how to stay on top of treatment.
- **Sleeping on your side:** Because sleeping on your back could impact the flow of blood and oxygen to the baby, sleeping on your side is the safest option. A pregnancy pillow does wonders for making this comfortable.
- **Aspirin:** Some believe that taking a daily baby aspirin can help prevent pregnancy loss in women with high levels of inflammation. But do not take aspirin without explicit instructions from your care provider.
- **Progesterone:** In some cases, progesterone can help prevent miscarriage in women who experience bleeding in the first trimester.
- **Low molecular weight heparin (LMWH):** The use of LMWH has sometimes been found to help minimize the chance of pregnancy loss.
- **Human chorionic gonadotropin (hCG):** Because hCG plays a critical role in the establishment of a pregnancy, it's believed that hCG injections might help prevent early pregnancy loss.

- **Steroids:** The steroid prednisolone has been found to reduce the amount of a type of cell called uterine natural killer (uNK). Women who have had recurrent miscarriages often have elevated levels of uNK.

- **Intravenous intralipid solution:** Much like prednisolone, intravenous intralipid solution therapy helps prevent natural killer cells from attacking a fetus. While not all women are candidates for this treatment, it's often beneficial for those with endometriosis, autoimmune disorders, connective tissue disorders, or rheumatoid arthritis, as these women are more likely to have elevated levels of active natural killer cells.

- **Immunoglobulins:** This is a type of antibody made by the immune system to battle bacteria, viruses, and other not-nice invaders. Injections of immunoglobulin are especially needed for immune-deficient patients, in addition to those with a negative blood type. While controversial, immunoglobulin therapy is sometimes used to help prevent pregnancy loss for a woman who has experienced recurrent miscarriages.

With all that said, I want to stress how important it is to avoid blaming yourself for your loss. While there are many ways we can promote a healthy pregnancy, a loss is often caused by circumstances out of our control. Give yourself credit for all you're doing to nurture your well-being, and do everything possible to release guilt and adopt trust in your body's ability to move through this pregnancy with ease.

If you're having a hard time enjoying this pregnancy because you're steeped in grief, it might be supportive to find new ways to honor your child who has passed. For example, instead of viewing your grief as the prime way to honor them, you can plant a memorial tree that you regularly meditate by, or write letters to the child. Whatever practice you're drawn to can help you connect to that child, assuring you they'll never be forgotten while also maintaining enough emotional space to give loving focus to your current pregnancy. Of course, you'll still have moments of regret, anger, and sorrow, but they'll no longer be the main channels of connection with your child who has passed on. You'll now have a new channel that fosters emotional relief and evolution.

14. I break out in a cold sweat every time I pee, in fear there will be blood when I wipe. Is blood a definite sign I'm miscarrying?

My husband Eric and I had just had sex, and I was going pee. I wiped, and froze. There was bright red blood on the toilet paper. I was ten weeks along, so according to a study published in *British Medical Journal* I had about a 9 percent chance of miscarrying. I know this because I imme-diately used my shaking hands to look up miscarriage stats. Then I did what any normal woman would do and called my mom while crying so hard I was snorting. She's an RN and always does a spectacular job of underreacting to most physical ailments. The first thing out of her mouth was, "Blood is not a definite sign you're miscarrying." Because we have no boundaries, I told her the blood came after sex. She assured me the blood was likely coming from my cervix, which bleeds more easily during pregnancy because blood vessels are developing in the area. Because of her aforementioned underreacting, I still made an emergency appointment with my OB, who seconded everything Mom said. I was fine.

So while it's never a bad idea to check in with your care provider if you experience vaginal bleeding, you don't need to panic like I did. Be-yond sex, there are many reasons why a bit of blood may flow out as your body moves through all these wild changes. For one, it's common to have light to medium bleeding as the embryo is implanting in the uterine lin-ing, about ten to fourteen days after fertilization. In addition, the cervix goes through a process called "cervical remodeling" that includes soften-ing, ripening, dilation, and postpartum repair. The softening begins in the first trimester and can cause bleeding in some women; the ripening begins a few weeks or days before you go into labor; and the dilating and post-partum repair stages are self-explanatory. Additional causes of bleeding include a vaginal exam and excessive exercise.

To assure you even more that bleeding is pretty normal, I'll cite a study, published in *Pediatric and Perinatal Epidemiology*, that found that 22 percent of women experience vaginal bleeding during pregnancy — and many of these go on to have healthy babies, even those that had some heavy bleeding. The study also reported slightly higher rates of bleeding in women of advanced maternal age, those with passive smoking exposure, or women who have had a prior preterm birth or multiple miscarriages or induced abortions.

While I'm here to uplift and not to freak you out, I'd be remiss if

I didn't mention the more alarming causes of vaginal bleeding, which include miscarriage, ectopic pregnancy, placenta previa (when the placenta covers part, or all, of the cervix), placental abruption (when the placenta separates from the uterus), and early labor. But know that these are much less common than the other mentioned causes of bleeding.

What to do

If your trips to the bathroom are shrouded in fear, take five long and slow breaths before sitting on the toilet. These breaths help to pull you out of fight-flight-freeze and allow calm, rational thoughts to return. You can also say an affirmation, like "I am on the exact path to motherhood I'm meant to be on" or "My self and my baby are glowing with health." Say whatever you need to return to a space of trust.

Then, if blood does appear when you wipe, repeat the process — five deep breaths and repetition of your affirmation of choice. Next, take note of the color and amount of blood, and check to see if any clots or tissue is present. If there is enough bleeding to require absorption, use a pad — never a tampon. Finally, give your care provider a ring to talk through the possible explanations for the bleeding, and then decide whether you need to be checked. All the while, keep breathing and reminding yourself of all the nonthreatening causes for a bit of vaginal bleeding.

After you've received the all clear from your care provider, they might still recommend the following: Netflix-ing and chilling, drinking more water, propping up your feet, backing off physical activity, and not lifting anything over ten pounds.

Anxiety Release Tool: To enhance that deep breathing and affirmation practice, try the tapping technique EFT, which stands for Emotional Freedom Technique. This can reset any fearful, chaotic energy running through your body. Instructions can be found on page 306. I recommend trying this technique before using the bathroom or moving into any activity that triggers negative emotions or physical responses.

15. I think kids are irritating. Does that mean I'll be a bad mom?

Nope. There are plenty of women who stiffen at the sight of kids but are still great mamas. You're allowed both. And if it's any comfort, I naively thought the fact that I love kids would make motherhood a breeze. I was mistaken.

For those who find comfort in a controlled environment where social norms are followed, kids can be jarring enigmas. If you're one of these people, you might feel like you're missing a part of the brain that allows you to relate to the littles, which could understandably make you uncomfortable interacting with them. And there is nothing wrong with feeling this way. We all have different things that make us tick and trigger discomfort. If kids are one of your discomfort triggers, it doesn't mean you're a monster; it means you're a human who finds it hard to relate to people who seem to be in their own world half the time, and who poop their pants.

Something that will have your back (and heart) as you get to know both your child and who you are as a mother is oxytocin, the "love hormone" or "social glue" that helps humans attach to their babies, even if that attachment takes a while. When you engage in common acts of mothering like feeding, holding, cooing, and smelling that yummy baby head, the pituitary gland releases oxytocin, which reinforces nurturing. So the more you nurture, the better you feel. And as you're reveling in this feel-good hormone, your baby will be doing the same. This love juice doesn't make you start loving all the babies, but it'll make you really like your own (at least most of the time).

If you notice a lack of pleasure when interacting with baby, your body might not be producing adequate levels of oxytocin. As this could be a sign of postpartum depression — which *is not your fault* — check in with your care provider to ensure you receive quality support.

In addition to oxytocin, there's also the little thing where motherhood cracks you open. It shakes up all your preconceived notions and turns you into a new version of your pre-pregnancy self. This new version might still find other kids irritating, but it will have a new skill set that helps you care for and relate to your little human. You'll also develop deeper empathy for the kid-crew as you gain insight into why they do what they do. For example, after you have a baby and hear another baby crying, you might find that you're no longer irked by the sound but instead recognize it as a request for a clean diaper or some boob. Realizing how much parenthood changes you can be equal parts overwhelming and fascinating.

The most drastic motherhood change I've seen took place in my friend, whom I'll call Clarissa. When a kid would run up to her, babbling about kid stuff, Clarissa used to recoil. She would give them a tight smile and excuse herself. The few times I saw her hold a baby, they would start crying — one time Clarissa started crying! So I was shocked when she became pregnant. Yes, kids freaked her out, but she said that because she and her partner came from small families they wanted people to hang out with as they grew old. Fair enough. But because her desire to have a baby was inspired by thoughts of what life would be like when the child was an adult, she had serious doubts and anxieties about her ability to care for a baby. She was so sure early motherhood would be awful that she asked her doctor to pre-emptively prescribe antidepressants. But she never needed them. When the baby was born, a switch flipped and her maternal skills turned on. She still finds other kids intolerable but adores her own. Her partner is in charge of "mommy and me" gatherings and kid parties, and Clarissa takes the reigns at home. It works for them.

That maternal-skills and all-consuming-love switch might not immediately flip for you, and that's okay. Even women who adore kids sometimes find it difficult to tap into mom mode. Be gentle with yourself, ask for support (professional support if you're really feeling blue), keep nurturing that baby even when it feels uncomfortable, and take care of your own needs, as they're still essential.

What to do

Remember that each mother and baby have their own way of relating. While these relationships may look similar on the outside, every mother and baby duo has a customized thing going. And you will find your thing as you navigate parenthood. You and your baby, and the rest of your tribe, will figure out the care systems and types of bonding that work best for you. It might not fall into place immediately, but continuing to follow your intuition regarding what feels right for you and your family will help you eventually find an individualized system that works. And don't worry if your system looks totally different from what other families are doing. All that matters is that you figure out a way of life that gives everyone involved the opportunities to be happy, healthy, and fulfilled.

Tip: Because it can feel really strange (and a little boring) to talk to a human who can't speak, begin practicing by talking to your baby while they're in the womb. As you practice this skill, know that you don't have to speak in simple sentences, or in a baby voice. Feel free to read aloud from the newspaper, sing along to your favorite opera, or talk to your belly about your thoughts on climate change. The point is to expose baby to your voice and language, so you might as well talk about things that interest you. This exercise will peel away one of the many layers of newness you'll experience during early motherhood, helping you feel a little more prepared for the unknown.

16. I thought about terminating this pregnancy. I now want the baby but am filled with guilt, and I fear that my initial ambivalence means I'll be a bad mom. How do I move past this?

Full transparency: This question came from my own experience. When I conceived Hudson, I was twenty-four, in a pretty new relationship with my now husband, Eric, and driving for work every day from Ojai to Los Angeles, over eighty miles one way. The conditions weren't great for a baby, but they also weren't horrible.

Eric was overwhelmed by the pregnancy but made it clear he would fully support whatever I wanted. My instincts told me this was the baby I was meant to have, but my mind, and my mom, told me I was crazy. My mom had worked in Planned Parenthood and saw firsthand that abortion was the best choice for many women in similar circumstances. However, I had a nagging feeling it wasn't the choice for me.

When I made the final decision to keep the baby, I felt both relieved and guilty. Despite my beliefs about a woman's right to choose, I thought, "If I'm meant to be the mother of this child, and I'm able to be a good mother, how could I have considered terminating?" And then I did something I never do. I got superstitious. I became sure that the invisible powers that be would punish me by causing a miscarriage.

Looking back, it's wild how hard I was on myself. I've supported friends through similar situations, and I had nothing but compassion for the journey they were on. I've loved friends through the sorrow and relief of choosing an abortion, and I've nurtured loved ones through the same guilt I was feeling over considering abortion when ultimately choosing to continue a pregnancy. I had held those women and with total honesty told them they had nothing to feel guilty about. I told them how much I admired their willingness to carefully and thoughtfully review all their options as they considered their ability to give a baby a safe and healthy life. Remembering those conversations was the first step in healing my guilt. The second step was realizing that guilt was a pointless emotion, at least in this case. It was sucking my attention away from enjoying and nurturing my pregnancy.

I've since had clients who navigated a similar start to their pregnancy. When they come to me drenched in guilt, the first thing I have them do is tune in to the emotions and physical sensations of compassion — whatever that means to them (more on that below). When they're in that softer, more forgiving state, I remind them that instead of guilt they deserve to feel pride. They didn't view pregnancy as something forced on them — something they had to do because they had no other options. They *had* options and chose pregnancy. When I finally came to this realization in my own experience, I felt my bond with my baby deepen. Our relationship wasn't being built upon a forced choice — we were in each other's lives on purpose.

What to do

Tune in to that aforementioned state of compassion. Sit in a private, comfortable space and close your eyes. Envision a warm light that represents compassion flowing into the top of your head and spreading through every nerve, cell, and muscle in your body. Feel your mind absorbing the compassion like a sponge. As you do this, take in long, deep breaths. In this state of calm, tune in to how you define compassion. What does that feel like in your body? What types of thoughts does the idea of compassion bring to mind? Feel yourself being bathed in those thoughts and feelings — become one with compassion.

As you float in this compassionate state, say over and over again, in your head or out loud, "I chose this baby, and that is amazing. I chose this baby, and that is amazing." Allow this mantra to remind you that considering abortion is not a betrayal of your baby. You went through the responsible process of looking at all your options and making a well-informed choice for your unique situation.

17. I smile and nod during my childbirth prep classes but don't really believe any of the tips will work. What should I do?

Most of the messages society gives us about childbirth boil down to, "It will be the most painful experience of your life…you'll hate your partner… you'll probably poop…and your vagina will never be the same." So, yeah, it's pretty hard to trust that anything short of narcotics will get you through.

When I was pregnant, I religiously practiced HypnoBirthing techniques and told everyone who asked that I believed this method would work. But I was doubtful, like *really* doubtful. Even while preaching its benefits, I would think, "How is a bit of breathing and meditation going to get me through the whole pushing-a-human-through-my-vagina thing without screaming for drugs?" But despite the doubt, I kept practicing. I kept asking, "Well…what if? What if this actually works?"

Watching HypnoBirthing birth videos actually chipped away at my doubt more than any other aspect of preparation. Witnessing these women have intense experiences with calm, and without drugs, helped me hold on to that "What if?": "If they can do it, what if I can too?" And then I went into labor. Holy guacamole, was it the most intense emotional and physical experience I'd ever had! But the childbirth prep techniques worked. I didn't use them all, but certain ones came to me at different times. It was like my body and subconscious mind were in cahoots to get me through the experience. I would be wondering what the heck to do, and all of a sudden an answer would come. "Keep doing your surge breaths…Sit on the birth ball and swirl your hips…Have someone press on your back…Tell Eric to stop sleeping because it's filling you with rage-envy…" The answers kept coming and held me in the space of knowing I could get through it. I did ask for an epidural, but everyone ignored me and I forgot about it when the next contraction came.

With all that said, my birth could have played out very differently, even with the same amount of preparation. I had a cervix that seemed happy to open, a uterus that really wanted to get the baby out, and care providers who didn't push intervention. I say this because I'd never want a woman to feel like she failed if she's vigilant about childbirth preparation but ends up needing interventions she hadn't planned on. And sometimes we change our mind during birth. We decide an epidural is the best thing for us, or that Pitocin is essential to get things going. None of that means all the work you put into childbirth preparation was a waste.

There is a common misconception that childbirth preparation classes, especially those more focused on unmedicated birth, have the sole purpose of getting you that unmedicated birth. I believe all childbirth preparation classes — at least those focused more on calm and empowerment than fear — help you do the following:

- Foster a greater bond with your baby during pregnancy.
- Develop a deeper understanding of your body and the process of birth.
- Receive tools to stay calm and focused whether you're having an unmedicated birth, a medicated birth, or a cesarean birth.
- Feel empowered to guide your birth journey, instead of feeling like you're at the mercy of others.

You don't have to have complete faith that the class you're in will get you an unmedicated birth. You just have to remind yourself that you're doing yourself and baby a huge service by putting thought and preparation into your birth experience, even though you have no idea how it will unfold.

What to do

Find a childbirth preparation method and a teacher you resonate with, as all methods and teachers are not created equal. You'll have a much better experience if you put time and effort into researching the various methods available and call up teachers you're considering. I recommend calling or video chat because it's easier to get an accurate read on someone when you're speaking with them. If you prefer online classes, look for a free introduction video you can watch before committing. You can find my online course here: udemy.com/course/childbirth-preparation-a-complete-guide-for-pregnant-women/.

Once you find the course for you, fully commit. Try all the techniques they recommend and continue practicing those that resonate with you. And remember, you don't need to believe that everything you're doing will guarantee an unmedicated birth. All you have to believe is that all this preparation will serve an important purpose, even if you don't know exactly what that is.

Sex and the Vagina

18. Are these kinky, kind of eerie sex dreams I'm having normal?

Heck, yes. When I was pregnant I had sex dreams about the guy that's always eating sandwiches outside our grocery store, the mysterious library clerk with dreadlocks, and some ex-boyfriends for good measure. Sometimes these were not-so-dreamy encounters, and I'd be trying to lock doors to stop the sex. I would wake up feeling relieved it hadn't actually happened, but also ashamed my mind had gone there. Other times, the dreams *were* dreamy, and I'd wake up in solidarity with preteen boys who need to sleep with tissue by their bed. I've heard women report sex dreams that involved family members, and even animals. Yup. Most of these women blushed as they whispered how turned on / embarrassed they were by these dreams. So you can be sure that however strange your sex dreams, and whatever your reaction to them may be, there's someone out there who has had a stranger one, and a similar response.

I also encourage you to really let this sink in: Our dreams don't make us miscreants unfit for motherhood. We don't need to shame our poor brain for the random stuff it cooks up when we're dozing, because those thoughts in no way mean we actually have a desire to engage in the acts playing out behind our eyelids, even if we wake up throbbing in all the fun ways.

Dreams should not be taken literally but instead viewed as representations of more emotional aspects of our life. For example, sexual dreams about people who aren't your partner are believed to represent breaking away from your old life as you near motherhood. And dreams about women, even if you're with a woman, are thought to symbolize feelings about your shifting body and identity.

Many of us actually have these bizarre dreams even when we're not pregnant — we just don't remember them. As you might have discovered, your sleep is much lighter during pregnancy, especially when your bladder is waking you every five minutes to pee out a few drops. Because of this light sleep, you remember more of your dreams. In addition, women have increased blood flow to the genitals and an influx of estrogen that ups vaginal secretions during pregnancy. These factors combine to make sex a common idea floating in your subconscious mind, and intense arousal a common response. Consider yourself lucky.

What to do

If you want to dive into the fascinating practice of dissecting your dreams, write them down, or make a voice memo when you wake up — even if it's the middle of the night. Then, take time later to examine the contents of the dream on your own, or with a therapist if you really want to get into it. Because dreams aren't a science, feel free to create meanings that feel good to you and that support the exploration of the changes you're experiencing. If you're still feeling uneasy about your mind-movies after this process, listen to this recording, which helps reduce the many forms of shame that crop up during pregnancy and motherhood: yourserenelife .wordpress.com/releasing-shame/.

19. I'm feeling so turned on and want to masturbate all the time. But when I do, I'm consumed with shame because I'm so aware of my baby being *right there*. Is there a way to stop the shame? Or should I just hold off on masturbation until after childbirth?

Do not, I repeat, do not deprive yourself of the deliciousness of masturbation during pregnancy. Because of the increased blood flow to the vagina I keep talking about, the surge of progesterone and estrogen upping your vaginal secretions, and uber sensitive breasts and nipples, your body is ripe for the pleasuring. Beyond being a totally normal activity during pregnancy, masturbation can actually elevate your health by soothing stress through a release of endorphins, improving blood flow, minimizing pregnancy pains, and helping you slip into a restful sleep. Baby also reaps rewards, as they can be comforted by the rhythmic uterine contractions triggered by orgasm.

It's important to remember that growing a baby does not cancel out your sexuality. You're still a sexual being who needs and deserves various forms of pleasure. However, as you explore your sexuality during pregnancy, you might find that different things turn you on. For example, I have a heterosexual friend who told me in whispers that one of the only things that turned her on during pregnancy were erotic stories about lesbian encounters. She said she wasn't attracted to women but found the stories so sexy during pregnancy. After she had the baby, I asked if the stories were still her thing. "Not really," she said. "I finally like my husband's penis again!"

If you prefer sex to masturbation but find that intercourse is uncomfortable, or have a partner who can't get over being so close to baby's temporary home, consider mutual masturbation. This allows you to share intimacy with your partner while bypassing everyone's discomfort.

Fun Fact: The beloved G-spot often becomes more accessible during pregnancy. And did you know you also have an A-spot and a U-spot? The A-spot is located above the cervix (so don't go there during pregnancy), and the U-spot encircles the urethral opening (go there).

In regard to baby being right there while the deed is being done, know that they have no idea what you're doing. They're busy floating in a warm waterbed and breathing in amniotic fluid. They couldn't care less what you're doing.

What to do

Masturbate! Find a comfortable, private space, pull out your inspiration materials or tools of choice, and go to town — downtown.

- If you have a hard time reaching that special spot, invest in a vibrator or dildo — just make sure they're clean before use by washing them with soap and water.
- Don't be shy about exploring various areas of your body — for example, those plump breasts.
- Before you begin the fun, minimize the chance of scratches during fervent rubbing by cutting and filing your nails.

If thoughts of baby trigger a flood of shame during masturbation, remind yourself that you're doing nothing wrong. It's healthy and natural. You can also close your eyes and envision floating away to another realm where only you exist — we'll call it Pleasure Town.

Note: If you have special circumstances, such as a risk of preterm labor, placenta previa, or uterine infections, confirm with your care provider that masturbation is a safe choice. And if you're embarrassed asking about this, know that they'll likely be relieved you trust them enough to ask this personal question, and that this is likely far from the strangest question they've received.

20. How do I become more comfortable having sex while pregnant? Is the baby aware of what we're doing?

Although sex is an essential component of conception (at least most of the time — love you, IVF!), I initially found postconception sex awkward, as I got all up in my head about baby being *right there*. I prayed he wouldn't start kicking during sex and tried to avoid wild rocking motions. I wasn't a lot of fun between the sheets that first trimester. Eric was even more unsettled, worrying about his penis poking the baby. We were missing the ingredients for a juicy sex life, until we learned something super helpful…

Babies have no idea what their parents are doing! They're floating in their warm fluid, pretty oblivious to what's happening around them. And sure, at around eighteen weeks' gestation, baby begins to hear sounds outside the womb, but they have no frame of reference for moaning or dirty talk. To them, it's all jumbled sounds. Regarding the penis-poke phobia, male partners need not worry, as the mucus plug securely lodged in the cervix prevents anything from getting into the uterus. And then there's those back-and-forth motions: baby might actually love this, as it creates a gentle sway in the womb that could help them get some sleep. And then, if you're the lucky duck who reaches orgasm, the flood of endorphins and rhythmic pulsations in the uterus soothes baby even more.

Yet, despite all the goodness prenatal sex can bring for all involved, it can still be strange to feel the little one move, or to suddenly start thinking of baby names when you're getting frisky. And the physical logistics of sex once your belly has bloomed can make it tricky to get baby thoughts out and bow-chicka-bow-wow vibes in. But because sex is such a wonderful way to maintain intimacy with your partner and enhance your mental and emotional health, we need to get you past these blocks.

What to do

Before you engage in sex, remind yourself and your partner of everything mentioned above. The baby doesn't know what's happening, couldn't care less about the sounds and motions, and has no idea that there's a penis afoot.

Something else that helps is making the sex *so good* — so in-the-present-moment-mind-blowingly-wow — that there's little room left for self-conscious baby brooding. Sprinkle some sexy fairy-dust on your libido by getting creative. Seek fresh inspiration in reading erotic stories together, investing in some new toys, taking your time with foreplay, or brainstorming other ways to get the juices flowing. For example, I never thought dirty talk was my thing until a need to spice things up exposed me to its naughty wonders in my second trimester. Suddenly I was so consumed by lust I had no awareness for anything but pleasure. "Baby who?"

Tip: If you're experiencing fatigue, get some nooky in the morning when your energy is likely at its peak.

If the logistics of sex are tripping you up (for example, maybe penetration is uncomfortable, or you can't find a user-friendly position), try out mutual masturbation or a pose that's suited for pregnancy, like doggy style, spooning, standing, seated, or cowgirl. Yeehaw, y'all!

With that said, if all you want to do is hold a trash bin in front of your face and nibble saltines, don't feel pressured to have sex. Your number one priority is taking care of your needs, so if sex isn't currently in your cards, don't beat yourself up. If your partner is yearning for hanky-panky, remind them that you love them and are turned on by them, and that your lack of desire for sex isn't personal — it's just not a good time. Then, when you're feeling better, you can check in with yourself to see if you're ready to engage in a pants-off horizontal (or vertical) dance-off.

Tip: If you've passed your due date and are trying to get things going, have a roll in that hay, as the hormone prostaglandin that's present in semen can stimulate the cervix and cause contractions. And the rest of you can rest at ease, knowing that sex shouldn't send a woman having a healthy pregnancy into preterm labor.

21. Could the rush of blood from an orgasm hurt my baby?

As long as you don't have a medical condition that creates a high risk for miscarriage, preterm labor, or bleeding (confirm this with your care provider), you're all clear to orgasm to your vagina's content. Heck, you might even find yourself reveling in multiple orgasms, as they can be more intense and easier to come by during pregnancy.

Regarding the rush of blood, it could actually benefit baby, as it sends more oxygen to the uterus. And the uterine contractions that occur during orgasm are like a massage for baby, while the surge of oxytocin fills both of you with happy feels.

What to do

If your pregnancy is free of special circumstances, orgasm away. If you're unsure whether you're at risk for a circumstance that could be triggered by sex or orgasm, check in with your care provider before heading to Pleasure Town.

It's also important to follow your instincts when it comes to sex and pleasuring yourself. If a position feels uncomfortable, move out of it, and if you'd prefer to skip penetration in favor of foreplay, speak up. And hey, girl, don't forget to take advantage of your alone time.

22. My vulva is so swollen you can see it through my pants. Why is it like that, and what can I do about it?

Been there. I even nicknamed myself Mama Moose Knuckle when I was pregnant. I was so embarrassed by my bulging vulva that I swapped my beloved yoga pants for sweats and skirts — until I discovered why the bulge was there, and that almost every other preggo lady was also hiding a puffy moose knuckle. Get this — to support the uterus during pregnancy, your blood volume increases by nearly 50 percent. This is caused by an elevation of the hormones estrogen and progesterone. In addition, as the uterus enlarges, it can block the flow of blood, intensifying swelling in the vulva and legs.

For many women, this surge of fresh blood can up your libido and create an almost constant state of arousal. After all, blood also rushes to the vulva and introitus (the lower area of the vagina), and it causes swelling when the body is preparing to orgasm. I'll trade my stretchy pants for that any day.

However, if you're experiencing pain, burning, or redness instead of pleasurable pulsations, check in with your care provider, as this could be a sign of infection, certain skin disorders, or low estrogen levels. In addition to the swelling, you might discover a web of varicose veins creeping across your vulva. Yay. These are also caused by the abundance of blood and will likely go away a few weeks after birth.

Another fun change this extra blood may cause is a darkening of the skin covering the labia. The skin could also develop a bluish or purplish tint. But as your blood volume returns to normal after birth, the coloring and swelling should minimize, or completely go away.

What to do

If you're one of the lucky ones experiencing throbs of bliss, relish it. But if you're not, check in with your care provider to ensure the discomfort isn't a sign of a special circumstance that requires attention. Then, try the following:

- **Soothe the ouch.** Slip back into comfort by applying a cold compress, elevating your hips, and wearing a compression garment (after getting the go-ahead from your care provider). To minimize varicose vein annoyance, take a warm bath, lie on your left side, and elevate your feet. Light exercise can also do wonders for many vaginal issues, as long as you remove that moist underwear and shower as soon as you're done.
- **Buy the right undies.** Lessen excess irritation by using 100 percent organic cotton, Goldilocks panties — not too loose and not too tight. And for the love of your crotch, skip the thongs.
- **Wear loose lower-duds.** Opt for roomy bottoms, as the friction from tight pants or skirts can increase discomfort — or constantly distract you with stimulation. (No judgment if you're intrigued by that idea!) Loose clothing also hides the bulge if you find it embarrassing. However, you don't need to be embarrassed. For example, a mom in one of my classes had the superpower of finding the chicest fitted maternity jeans. These jeans showed off everything — her toned legs, juicy booty...and enlarged vulva. But she didn't care, saying, "It's a product of this amazing process that's happening inside me, and I have no desire to hide it. And I get a kick out of seeing people's faces when their eyes land on it."

23. Why does my vagina smell weird?

Because my husband Eric and I have no boundaries, I would fill him in on the various scents my vagina would emit during pregnancy. He loved it. Some days it would be Scent of Asparagus. Others would be Cabbage with a Splash of Dirty Socks, and on the really special days I got to enjoy the aroma of Expired Fish with Undertones of Ammonia. (I should patent these scents before someone tries to steal them out from under me.)

Luckily, Eric had no idea what I was talking about, because only my nose was lucky enough to pick up the scents. I had developed something called hyperosmia, which is a heightened sense of smell (the worst super-power ever). This increased nasal sensitivity meant I picked up every fragrance my vagina was dropping. Asking the smart medical people I know about these smells revealed that (most of the time) they don't actually emanate out of the interior of the vagina; instead they are primarily caused by leftover urine in and around the vulva. While these leftovers don't have much of an aroma when you're not pregnant, pregnancy pee can take on strong scents for any of the following reasons:

- **Dehydration:** When you're dehydrated, urine will be more concentrated, meaning its aroma will also be more concentrated. More water = less-stinky pee. This is an amazing motivator to stay hydrated if I've ever smelled one.
- **Diet:** When you're pregnant, it's not just asparagus that stinks up your flow — Brussels sprouts, garlic, and onions also do a number on your Vagina Eau de Parfum. I craved all of these. Brussels sprouts barbecued with maple syrup, sautéed onions on top of chicken potpies, and garlic in everything. No wonder oral sex wasn't a thing during my pregnancy. Other foods that can tinker with urine include broccoli, cauliflower, curry, fish, and cumin.
- **Vitamins and supplements:** Vitamin B6, calcium, and vitamin D can all make urine smell fishy. Because most prenatal vitamins contain all three, you can expect slightly (or not so slightly) fishy pee.

In addition to all of the above, the increased blood supply during pregnancy can impact the pH balance of your vagina, sometimes causing it to become more acidic. You'll likely also experience more discharge; this shouldn't have much of a smell, but when mixed with urine it might take on a more pungent odor.

What to do

Tell your care provider. While a fragrant vagina is often caused by the issues above, it can also be a sign of a yeast infection, urinary tract infection, bacterial vaginosis, sexually transmitted disease, or other issues. While I understand the embarrassment that comes with a smelly vagina, your care provider has smelled it all and will just be glad you're comfortable enough asking whether you should be concerned. After you have the clean bill of health, try the following to deodorize your petunia:

- **Wipe well.** Kill the number one culprit of vagina stink, leftover urine, by wiping with unscented, organic cotton intimate wet wipes.
- **Wear organic cotton underwear.** The sweaty crotch we talked about in the last question can contribute to vaginal odors. By wearing breathable cotton panties you can minimize nether-region odors.
- **Drink apple cider vinegar.** Because this type of vinegar makes your urine a bit more alkaline, it also makes it smell better, as more acidic urine smells more like ammonia. After checking with your care provider, aim for mixing one to two tablespoons of apple cider vinegar into your smoothie or juice, up to two times a day.
- **Use essential oils.** While I can almost guarantee that no one else can smell your vagina, you can keep it from bothering you by rubbing two to three drops of an essential oil — mixed with a carrier oil like jojoba or almond oil — into your inner thighs, being sure not to get it on the vagina. Use only mild oils that are safe to use on the skin, like lavender, frankincense, or sandalwood. With the exception of these oils, stay away from all scented feminine hygiene products, as they could cause irritation.

24. My vagina occasionally feels like a bolt of lightning is hitting it. What's up with that? How can I make it stop?

Well, my friend, you are experiencing what's aptly called *lightning crotch.* You sometimes feel like you're getting an electric punch to the crotch because baby is pressing on or kicking a nerve, or their head is dropping down in preparation for B-Day and pressing on nerves around the cervix. Because of this, lightning crotch (so fun to type!) often occurs in the third trimester.

These bolts of ouch can also be caused by round ligament pain, which happens when the ligaments that support your pelvis and uterus stretch too far and too fast because of an influx of the hormone relaxin. While lightning crotch could be a sign that your body is preparing for labor, it's not usually a symptom of early labor.

What to do

Make sure you're getting enough magnesium, as this mineral is essential for nerve function. To discover if you have a deficiency, ask your care provider to order a magnesium RBC blood test. If you are deficient, ask them about the best ways to get the recommended dose of 350–360 mg of magnesium per day. They'll likely recommend a supplement or eating more magnesium-rich foods, like almonds, spinach, chard, avocados, bananas, and pumpkin seeds.

In addition, spinal manipulation and myofascial release by a chiropractor trained to work with pregnant women, as well as acupuncture, could reduce nerve pain. But get the go-ahead from your care provider before seeking these treatments.

Beyond magnesium and bodywork, you can minimize the discomfort of what one of my friends lovingly refers to as "electro puss" by whipping out those pain-relieving techniques you're learning in childbirth prep class. For example, taking deep breaths, changing positions to get baby off your nerves, and relaxing your body can alleviate those jolts of pain. In addition, wearing a belly support garment could potentially lift baby off the nerve, or nerves, they occasionally press on.

25. My discharge is grossing me out. Why is there so much of it? Is it ever a sign of a problem?

One of my childbirth prep class mamas once told me she felt like she had a bottle of "drippy glue" leaking out of her vagina. "It's everywhere down there — all the time. I go through like ten pair of underwear a day. WTF?"

I'll tell you what I told her: Vagina-glue is a sure sign your child will be an arts and crafts savant. Just kidding. But for real, this is an incredibly normal by-product of pregnancy, and it has a fun name! Leukorrhea. Okay, maybe not so fun.

This abundance of goo is caused by an elevation in estrogen, which increases the amount of blood pumping to the pelvis area, which stimulates the mucous membranes, which makes your vagina a discharge factory. It can be icky, but it serves many purposes for the vagina, such as wiping away dead cells, helping its bacteria levels find equilibrium, and guarding the birth canal from infection.

While leukorrhea is usually thin, odorless, a little sticky, and clear or white, its color can range from green, yellow, pink, or red, to white, brown, or gray, depending on what's going on within your body.

Here's a discharge color guide:

- **Clear to white:** This is what normal discharge usually looks like.
- **Green or yellow:** These hues could signal the presence of the STD chlamydia or trichomoniasis.
- **Pink:** A bit of pink discharge in early pregnancy could appear when the embryo implants in the uterus. When you're nearing your due date, thick gobs of clear discharge tinged with pink or red could occur when your mucus plug dislodges in preparation for birth — this is also called *bloody show*.
- **Red:** Tinges of red in discharge can be normal in early or late pregnancy, because of the implantation and mucus plug mentioned above. A touch of red discharge may also appear after sex. However, if you experience so much red that it's more blood than "red discharge," reach out to your care provider immediately, as this could be a sign of a complication.
- **Brown:** Brown discharge is common in early pregnancy, when old blood is clearing out of the uterus. Alert your care provider if you experience dark brown discharge, as this could be a sign of miscarriage, ectopic pregnancy, or an issue with the placenta.
- **Gray:** The vaginal infection bacterial vaginosis could cause gray discharge. It's caused by a bacterial imbalance in the vagina that can be rebalanced with antibiotics.

In addition to color, the odor, consistency, and accompanying symptoms of discharge could be signs that something is off:

- **Fishy:** In addition to gray discharge, a fishy odor is a common calling card of bacterial vaginosis.
- **Cottage cheese:** If food aversions haven't already put you off cottage cheese, know that the vagina equivalent of this dairy dish may appear on your toilet paper if you have a yeast infection.
- **Itching or burning:** Another joy of a yeast infection is itching, burning, an inflamed vulva, or my favorite, all of the above!

If you experience discharge that indicates an infection or other issue, tell your care provider. While you're likely qualified to diagnose a yeast infection, for example, it's still best to get the green light before using over-the-counter or homemade treatments.

What to do

Because pregnancy doesn't need any help being uncomfortable, here are a few ways to minimize the wet and yucky feeling of normal discharge in your unders, and the bevy of discomforts caused by not-normal discharge:

- **Wear unscented, organic cotton panty liners.** These are a safe way to prevent discharge from soaking through your panties and making you feel like you wet yourself a little.
- **Don breathable cotton undergarments.** Beyond being comfortable, not-too-tight underwear made from a breathable fabric like cotton helps prevent excess moisture — which is like a breeding ground for yeast infection–inducing bacteria.
- **Say no to tampons and douching.** Beyond a penis, your fingers, a sex toy, or your care provider's vaginal exam devices, nothing should be going up your vagina during pregnancy. As tempting as it can be to use a tampon to thwart your discharge's descent, tampons can introduce harmful bacteria. And you don't want to douche, as it could disrupt the balance of micro-organisms in your vagina and potentially cause bacterial vaginosis.
- **Use unscented personal care products.** As the chemicals used for many scented products can disrupt the sensitive vaginal ecosystem,

resist the temptation to purchase perfumed toilet paper, soaps, oils, or anything else that might touch your vagina.

• **Honor the wiping rule.** When we were potty trained, many of us were taught to wipe front to back, to prevent fecal matter from entering the vagina. This is especially important during pregnancy, as not abiding by this golden rule could lead to a urinary tract infection (UTI).

• **Get those probiotics.** Eating unsweetened yogurt, kefir, sauerkraut, and other probiotic-rich foods infuses the vagina with healthy bacteria, helping to prevent unpleasantries like yeast infections and bacterial vaginosis.

• **Avoid sugar.** As yeast loves sugar, eating too much of the sweet stuff can cause an overabundance of yeast in the vagina, which leads to... you know.

Skin and Appearance

26. I've heard so many women talk about loving their pregnant body, but I can't stand mine. I can barely look in the mirror, and I feel so unsexy. My body shame is even making me resent my baby. Is there something wrong with me?

With a culture that has historically valued a flat stomach and slim thighs above all else, it's so normal for pregnant women to feel uncomfortable and unattractive as their body shifts. Even women who never had body issues can have physical insecurities triggered during pregnancy.

The cause of much of this insecurity is the speed at which the changes are happening. We barely have time to integrate with what's happening. It's like, bam! — one morning we wake up and it looks like someone drew a line down our belly with a brown Sharpie. Then bam! — our fingers are too pudgy for our rings and our nose has gotten wider and squishier. And oh look — now our favorite clothes don't fit, parts of our body we didn't think would bulge are bulging, and our feet feel like they were injected with Play-Doh. And the changes don't stop for at least twelve months. I mean, come on! Who wouldn't be thrown by these almost constant shifts in appearance?

If you're thinking, "Um, those ladies who are always waxing lyrical about their pregnant bodies don't seem bothered by the same changes I'm experiencing," I hear you. But while those I've-never-felt-so-radiant wenches (just kidding, I'm just jealous!) probably aren't lying, I can almost guarantee they have moments when they look in the mirror and feel a jolt of insecurity when they notice how wide their hips have become or see the fresh stretch marks on their thighs. It can be a shock for anyone — even if they're not talking about it.

But this shock can feel really big if you, like me, have struggled with body image. When I was in high school, I was convinced that if I were just skinny enough, everything I ever wanted to happen would happen — like my skinny body would be my fairy godmother. So in pursuit of this totally logical dream I would starve, then binge, starve, then binge. After lots of therapy I got it under control and began loving my body (most of the time)…but then I conceived Hudson.

When I began showing, all I could focus on was the spreading and softening of the faint outline of abs I had worked so hard for, and my butt, which had always been a pancake, becoming a lumpy pancake. I felt like the most unsavory pregnant lady in the history of pregnant ladies. This led me to believe Eric would never ever want to have sex with me again. He tried everything to convince me otherwise, but nothing worked. I felt horny (because pregnancy hormones can cause mega-arousal) but didn't act on it because I was sure my body was incapable of inspiring lust and would probably horrify Eric if he saw it naked.

This all made me feel discouraged and resentful. *Especially* resentful. I was resentful that my husband got to have a baby without dealing with any physical changes or feeling like he'd lost his sex appeal. I was also resentful that I was giving up what felt like every fiber of my body and desirability for my baby.

While I didn't feel too bad about resenting my husband (I mean really, why can't nature make them feel a few contractions?), I hated that the shock of my body changing made me feel even a tinge of resentment against my baby. That I could feel anything but total love for him devastated me. So, yeah, a majority of my first trimester was spent in a sexless pit of resentment and guilt. Fun, right?! But mamas, I got out.

Bolstered by the brighter perspective brought on by the body image–enhancing tools of working out, therapy, and the weird stand-naked -in-front-of-a-mirror exercise I outline below, I finally realized that unconditional love for my child can live in harmony with a splash of resentment and a sprinkle of annoyance. Thoughts of our children are not always going to cause hearts to pop out of our eyes — and that's okay.

You will save yourself a world of self-inflicted emotional torture later down the road by giving yourself grace *now* for having feelings about your baby that aren't all rosy. (Of course, if those thoughts turn violent in any way, alert your medical care provider.) If you're feeling irked that baby's making your skin ripple with stretch marks and your sexy time turn into "just rub my feet" time, it's all good. You're not alone. You're part of a tribe of strong, radiant, multilayered women also feeling so many feels about their body and baby.

What to do

While training your mind to sprinkle grace over the whole range of emotions about how baby is impacting your body image and sensuality, give yourself physiological support by talking with your care provider about starting (or continuing) an exercise program. Exercise not only strengthens the body for birth but also releases endorphins that elevate your mood and help you see yourself in a more attractive, sexy-time glow. Up the exercise benefits by being active outside, as the combination of fresh air, vitamin D, and movement is magic.

In addition to discovering a movement plan that works for you, try this:

- **Eat mindfully.** Think about what you're eating, as certain foods can exaggerate the anxiety and depression sometimes triggered by body image stressors, while others can enhance your energy and mood. Soda and other high-sugar drinks, pretty much anything with high-fructose corn syrup, white bread, too much coffee, and fried foods are major culprits when it comes to making you feel blah. On the flip side, whole grains; chickpeas; Brazil nuts; eggs; omega-3 fatty acids; foods high in antioxidants, like berries; and probiotic-rich nosh, such as yogurt and kefir, can all help your mind and body smile. Make sure your diet supports any special circumstances you might have by running it by your care provider.
- **Get naked in front of a mirror.** Release body shame and up your feelings of sexiness by standing naked in front of a mirror and finding one area of your body that you love. After you find that area (and it can be as small as your lips or a smooth patch of skin at the base of your neck), really focus on it. Allow yourself to fill with thoughts about how beautiful that area is and how appreciative you are that it's nourished by blood and oxygen and all the other miraculous functions of the body. Each time you do this exercise, find a new area to focus on.

  The point is to start training the mind to shift focus from the parts of our body we don't like — the parts we usually obsess over — and realize that our body is actually covered in beauty. Know that this exercise can feel super uncomfortable in the beginning, as the act of immediately homing in on cellulite or extra padding is ingrained in us. But if you commit to pushing past the discomfort and the inclination to body-shame, you'll slowly move into a space of adoration for your body that can create a whole new body. Pretty cool!

• **Seek therapy.** For those who have struggled with eating disorders or exercise addiction, pregnancy might reignite old thought patterns. Give yourself the customized emotional nourishment you deserve by finding a therapist you trust and connect with. A good therapist can offer wonderful support for integrating with your changing body and figuring out how to fall in love with it, or at least come to terms with it. They can also help you work through the feelings toward your baby these changes might trigger.

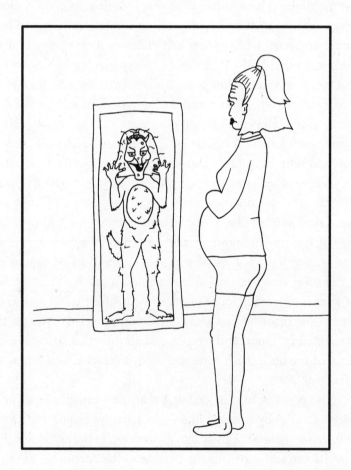

27. Why does it look like a crimson, white-capped mountain range has sprung up on my face?

Throughout my pregnancy, topographical maps of the Sierra Nevadas would pop up along my jaw and the edge of my nose. Everest even made an appearance once. I felt like a prepubescent boy. And I'm not alone. Many of the mamas I work with come into childbirth prep classes horrified that the clear, dewy skin they'd worked so hard to maintain had reverted to red, bumpy chaos. The main reason for this is…wait for it… wait for it…you guessed it! Hormones! Increases in the hormone androgen can incite acne, as it causes oil glands to become overeager producers.

The good news is that for most women this condition will resolve after childbirth, when androgen levels drop. And hey, girl, throughout it all, remember that you are a gorgeous-baby-making goddess, regardless of what your skin is up to.

What to do

Combat that acne with the following:

- Be hypervigilant about skin care. Wash with an organic facial cleanser — made specifically for acne — every morning and evening, and after heavy sweating.
- Avoid washing too often, as this can actually cause more oil to develop.
- After washing your face, use an organic anti-acne toner. You can also make toner with one part raw, unfiltered apple cider vinegar and three parts distilled water. Follow this with an organic moisturizer that doesn't contain retinol. Some effective moisturizers made specifically for acne include ingredients like raw shea butter, aloe vera, and manuka honey.
- Wash your hair regularly, and keep it out of your face. Oily hair rubbing on your face could exacerbate acne.
- Use the speaker feature, or headphones, when talking on your phone, as the screen is often covered in oil and dirt. Cell phones are way grodier than they look.
- Staying on the theme of keeping gross stuff off your face, wash your

pillowcase once or twice a week. On a side note, experts (aka my grandmother) believe silk pillowcases reduce the development of wrinkles.

- If the acne is out of control and it's stressing you out, ask your care provider for a dermatologist referral.
- While it's tempting to use medication or chemical-laden treatments, these often aren't advisable for pregnant women. Many experts also advise against topical treatments containing salicylic acid.
- Wear makeup only when you feel it's absolutely necessary. And make sure you're using oil-free products.
- Drink plenty of water, and avoid refined sugar and processed foods.
- And here's the one that is near impossible for me — do not pop those suckers. While it's one of the most satisfying feelings in the world, it could leave scars.

28. Why are there dark spots all over my face?

You have what's called melasma (aka the pregnancy mask), which is caused by an elevation in progesterone that prompts pigmentation levels to increase. This results in dark, discolored patches on the skin, and it's incredibly common in pregnant women. The good news is, it isn't accompanied by other symptoms and isn't dangerous for you or baby. It should fade after childbirth, when progesterone levels drop.

What to do

Check in with your care provider to confirm the patches aren't a sign of another skin condition. After melasma is diagnosed, apply organic zinc oxide sunscreen every morning, and reapply as needed, as sun exposure can darken the patches. You can also avoid excess sun by becoming a hat lady and using your melasma as an excuse to skip that hike in favor of a cozy book-reading sesh in bed.

29. I've turned into Sasquatch. Why am I so hairy?

My tummy, upper lip, back, and bum took to growing extra hair (à la an elderly man) during pregnancy. And it wasn't peach fuzz…it was dark, shockingly long hairs. Eric once caught me mid–tummy shave. Not cute. Unsurprisingly, an increase in hormones are to blame, specifically androgen and, wait for it, wait for it…estrogen! These hormones not only induce hair growth but also prevent hair from shedding. This is a big reason your locks become so lustrous — the hundred or so strands that typically shed each day stay put when you're growing a baby. An increase in your metabolism and blood circulation also play a part in all this, as they keep the hair pumped up with nutrients. Regarding the darkening of body hair, this is caused by the extra melanin — a pigment that impacts the color of hair, skin, and eyes — your body makes during pregnancy.

Androgens, primarily composed of testosterone and androstenedione, are a main cause of hair growth during pregnancy in places usually reserved for male hair growth. They've been nicknamed "male hormones" because — while they're present in both men and women — men typically have higher levels of them. In the female body, most androgens are converted into estrogens. Androgens were likely to blame for the coarse, curly, and black nipple hair my friend Chelsea reported during her pregnancy. She said she had more of it than her husband. I took her word for it.

In rare cases, excessive body hair can be a sign of hyperandrogenism, which is an overproduction of androgens. This condition can cause high blood pressure, acne, weight loss, and other not-great side effects. If you feel your body hair is out of control, let your care provider know.

What to do

If all the hair really bugs you, go ahead and shave. Hair removal products aren't recommended, as the chemicals leach into the skin. And while waxing is safe, it usually isn't advised because hot wax can irritate extra-sensitive pregnant skin. If the hair only kind of irks you, consider making peace with it and saving yourself major time in the shower. You can really make friends with it by rubbing almond or jojoba oil all over after showering, softening the hair and minimizing the development of stretch marks. And take heart in the knowledge that your Sasquatch traits will almost entirely disappear by six months after birth.

30. My boobs are so itchy I feel like sticking sandpaper in my bra. Why are they itchy, and how can I soothe them?

If you walked through a Target parking lot in Los Angeles, summer of 2012, and saw a pregnant woman with her hand down her shirt and a "scratching that itch" face…that was me. (Target was my spot for napping and boob itching before making the long drive home from work.) My breasts — nipples especially — became so insatiably itchy during my last trimester that I was itching my upper privates anytime I wasn't in public. When I was home, I slathered cream all over them and walked around topless. It wasn't cute.

There are numerous reasons for the tickling-teats phenomenon:

- **Hormones:** Those dang hormones. As they build, they can create increasingly itchy skin, especially in the bosom.
- **Stretching:** As if the visual of stretch marks weren't irritating enough, stretch marks also exaggerate itchiness, as they cause the skin to dry out. Talk about adding insult to injury!
- **Eczema:** The most evil of all itchy-booby culprits is pregnancy-induced eczema. This skin condition can make you feel like a body's worth of chicken pox is condensed on your boobs. Not cool.
- **Prurigo of pregnancy:** As the immune system adjusts to all the changes pregnancy throws at it, itchy, bugbite-like bumps, called prurigo, might appear on the skin.
- **PUPPP.** Pruritic urticarial papules and plaques of pregnancy (say that five times fast) can cause bumps or hive-like rashes anywhere from the stomach to the boobs. If the sight of it weren't fun enough, it's also itchy. It will go away after pregnancy.
- **Intertrigo.** Essentially, this is just an underboob rash caused by the three amigos heat, moisture, and friction.
- **Yeast infection.** While yeast infections usually just party in your pants, they occasionally make trips up north, especially during pregnancy. Its party favors are usually dry, flaky skin and possibly bright red nips. If you suspect this is what's going on, contact your care provider.

What to do

Stick that sandpaper in your bra. Just kidding. There are kinder ways to calm the itch:

- **Drink more water.** Consuming your body weight in ounces of water (e.g., if you're 140 pounds, strive for 140 ounces of water) every day will soothe many of these skin ailments, in addition to clearing up clogged bowels and a slew of other pregnancy annoyances. While this water recommendation is higher than most, it takes into account increased sweating, vomiting, and those days when you forget your water bottle.

- **Consider your boob hammock.** A too-tight bra or one made of synthetic material could aggravate itchiness. Opt for a bra that's done away with underwire and dye and can grow with your expanding melons. You can even start wearing nursing bras early, as they're often mega-comfortable. In addition, make sure your bras are made with natural fibers like cotton or bamboo, which is more comfortable than it sounds.

- **Butter up your boobs.** Alleviate the itch by applying shea or cocoa butter, lanolin cream, or jojoba or olive oil. Heck, straight-up butter would even help. Keep your anti-itch agent of choice in your purse so you can slather on the go. (Target parking lots are excellent for this activity.)

- **Don't itch.** I hate typing that because I hate when people tell me that. But alas, people are right. While it's heavenly in the moment, scratching often intensifies the itchies and can make skin so raw you're then itchy *and* in pain. Instead of scratching, pull out that boob butter.

- **Spring for organic, unscented detergent and skin products.** As the chemicals in detergent, bodywash, and lotion can all intensify the itch, switch to products that are organic and unscented.

- **Humidify.** Because dry air almost always exaggerates itchiness, moisten the air by placing a humidifier in your bedroom and any other room where you spend ample time. There are amazing portable humidifiers (about the size of a water bottle) that help ensure you're never without a dewy draft.

Fluids and Other Bodily Emissions

31. Why am I sweating so much?

During my third trimester I would frequently awake to a pillow so drenched with sweat it was squishy. (And it made all the squishy sounds.) My night sweats and, heck, my all-day sweats were out of control. I looked, smelled, and felt like a Swamp Mama. It was really sexy.

Not surprisingly, it's believed the intense sweating many women experience during pregnancy is due to the spike in estrogen and progesterone. (Those buggers seem to tinker with everything.) In addition, an increase in body temperature and blood flow to the skin contributes to the pregnancy glow, or for ladies like me, the pregnancy drench.

What to do

Let you care provider know. Although the sweats are likely just a side effect of growing a human, it's wise to rule out circumstances like infection or thyroid issues. After you've determined all is well (besides the whole waking up in a swimming pool thing), minimize your excessive glisten by trying the following:

- **Exercise.** It seems counterintuitive, but whether you're pregnant or not, exercise has been found to reduce sweatiness (at least after the exercise).
- **Stay hydrated.** While drinking water won't make you sweat less, it will minimize overheating. It also helps you replace all the fluids you're losing, which is crucial, as those fluids impact amniotic fluid levels, blood volume, new tissue production, nutrient delivery, digestion, and removal of wastes and toxins (bye, constipation). Hydration is crucial.

    To ensure your sweating doesn't impact your vitality, shoot for drinking your body weight in ounces every day. For example, a woman who weighs 140 pounds would drink 140 ounces every day. It's a lot. But if you're a sweating-overachiever, the extra fluids will be worth the effort. If your care provider is concerned about the electrolytes you're losing via sweat, consider getting some of your fluids from coconut water and noshing on bananas, watermelon, and avocado. You can also put a dash of pink Himalayan sea salt in your water.

- **Be cool in the bedroom.** Minimize night sweats by lowering your thermostat to around 65 degrees Fahrenheit, turning on a fan, having a cup of cold water by the bed, and sleeping in sheets and pajamas made with breathable natural fibers like organic cotton, linen, or bamboo. (Cotton percale is an especially cool option for sheets.) In addition, have an extra pair of pj's and a clean sheet you can lay on top of your half of the soiled sheet at the ready, in case you still wake up soaked in the middle of the night.
- **Wear loose, breathable clothing.** Nothing inspires sweat glands like a tight polyester dress or some snug rayon pants (hello, sweaty crotch). Do yourself a favor and swap the tight for the flowy, and the impermeable for the breathable. And just like the pj's mentioned above, look for duds made with organic cotton, linen, or bamboo.
- **Powder your undies and thighs.** You can prevent the heat rash or chafing that can be caused by an abundance of moisture in your nether regions by sprinkling organic talc-free powder (or cornstarch!) in your undies and dabbing some on your thighs before putting on your bottoms. While there's no evidence that talc-free powder in the vaginal area is harmful, it's still wise to check with your care provider before your inaugural sprinkle.
- **Carry a folding fan.** Look like the chic lady you are by keeping a folding fan in your purse and whipping that baby out whenever you're feeling flushed.

32. My various body odors and breath have gotten out of control. Is that normal? What's a safe way to mask the stinks?

This smelliness is totally normal, but as I'm sure you're tired of hearing from me, you should still tell your care provider just in case it's an indicator of a special circumstance. But it's probably related to the following pregnancy phenomena:

- **Dragon breath:** Progesterone can impact the slant between your esophagus and stomach, causing smelly gastric juices to bubble up. In addition, many women develop pregnancy rhinitis (fancy term for a chronic stuffy nose), which can lead to mouth breathing, which dries out the saliva that staves off the buildup of pungent bacteria.

- **Underarm funk:** The increase in your basal metabolic rate causes an increase in your blood supply and body temperature, prompting sweat glands to go into overdrive.
- **Shift in vaginal fragrance:** This is caused by a change in the vagina's pH balance, which produces a sweet scent that's often compared to the aromas of glue or dough. Sometimes an odd smell can be created by a yeast infection, which is often accompanied by redness, itching, burning, or strange discharge. If you have bacterial vaginosis, a fishy, ammonia-like aroma will waft about.

What to do

Know that you're probably the only person who thinks you're stinky. Because your nose is seriously sensitive to smell during pregnancy, the aromas floating up from your mouth, pits, and vagina are exaggerated by your smell receptor. However, we don't want you gagging over your odors. Try out the following to soothe the stench:

- **Do hygiene on the go.** Keep organic, unscented feminine hygiene wipes to freshen up your vagina and armpits when you feel the moisture collecting. In addition, always have organic deodorant on hand. And since food stuck in the teeth and bacteria on the tongue can get stinky, store dental floss and a tongue scraper in your bag.
- **Shower on the regular.** Start your day with a shower that ends with a cool rinse, so you don't start sweating before you're done toweling off. If you find yourself sweaty, sticky, and stinky later in the day, don't be shy about taking shower deux.
- **Use natural antibacterial products.** After showering, minimize a buildup of bacteria by wiping an apple cider vinegar toner (mix one part apple cider vinegar with two parts filtered water) on areas that collect sweat. And as honey, coconut oil, cinnamon, and cloves also have antibacterial properties, using body oil or lotion infused with these ingredients can minimize unpleasant odors.

    In addition, friction removes bacteria — so use a coconut sugar scrub once a week. To make, melt one-half cup coconut oil in the microwave for about forty-five seconds, or until completely melted. Then, mix in one cup white sugar and transfer mixture into a mason jar.

- **Wash clothes with distilled white vinegar.** Pour a half cup of distilled white vinegar into your washing machine during the rinse cycle, as this liquid is great at deodorizing clothes.
- **Drink water.** As a dry mouth is a mega-manufacturer of bad breath, drink water on the regular. Add to the freshness by mixing in a few sprigs of mint and a squeeze of lemon.
- **Snack out the stink.** Noshing on leafy greens, celery, cucumbers, pears, apples, pineapple, cherries, melons, citrus fruits, parsley, basil, and spirulina (stick it in a smoothie to mask its taste) can help erase funky breath. In addition, staying away from too much garlic, onion, and curry reduces your pungency.
- **Avoid scented products.** As tempting as it is to mask smells with perfumed lotions and sprays, many chemically produced scents can irritate skin. If you really want to conceal the scent, mix one drop of organic lavender, rose, ylang ylang, grapefruit, sweet orange, or lemongrass essential oil with one teaspoon of a carrier oil like almond or jojoba oil, and rub on pulse points.

33. I sometimes open my mouth to talk and a burp comes out instead. Why? And what's up with my constant constipation and uncontrollable farting? Is there a way to minimize all this gas? Or to at least feel less embarrassed when it happens?

Thanks to progesterone, your intestines relax during pregnancy, making digestion less efficient and increasing the time fecal matter stays in the intestines by up to 30 percent. The pressure of the uterus on the abdominal cavity also slows digestion. This can all cause constipation, which leads to a buildup of gas that can burst out your northern or southern orifices — sometimes smelling like sulfur. Female gas actually tends to smell more sulfur-y than man-gas because our farts have a higher concentration of hydrogen sulfide. Adding to our lady-luck is the fact that even if we're not constipated, those relaxed bowels make it tricky to control gas leaks. During my pregnancy naps, I was often awakened by belly-rumbling sulfur toots so smelly I would sometimes lose my lunch. Who says pregnancy isn't glamorous?

While all the gas can make you blush, it also has some benefits:

- It's a sign you're staying on top of your fruits and veggies.
- The slow moves of your intestines allow more time for your body to absorb nutrients from food.
- Farting and burping in front of your partner — or other loved ones — can be a strangely bonding experience, as it's an ultimate sign of comfort.
- Letting it rip with abandon actually makes your kisser more desirable, as holding in farts can make the breath stink.

What to do

Despite the benefits of passing gas, having too much of it gurgling around can be uncomfortable. The primary way to lessen that discomfort is revving up digestion. There are numerous ways to do that:

- **Move it or snooze it.** A stagnant body usually leads to sleepy bowels. Get things going by talking to your care provider about an exercise plan that's safe for your unique circumstances. Getting in thirty minutes of exercise every day is often enough to keep the intestines chugging along at a gas-minimizing rate.
- **Investigate your diet.** If you notice that your gassiness intensifies after eating certain foods, consider eliminating them from your diet, or at least decreasing your intake. Foods that are especially gas-inducing include broccoli, cabbage, Brussels sprouts, artichokes, asparagus, onions, lentils, pork, fried foods, and artificial sweeteners. Many people also experience gas after consuming dairy or gluten. To support this recon mission, keep a food journal for a week, recording which meals made you burp or fart. Also know that you may experience more gassiness after taking your prenatal vitamin.
- **Soften your stools.** Hard fecal matter leads to constipation, which

leads to all the fun I've been outlining. Prevent brown bricks and pebbles from forming in your intestines by drinking plenty of water and consuming twenty-five to thirty grams of fiber every day, as fiber infuses the intestines with water. Prunes, bananas, figs, flax and chia seeds, blackberries, avocados, leafy greens, pears, and apples are all fiber-full. Fiber supplements can also provide a quick fix. Because I'm a lady blessed with lazy bowels with or without a bun in the oven, I start every day with prunes and Metamucil. My morning sex appeal is almost too much to handle.

- **Chew your food.** As one cause of gas is bacteria in the large intestine breaking down food that wasn't fully digested by enzymes in the stomach, adding to your chew count can lower your burp and fart count. Aim for chewing each bite of soft foods at least ten times, and denser foods at least thirty times.

  In addition, slowing down your chewing (and drinking) and minimizing talking while eating can help limit the amount of air you swallow.

- **Eat smaller meals.** Noshing on six small meals, instead of three big ones, spreads out the load your digestive system has to work through, minimizing backlog.

- **Sleep on your left side.** This position aids digestion, helping you wake up ready to poo.

- **Say yes to the muumuu.** Staying away from tight clothing — especially articles that squeeze the waist — allows your bowels to pulsate without restriction. In addition, loose clothing can reduce discomfort from bloating.

- **Filtered panties.** That's right folks, filtered panties are a thing, and a thing that can alleviate fear when feeling a big one coming on and thinking, "Will it, or will it not, be a stinker?" If you're worried about the sound: A trick I often utilize is pretending like I'm talking to someone on my cell phone and letting out a laugh as I simultaneously let out the toot. You're welcome.

- **Air freshener.** If you're still concerned with the smell after donning those filtered panties, do as I did and carry around an on-the-go bottle of an essential oil air freshener.

- **Seek professional care.** If you experience constipation or abdominal pain for more than a week or feel like you're rarely able to have a complete bowel movement, alert your care provider.

Let it be known that even if your bowels are always on their A-game, you're still going to burp and fart, sometimes without warning. While it can feel embarrassing, know that it matters to you way more than it does to other people. Sure, others may clock your toot or belch, but they'll likely spend only a second considering it, thinking, "Oh, so-and-so just farted/burped. But who cares? They're pregnant." Even when you're not pregnant, who cares? We all do it. It's been found that, on average, many people produce four pints of gas and fart up to twenty times every day.

General

34. I succumbed to sushi and a glass of wine. Am I the worst pregnant lady ever?

No way, mama. While I certainly wouldn't advise downing alcohol and raw fish on the regular without your care provider's go-ahead, that fish with a side of red wine can actually help reduce anxiety. A plant compound found in red wine, resveratrol, creates anxiety-soothing effects by blocking the expression of an enzyme that controls stress in the brain.

And then there's the sushi. A study published in the peer-reviewed journal *PLOS One* found that pregnant women who ate oily fish high in long-chain essential n-3 polyunsaturated fatty acids (PUFA) and docosahexaenoic acid (DHA) had lower levels of anxiety than their vegetarian peers, as these compounds are essential for optimal neurological function and impact mood changes. The study also reported that because baby is taking many of those happy compounds, the mom can easily become depleted, meaning she really needs to stay on top of her fish intake. Two to three servings of low-mercury, fatty fish each week is recommended.

With all that said, there are still concerns about drinking too much alcohol and eating fish raw. So what's safe, and what should be avoided? Concerning alcohol, there is no evidence proving light consumption (up to two glasses a week) is harmful to the fetus. But because heavy drinking can be incredibly harmful, many care providers recommend abstaining "just in case." Essentially, the light-drinking-while-pregnant question is still a bit of a gray area, but almost any care provider will tell you that having a few (very spread out) glasses of wine during your pregnancy shouldn't be an issue.

Now let's debunk the belief that raw fish is the enemy of a healthy pregnancy.

- A primary fear about raw fish is that it will expose you to parasites. However, most fish is flash frozen before shipment, which kills parasites.
- If salmon is your fish of choice, it's likely farmed instead of wild, making it much less susceptible to parasites.
- A study published in *Obstetrics & Gynecology* reported "sushi that was

prepared in a clean and reputable establishment is unlikely to pose a risk to the pregnancy."

- What you want to stay away from, more than that salmon roll at your local sushi spot, are fish dishes (cooked or not) that are high in mercury. King mackerel, marlin, swordfish, tilefish, ahi tuna, and bigeye tuna are all fishies to steer clear of.
- According to a study published in *Clinical Microbiology Reviews*, most seafood-related illnesses are caused by shellfish, not fish.

What to do

If you're mourning the loss of your vino and rainbow rolls, talk with your care provider about what would be safe for you to consume in your unique situation. You might find that because of certain special circumstances, it's best for you to stay away from alcohol and raw fish most of the time. But if you're having a healthy pregnancy, your care provider may surprise you by giving the go-ahead for a glass of wine and some sashimi once a week, for example. The answer you get will likely depend on the research the care provider has been exposed to and how conservative they are. If they give you an answer that feels off, don't hesitate to dig deeper, asking them about their reasoning for the answer they provide. And if you really want to get a breadth of opinions, reach out to other care providers — making sure to throw some midwives into the mix.

If you're cleared for intermittent treats, make sure to select the healthiest options. For example, if you can have wine from time to time, opt for an organic brand. Regarding sushi, only go to restaurants that provide super-fresh fish and have glowing reviews. Many cities have a public grading system for restaurants, helping patrons know which eateries passed their food and hygiene inspection with flying colors.

35. I'm over thirty-five, and when people refer to my pregnancy as "geriatric" I want to scream. How can I ask them to use a different term? And how can I shift my own beliefs around being an "old mom"?

Ugh. Whoever came up with the term *geriatric pregnancy* should be sentenced to a month of watching nothing but infomercials. I mean really,

I can't think of a better term to make a woman feel like her body is ill equipped to carry a healthy pregnancy. While science has shown us that as women (and men!) age, their fertility declines and rates for various special circumstances increase, it's absurd to make every pregnant woman who is thirty-five or older join the Geriatric Pregnancy Club. In many ways, factors such as lifestyle, physical and mental health, and genetics play a much bigger role than age in how a woman's body handles pregnancy. If you rock a healthy lifestyle, you likely have a much better chance of having a thriving pregnancy than a twenty-five-year-old who smokes, drinks, and thinks healthy eating is getting sliced strawberries on top of a funnel cake.

Understanding the offensive nature of the term *geriatric pregnancy*, many now slap the label *advanced maternal age* (AMA) on pregnant women thirty-five or older. But that's not much better. Why do we need to label these women at all? Why can't care providers just look at each pregnant woman as a unique human? Why can't we look at her personal and family medical history, current health, and other personalized factors to determine what testing she should have and what circumstances she might be at risk for, instead of automatically treating her as a geriatric, and therefore high-risk patient?

To be fair, many care providers do treat women thirty-five or older in this customized manner, understanding that just because she's been on Earth for a set number of rotations doesn't mean she needs to see a high-risk doctor, get that amniocentesis, and schedule a C-section (something three of my clients were told they should have, simply because they were in their early forties). These are the care providers you want to find, primarily because if you're seen by a care provider who perceives you as high risk only because of your age, you might have a higher chance of receiving unneeded interventions because their misguided perceptions color their recommendations.

More and more research is also showing that women of AMA aren't actually at much higher risk for many of the special circumstances often attached to "geriatric pregnancies" than their younger counterparts. For example, a study published in *Scientific Reports* found that pregnant women over the age of thirty-four had only a slightly increased risk for gestational diabetes mellitus and hypertensive disorders than younger women. These researchers also found no increased risk of postpartum hemorrhage, preterm birth, low APGAR scores, or NICU admission for the babies of AMA women. And according to a study published in the journal *Human Reproduction*, women aged eighteen to thirty-four had a stillbirth rate of 0.47%, while women between thirty-five and forty had only a slightly higher stillbirth rate, at 0.61%.

So enough with the derogatory labels. It's time for a change.

What to do

Minimize the anxiety that's often produced by all the chatter about a geriatric pregnancy by trying the following:

- **Find a care provider who doesn't make you feel like a dusty china doll.** There are a ton of amazing care providers who also roll their eyes at the term *geriatric pregnancy*. Put in the effort to find one. Ask friends and family members (especially those who had a baby after the age of thirty-four) for recommendations, and have a consult with your top choices. Ask them what their views are on women having babies after thirty-four, then hire the care provider who makes you feel most empowered about your ability to have a healthy pregnancy and birth experience, regardless of your age.
- **Ask for a reframe.** If the care provider you eventually choose or someone who works with them drops the term *geriatric pregnancy*, or even *advanced maternal age*, when referring to your unique pregnancy, ask them to stop, and tell them why. For example, if these terms replace your confidence and trust in your body with fear and doubt, explain that to your care provider. You can tell them you're fine hearing about the tests and precautions they recommend (unless of course you're not), but you'd like to keep labels out of the discussion.
- **Remember that you're a one-of-a-kind woman, not a statistic.** Viva the cliché "Age is just a number." It truly is just a number and means very little when it comes to how healthy your pregnancy will be. For example, my client Ava had her first baby in her early twenties, when she was a self-proclaimed "fast food addict." She felt bloated, tired, and "fuzzy minded" during that pregnancy, which ended in an emergency C-section because of pre-eclampsia. When her thirties began, she cleaned up her lifestyle, and she became pregnant again at thirty-three. She loved this pregnancy, which came with ample energy, mental

clarity, and no special circumstances. She had a complication-free vaginal birth after cesarean (VBAC). I saw pictures that proved she also looked younger in her thirties than she had in her twenties.

So if all the lame geriatric labels are getting to you, remember that how you feel is much more important than the date on your birth certificate.

- **Work your plan for healthy eating and exercise.** Taking those prenatal vitamins and omega-3 supplements; loading up on fruits, veggies, and other nutritious fare; drinking lots of water; moving your body; and sleeping at least seven or eight hours a night will do wonders in helping you have a healthy pregnancy.

- **Be curious about all the recommended tests.** When you reach the age of thirty-five, care providers often recommend a heap of tests. If you feel good about all of them, great. But if you feel unsure about what is actually necessary, ask questions until you feel satisfied with the quality and clarity of the information you're receiving. In addition, doing your own research can fortify you with information that may have been left out because of your care provider's biases. However, make sure your resources are reliable. Studies published in peer-reviewed journals are a good place to start, and many can easily be found online.

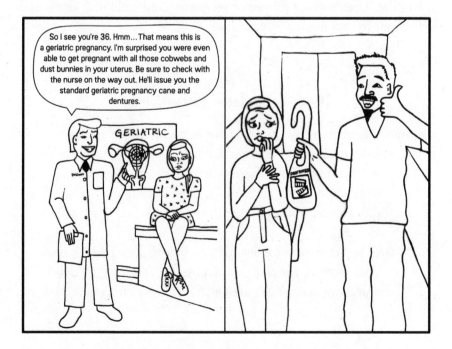

36. I smile and nod when my care provider is talking, but I have no idea what half the terms or tests they're mentioning mean. Can I have a crash course on the words coming out of my care provider's mouth?

You got it, toots. Being pregnant can feel like entering an alternate universe where everyone is speaking in baby-tongue, and you just smile and nod because it's too overwhelming to stop all the baby people every twenty seconds to ask for a definition and explanation. When I went to prenatal appointments, I begged my mind to become a steel trap that could capture all the words my care provider said that I didn't understand, so I could later ask Google. Why didn't I just ask my doctor questions, or write down a list in the moment, you ask? Because I was petrified of being seen as illiterate in pregnancy and birth talk. Looking back, I feel so bad for that version of myself. Of course I didn't know all that stuff — I had never been pregnant before! I wasn't yet part of that world.

So that's my long way of saying, when your care provider starts rattling off gibberish, don't be afraid to pipe up and say, "I actually have no idea what you're talking about. Please rewind and explain." To help you out, here are some of the more uncommon terms your care provider might use. There's also a full list of pregnancy and childbirth terms and definitions in the glossary on page 318.

Pregnancy Term Cheat Sheet

amniocentesis: A test typically done between sixteen and twenty weeks' gestation to test for developmental abnormalities in the fetus. To perform the test, the care provider inserts a hollow needle into the uterus to retrieve a sample of amniotic fluid. This is most commonly done for women thirty-five and older.

APGAR score: A measurement of how baby is handling life outside the womb. The care provider usually performs this evaluation about one to five minutes after birth by rating the baby's color, heartbeat, reflex, muscle tone, and breathing (which is what APGAR stands for: appearance, pulse, grimace, activity, and respiration). The score ranges from 1 to 10.

birth doula: A person trained in childbirth who provides emotional, educational, and physiological support before and during childbirth. They do not provide any medical assistance, but instead support mom with tasks like the creation of birth preferences, navigating choices during childbirth, utilizing pain- and fear-relieving techniques, and overall helping mom have a calm and empowered birth experience. Birth doulas often support the woman's partner as well.

cerclage: A procedure sometimes done for a woman with an insufficient cervix (the cervix opening too early). In this procedure, stitches are used to close the cervix. They will be removed near the end of pregnancy.

colostrum: The first substance that comes out of a woman's breasts after birth. Nicknamed "liquid gold," colostrum often has a yellowish color and is filled with high levels of protein, salts, fats, and vitamins. Many consider colostrum a superfood for newborns, as it boosts their immune system, coats the stomach and intestines to help prevent illness, acts as a laxative, can prevent jaundice, and lowers blood sugar. You'll only produce about one to four teaspoons per day, and it will be replaced when your milk comes in about two to five days after birth.

cord blood banking: The process of collecting blood from the umbilical cord and placenta after the cord is cut, freezing it, and storing it in a cord blood bank. Some parents elect cord blood banking because the blood contains hematopoietic stem cells that can be used to treat diseases like leukemia and lymphomas, in addition to some disorders of the blood and immune systems, such as sickle cell disease and Wiskott-Aldrich syndrome. The stem cells can benefit the child or their first- or second-degree relatives.

cord prolapse: A rare, serious complication that involves the umbilical cord dropping through the cervix and into the vagina, before the baby. If you can see the cord (which is not always the case), call 911 and lift your butt into the air, to get the weight of the baby off the cord.

delayed cord clamping: The practice of allowing the umbilical cord to stop pulsating before it is clamped and cut. This allows blood from the placenta to be transported into the baby, sometimes increasing the baby's blood volume by up to a third, minimizing iron deficiencies and supporting brain development.

dinoprostone (Cervidil): A medication, usually administered as a vaginal insert, used to soften the cervix. One of the mildest forms of induction medication, dinoprostone is often utilized before misoprostol (Cytotec) and synthetic oxytocin (Pitocin). A woman must remain in bed for two hours after insertion; it is removed after twelve hours, or when labor is established.

effacement: The thinning of the cervix. The cervix starts out being about three to four centimeters long, and as labor progresses it gets shorter, thinner, and wider (dilation).

engaged head: The settling of the baby's head into the pelvis. This generally happens during the end of the third trimester when you're nearing labor. When this happens, you'll typically be able to breathe easier, as there's less pressure on your diaphragm. You might also feel increased pressure in your pelvis.

external cephalic version (ECV): A process used to turn a breech baby into the head-down position for birth. In an ECV, the mother is typically given a medication (via IV) that relaxes her uterus, and then a care provider strategically presses on various areas of the abdomen, trying to turn the baby. An ultrasound is sometimes used to guide the process, and the baby's heart rate is closely monitored. And will it hurt? Probably. If you need an ECV, use it as practice for childbirth by putting your breathing techniques and other relaxation tools to work.

fontanelles: The two spaces between the baby's five skull bones where the sutures (soft membrane gaps) intersect. Also known as "soft spots." The fontanelles are covered by strong membranes that protect the brain. They are located near the front of the skull and on the crown. While many new parents are terrified they'll poke a hole in baby's head if they accidentally touch one of these spots too hard, you won't — they're a lot tougher than they look (both the spots and the baby as a whole). They should usually close by baby's twentieth month.

group B strep (GBS): Naturally occurring bacteria that can cause serious illness in newborns. When I tested positive for this, I logically thought it meant pregnancy had given me an STD. But no. GBS is a bacterial infection found in the vagina or rectum of about 25 percent of women. Between weeks thirty-five and thirty-seven of gestation, a swab test will be used to determine if you have GBS. While it typically does not cause symptoms in the mother, it can be dangerous if passed to the baby during delivery. Because of this, care providers often recommend that women who test positive be given IV antibiotics at the onset of labor and then every four hours until baby is born.

lanugo: Fine, soft hair covering the newborn in the womb and helping a protective layer of vernix stick to the skin. The hair usually sheds around month seven or eight of gestation, but it sometimes sticks around for many weeks after birth. Lanugo is most commonly seen on babies born prematurely.

lochia: Vaginal discharge present after birth that contains blood, mucus, and uterine tissue. It typically lasts for four to six weeks, but usually it isn't too heavy after the first week.

misoprostol (Cytotec): A medication (pill) used to induce labor, administered orally or vaginally. The use of misoprostol is controversial, as it can cause hyperstimulation of the uterus

and other potential complications, according to a study published in the *Journal of Perinatal Education.*

nonstress test: A test done in the hospital or birth center to confirm baby's health in the womb. It's noninvasive and only
consists of baby's heart rate being monitored. Care providers
specifically want to see how baby's movements impact their
heart rate, as their heart should beat a bit faster when they
move. It usually can't be done before week twenty-six of gestation.

nuchal cord: An umbilical cord that is wrapped around baby's
neck. While it sounds scary, nuchal cord is rarely dangerous.
According to a study published in *Maternal Health, Neonatology and Perinatology,* 10 to 29 percent of fetuses experience
nuchal cord. My son had this.

nuchal hand: When baby's hand is by their face when they're
born. Also called *compound hand.* My son did me the favor
of being in this position as I pushed him out. Nuchal hand
is likely what made that stage of labor take longer, and made
it so hard I sounded like a constipated boar whilst pushing.

placenta abruption: A rare occurrence where the placenta prematurely detaches — either partially or completely — from the
wall of the uterus, sometimes causing heavy bleeding and a
lack of oxygen for the baby. If this happens early in pregnancy,
the baby will be closely monitored through ultrasound. If it
occurs later in pregnancy, the baby will probably be delivered
through C-section.

placenta accreta: When the placenta grows too deeply into the
uterine wall. This often prevents the placenta from detaching
completely from the uterus after baby's birth, which could
cause hemorrhaging. In this situation, the baby is usually delivered through cesarean. And in severe cases, a hysterectomy
(the surgical removal of the uterus) may be required.

placenta previa: When the placenta is covering part or all of the
cervix. The primary symptom is vaginal bleeding (often
with bright red blood), unaccompanied by pain. Sometimes,

placenta previa resolves itself. When it doesn't resolve by the time a mother is full term, the baby is often delivered via cesarean.

postpartum doula: What I like to call an "Earth angel" — an individual trained to swoop in for a few hours each day, for the first few weeks of baby's life (or more!), to provide support with breastfeeding, infant care, and mama's emotional and physical recovery. In addition, postpartum doulas often help with housekeeping, meal prep, errands, childcare for siblings, and pretty much anything the parents and baby need.

prodromal labor: The frustrating phenomenon of early labor that feels like much more than Braxton Hicks contractions but isn't actually doing much to dilate the cervix. However, this type of labor isn't totally pointless, as it can help baby get into the ideal position and prep the muscles, pelvis, and your brain for active labor. This is different than early labor because the contractions often start and stop (for example, you might have them only at night), instead of progressively getting longer, stronger, and closer together, as often happens when a woman is experiencing early labor that transitions into active labor. I recommend using prodromal labor as an opportunity to get into the groove of birth by practicing pain-relieving techniques, even if the contractions aren't intense.

Rh factor testing: Ready for a science lesson? Here goes. Rh is a protein found on the surface of red blood cells. If you have the protein, you're Rh positive. If you don't, you're Rh negative. Most people are Rh positive. During your first prenatal visit, your care provider will likely order a blood type and Rh factor screening test to see what blood type you're working with. If you're Rh negative, the baby's father will be tested. If the man is Rh positive, it's likely your babe is also Rh positive, which means the two of you are Rh-incompatible. In this case, your care provider will likely recommend the RhoGAM shot.

Rh immunoglobulin (RhoGAM): If you and your baby are Rh-incompatible, you'll get a shot of Rh immunoglobulin (brand name RhoGAM) during week twenty-eight of pregnancy, and within seventy-two hours after delivery if it's confirmed that baby is Rh positive. The shot prevents your body from making antibodies during your first pregnancy that could attack the fetus during subsequent pregnancies. Without the shot, your immune system would detect the foreign proteins on baby's blood cells (foreign only if you're Rh negative and they're Rh positive) and create antibodies so it could attack the foreigner should it show up again — which it would if you get pregnant again with an Rh positive baby.

transverse: When baby is lying sideways, instead of head down. Most babies transition into head down, but if they don't by around thirty-six weeks' gestation, your care provider might recommend an ECV.

vernix caseosa: A waxy, cottage cheese–like coating on baby's skin that protects them from the "pruning" effects of amniotic fluid. In addition, when baby swallows vernix caseosa in utero, it can help develop their gut bacteria, serves as a lubricant during birth, protects baby from bacterial infections after birth, and helps heal vaginal tears, as the vaginal opening is exposed to it as baby emerges. Because of these postbirth benefits, the World Health Organization recommends waiting six hours before giving baby a bath. If you want to maximize these benefits, request on your birth preferences that baby not be wiped off after birth, and that their first bath be delayed.

vertex: When a baby in utero is positioned head down.

What to do

Review these phrases, but don't be afraid to ask questions when someone starts talking in terms (or recommends tests) you don't understand. People love to feel smart and impart wisdom to others — so you're giving them a gift by asking the questions.

37. I've been craving inedible items like clay and dirt. What the heck is going on?

A craving for nonfood items does not mean you're losing your mind; it means you're likely experiencing a type of eating disorder called pica. While rare, pica can crop up during pregnancy, surprising women by summoning the desire to eat clay, dirt, cornstarch, laundry detergent, and other inedible items. And although ice isn't inedible, a regular craving for it could also be linked to pica. For some women, pica pushes them beyond cravings, causing them to actually eat their substance of choice.

These cravings are often caused by a deficiency in iron, zinc, iodine, calcium, thiamine, vitamin C, or other nutrients. Pregnant women, especially those with pre-existing conditions or chronic morning sickness, are prone to these deficiencies. I had an intense desire to chow down on snow during my pregnancy. Come to find out, I was anemic.

Pica requires immediate attention, as a lack of nutrients can cause uncomfortable symptoms and impact fetal growth. In addition, ingesting inedible items could be toxic for the mother and baby.

What to do

See your care provider ASAP. They will likely order tests to see if you're deficient in iron, zinc, iodine, or other nutrients, in addition to performing other evaluations they deem necessary. When nutritional deficiencies are found, care providers typically recommend diet changes or supplements. If they suspect a part of the issue is psychological, they might refer you to a mental health specialist.

Birthing

Doesn't it feel a little (or a lotta) inconceivable that a human will come out of your body? I couldn't wrap my head around how my body would make enough room for another head to fit through a path that seemed no wider than a toilet paper roll opening…on a good day. This perplexed feeling can trigger a slew of other concerns and what-ifs that, if left unattended, can send a woman into labor tense and afraid. That's no way to move into one of the most significant experiences of your life.

Instead, I want you to get more and more excited as you near the birth of your baby, feeling confident in mind and strong in body. Sure, there will still be some nerves and unknowns, but overall, I hope you feel prepared and pumped! One way to get to this place is to acknowledge that you have questions about birth that feel like too much to handle. You have questions that you're afraid to acknowledge because that might make you feel "other than." Instead of pushing these questions down, invite them up. Bring them into the open. The questions in this section are a good place to start.

The cool thing with the format of this book is that it provides a soft entry into these questions and their answers. You can read them all, even the ones you don't think apply to you, and discover what's really going on inside you without having to tell a soul. After you realize you're not the only one and begin discovering the reasoning behind your murkier thoughts around birth, you might feel emboldened to strike out and share. Or not. If this is your private oasis to explore and hold things close, that's cool too. This is all for you, and I support you in navigating the path that feels most nurturing. Here we go.

Relationships

38. I don't want my partner at our child's birth. Is there something wrong with me? Should I just get over this feeling? Do I even have a say in whether they're there or not?

Oh, partners. They can be lovely, but they can also fudge things up during birth. So it's more common than you'd think for women to not want their partner present during childbirth. However, few women admit it, even to themselves, because not wanting a partner present at birth makes many moms-to-be think there might be something fatally wrong with their relationship. But not wanting your special someone there while you birth your other special someone doesn't mean your relationship is doomed.

I've heard numerous reasons why women want to have only a doula, or maybe their mom, sister, or nursing staff, present at birth. One mom I worked with (we'll call her Emily) had a hubby who got seriously squeamish in hospitals and once passed out after seeing blood from a cut. Emily was worried that instead of supporting her, the medical team would end up caring for her husband. Another mom (we'll call her Yvonne) had a partner who never wanted her to be uncomfortable. If Yvonne were sick, her partner would fuss over her until she had to ask for space. Yvonne worried that her partner's overattentiveness might be distracting during birth. The other woman who comes to mind (we'll call her Cassandra) had a boyfriend who was adamant that she not get the epidural, but she wasn't sure how she felt about the epidural. This sparked discord.

I worked with these moms on plans for discussing these concerns with their partners. In the first two cases, the couples decided to have the partner present only at the very end, when the baby was emerging. And for Squeamish Dad, a nurse was assigned to him in case he got woozy. Regarding No Epidural Dad, when Cassandra determined the epidural was the right choice for her, he couldn't support her, and they decided it would be best for him to join her after their baby was born.

There are numerous reasons women might want their partner to support them from a distance during labor — and they're all totally legit and worthy of attention. While your partner is of course an important part of the equation and will likely be a huge part of the child's life, childbirth is all about what makes you feel most comfortable. While it's monumental in many ways, birth is also a drop in the ocean of the child's life; if your partner isn't there, it doesn't mean their connection with the baby will be scarred.

What to do

If you're feeling like you might not want your partner with you during labor and delivery, do this…

- **Spend time exploring the reasons behind this feeling.** To start, ask yourself, "In what scenario would I be most relaxed?" Then, through good ole meditation, journaling, or talking with a trusted friend whose eyes won't widen when you tell them your thoughts, get clear on what that optimally relaxed scenario will look like. Who is there? Where are you? What does the room look like? How are you being supported?

    As you explore this scene, pay attention to whether or not your partner is there. If they are, how does their presence make you feel? What are they doing that does, or does not, make you feel relaxed? If you don't see them there, examine and write down the reasons behind their absence.

- **Talk to your partner.** If the previous exercise makes you realize you don't want your partner at the birth, or want them present only during a certain phase of labor, summon the courage to talk to them. While this may feel like the last thing you want to do, know that having this conversation will seriously lighten your emotional load and help you have a more positive birth experience.

    If the reasons you don't want your partner at the birth strike deep chords in your relationship, it could be beneficial to have this discussion with the support of a counselor. You can even see the counselor alone first to talk through your concerns and make a game plan for how this request for nonpresence will be presented to your partner.

    However, if your reasons are more basic, as with the queasy husband or overattentive partner I mentioned, you're probably safe just having a sit-down with your person. You can start the conversation by asking, "Have you thought about how present you want to be at the birth?" See what they say. You might find that they're also hesitant about being there. Or they might be full of ideas about how they'll coach you through breathing and get you into squats. Either way, exploring this topic together will either help you become more resolute in your decision to not have them there, or dissolve many of your initial concerns. After the first phase of this discussion, decide whether you're good to move forward with the "This is what I want to happen during birth" portion of the talk, or need time to process what was shared.

- **Make a plan for partner's involvement.** When you're clear on what you need from your partner, make a plan for how involved (or not involved) they'll be during birth. While it might be tempting to make concessions in favor of their feelings, make sure to not make compromises that limit your comfort. This conversation could be uncomfortable on the front end, but you will feel so much better when it's all out in the open and you can move forward.

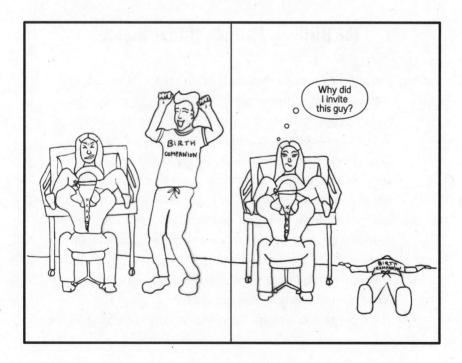

Medical Care Providers

39. What are my rights during birth? Do I have to do everything my care provider says?

You have a lot of rights. Essentially, you have the last word on every facet of your care, and you don't have to do anything your care provider suggests if you feel it's the wrong call. But that's where the water gets murky. Although you should be the key decision-maker during your pregnancy, childbirth, and postpartum experience, the people around you — specifically, your medical care provider — often hold ample sway in how things unfold. Intentionally or unintentionally, these people may manipulate your decisions based on legal or timing considerations, a hospital's (possibly outdated) culture, or their personal biases. Fortunately, there are ways to get around this — the first being to know your rights. These include the following...

The Birthing Mother's Bill of Rights

- **The right to receive thorough information about any intervention being recommended:** You have a right to ask your care providers questions until you're satisfied with the answers and feel you have enough information to make an informed decision. They should explain — in easily understandable terms — the risks and benefits of anything they're recommending. You can also ask what information is evidence-based and what is just coming from their personal experience. And you can ask about the cost of everything, down to the stool sampler they're offering you in that little white cup.
- **The right to request options:** If you're unsatisfied with a proposed course of action, you can ask for other options.
- **The right to turn down interventions:** After receiving all the

information, you may feel that an intervention is unnecessary. If this happens, it's your right to turn it down. While you might not be a medical expert, you are an expert on what feels intuitively right for your body and baby. If everything in your being is screaming "No!" you get to listen.

And just because you (likely) signed a consent for care form when you were admitted doesn't mean the care providers don't have to obtain your permission before moving forward with any procedure.

The following are procedures that my clients are usually surprised are *not* obligatory:

- **Vaginal exams:** While it can be nice to know how dilated you are, it's not an essential part of childbirth. So you don't have to let anyone perform a vaginal exam if they make you uncomfortable.

- **Heparin lock:** Many hospitals strongly encourage women to accept a heparin lock — a catheter that is placed in a vein with a drop of heparin to prevent blood clotting and is then locked off — so they have an open vein should they need to hook you up to an IV. But you don't have to agree to it.

- **The right to ask for a second opinion and/or change care providers:** If you feel your care provider isn't providing all the information or is leading you in a direction you feel uncomfortable with, ask to see another care provider. While the current care provider might push back, you're doing nothing wrong by making this request.

- **The right to move around:** If you want monitors, tubes, IVs, and so on removed so you can freely move around during labor, you can ask hospital staff to remove them. Your care provider might recommend staying connected to certain apparatuses because of medical needs, but they can't force you to do so. You also have the right to get into the position of your choice when delivering your baby.

- **The right to privacy:** No one gets to decide who is in your birthing space but you. If you want someone to leave the space, they have to comply, even if they work there. I once was a doula for a mother who felt unsafe around her OB-GYN. When the baby was being delivered, she demanded that he leave and send in the on-call midwife. He was beside himself but had to do what she said.
- **The right to know who is in your birthing space:** You have the right to know the identity and qualifications of any person in your birthing space.
- **The right to check out of the hospital:** I've worked with many women who didn't know they could check themselves out of the hospital "against medical advice." If you don't feel like you're being treated well, you can leave the hospital and check into a new one. The hospital won't make this easy, but what you're doing isn't illegal.
- **The right to receive records:** You have the right to request copies of your medical records at any time, and to receive a comprehensive explanation of the contents.
- **The right to speak with hospital administration:** If you feel your rights are being violated, you can ask to speak with a supervisor.
- **The right to be treated like the empowered, intelligent woman that you are:** No one has a right to talk down to you, or make you feel like you're not equipped to make well-informed decisions about your body and baby. If someone treats you without respect, you can turn around and demand it.

Note: Demanding your rights in some of these situations may require you to go against your care provider's recommendations. If the doctor feels strongly enough about a recommendation, you may be required to sign a document confirming your choice to refuse care.

What to do

In addition to understanding your rights, there are numerous ways to ensure that you have care providers who not only honor your rights but encourage you to stand up for those rights. And if you end up being cared for by individuals who don't respect your rights, despite your valiant efforts (it happens to the best of us!), here are some tools for those situations:

- **Find a care provider who believes in "patient autonomy."** See "Essential Tips for the Journey" on page 302 for more information.
- **Create a thoughtful list of birth preferences.** I love me some birth preferences. Not only are they a golden opportunity to pour positive intention into your birth experience, but they also allow you to clearly state how you expect to be treated. While all care providers should be well informed of your rights, your birth preferences serve as a clear reminder of what those rights are, and which ones are of particular importance to you.
- **Hire a doula.** While most doulas won't be your voice during birth, they can be the Birthing Angel on your shoulder, letting you know if someone is not honoring your rights. They can also provide ideas for how you and your birth companion can advocate for those rights.
- **Take two childbirth preparation classes.** If you're planning on giving birth in a hospital, I recommend taking both the childbirth prep class offered by the hospital and a class not affiliated with the hospital. I encourage you to take the hospital class first to gain insight into the hospital's birth culture and what rights you might have to advocate for. This class is largely for recon, and I suggest keeping a running list of questions and concerns about information shared there.

  Then, take this list to a childbirth preparation class that's aligned with your personal birthing philosophy — for example, HypnoBirthing or Lamaze — and share it with the instructor. The instructor can likely help you determine whether there are any red flags that suggest you should find a new hospital, or provide guidance on how to navigate aspects of the hospital's birthing culture that might go against your own. Both classes will likely help you become more informed and equipped to have an empowered birth experience.
- **Be clear when refusing treatment.** If you ever need to go against your

care provider's recommendation, make it explicitly clear that you're doing so. You might even need to request they provide verbal confirmation that they understand your decision.

- **Research the laws in your area.** Because each state has their own laws when it comes to childbirth, it's wise to email the American College of Obstetricians and Gynecologists Resource Center at resources@acog .org and ask for guidance finding the most up-to-date regulations for your state.
- **Fortify your courage.** Advocating for your rights can be difficult, especially in the face of a strong-willed care provider adamant that you follow their lead. But you are so much stronger than you realize, and pushing yourself to call on that innate power during one of the most important experiences of your life will likely transform the experience. Listen to this guided meditation to tap into your inner power source: yourserenelife.wordpress.com/birthing-rights/.

40. Does anybody actually pay attention to birth preferences?

Yes! There's an annoying misconception that medical staff snicker behind a pregnant woman's back if she presents birth preferences. If you've found a care provider you trust, they should fully respect your right to set intentions for your birth — which you can do with birth preferences. During my son's birth, the nurses respected my preferences so thoroughly I had to ask them to ignore some of them when I changed my mind.

However, some care providers do see birth preferences as a threat to their position of power and as someone trying to tell them how to do their job. But the thing is, you're not a patient coming in for a standard procedure. You're a healthy woman moving through a natural, biological process that requires the expert knowledge of a doctor or midwife only if a special circumstance comes up, or if *you* decide you want intervention. You're not there to receive the care provider's standard protocol. You're there to cocreate an everyday miracle with your baby, body, care provider, and birth companions. And you deserve to be at the helm. No one else does. Your birth preferences are a way to plant a flag that says, "Unless my health, or my baby's, becomes tenuous, this is how I want my birth to unfold. And I reserve the right to change my mind at any moment."

What to do

Remind yourself over and over again that it's your prerogative to take a stand regarding how you and your baby are treated during and after birth. This is a sacred experience that *you get to guide*. Once you've tapped into your confidence about your right to lead your birth experience, do the following:

- **Create your preferences.** Contemplate each aspect of the birth experience (e.g., onset of labor, active labor, baby's descent and emergence, baby's care, and your care after birth) and write out how you'd like it all to play out. My book *Feng Shui Mommy* has a chapter devoted to birth preferences and includes a sample list you can find here: your serenelife.wordpress.com/birth-preferences/. This list is a good place to start if you're feeling overwhelmed by the prospect of creating this document.
- **Phrase preferences in a positive tone.** Help prevent defensiveness in your care providers by writing what you *do* want them to do, instead of what you *don't* want them to do. For example, you could write, "I would prefer to labor without medication" instead of, "Don't offer me medication."
- **Keep it to one page.** Your care providers are more likely to read all your preferences if you fit them all on one page. This often means that only the most important preferences make the list. You can always verbalize minor preferences.
- **Share preferences with your care provider.** Take your preferences to a prenatal appointment at least six weeks before your due date. Have your care provider go through each preference with you. If you'll be delivering in a hospital, ask if any of your preferences go against hospital protocol. If they do, you could decide to change the preferences, or prepare yourself and your birth companion to advocate for the preferences the hospital may push against. It's also important to acknowledge that in the event of an emergency, you're willing to let go of preferences that would inhibit quality care.

    If your care provider seems exceedingly unsupportive of your birth preferences, consider hiring someone else. For guidance, see question 10 in this book, about changing care providers.

- **Have extra copies.** While the list of birth preferences you gave your care provider should make it into your chart, it may not. Ensure the list is at your birth by bringing at least two copies with you to the hospital or birthing center. And when you arrive, make sure everyone is on the same page by going over the preferences with support staff.
- **Adopt an attitude of adaptability.** Remember that just because you wrote the preferences doesn't mean you will have the exact birth they outline. The unexpected does happen, but the combination of understanding that possibility and still creating preferences sets you up for an empowered and satisfying birth experience.
- **Be thoughtful about the preferences you let go of.** If someone besides you suggests pushing aside a certain preference while you're in labor, think it over before agreeing (unless it's an emergency situation). It can be easy to just say yes to whatever's suggested when we're on the wild journey of birth, but pausing, asking questions, contemplating, then making a decision that feels intuitively right for you allows you to write the story of your birth, instead of being a passive participant.

One mom I supported ended up changing her mind about almost all her birth preferences because of various circumstances that came up. But because *she* was the one opting to let the preferences go, instead of being forced into the decisions, she has positive memories of her birth experience. She felt confident in making the preferences, and confident in breaking them.

An article in the *Journal of Perinatal Education* found that a woman's positive and negative perceptions of her birth experience are more connected to her feelings and ability to exert choice and control during birth than to the specific circumstances of the birth.

41. What if I don't like my labor and delivery nurse? Do I just have to deal with them?

Heck, no. If a nurse makes you feel uncomfortable, you get to "bye, Felicia" them. As the nurses assigned to you are the primary care providers you'll have during birth (doctors usually just show up to help deliver the baby), you want them to make you feel safe and heard. If you cringe every time a certain nurse comes into the room, that's a clear sign you need to request a different one. Many women don't realize it's even an option to ask for a different nurse, but it definitely is, and you won't be the first person to utilize this right.

The thing is, not every nurse is a great fit for every mother. It's not personal — it just means their vibe doesn't jive with your vibe. If you're wanting an unmedicated birth, for example, and you see the nurse roll their eyes when reading your birth plan, it's clear their presence is not going to fill you with confidence or empowerment. And you deserve to feel confident and empowered. You deserve nurses who enhance your experience.

What to do

If a nurse makes you uncomfortable, think about what type of personality you would prefer. For example, do you want someone supportive of unmedicated births? Someone with a gentler energy? Someone who is direct and open with information? Someone with a good sense of humor?

Once you've determined what type of nurse you *do* want, ask your birth companion or doula to go to the nurses' station and request to speak with the charge nurse, as they have the power to assign a new nurse. Your birth companion doesn't have to go into detail about why you want a nurse reassigned, they can simply say something along the lines of, "My partner and I don't feel that [insert nurse's name here] is a good fit for us. We would prefer someone who is more [insert the traits you would like your new nurse to have]."

There's no guarantee you'll get the exact type of nurse you want, but chances are they'll be a better fit than the last nurse, especially because they know you're willing to advocate for yourself and are paying attention to how you're treated.

While some women feel that requesting a different nurse is being dramatic, I think it's one of the most empowered decisions you can make during birth. The people in your birthing space have a profound impact on how your birth unfolds, and you deserve to have the final say over who is and isn't welcome. This is just another day of work for them, but it's a monumental experience for you. You get to be as picky as you want. In addition, I wouldn't worry about hurting anyone's feelings — you're not in the hospital to make friends, you're there to have the happiest and healthiest birth experience you can.

Come prepared: Another option is to ask your care provider if they know of any nurses at the hospital where you'll be delivering who they think would be a good fit for you. You can then ask for them by name when you check in. If those nurses aren't available, ask if there's a nurse who shares your general birth philosophy. For example, if you're hoping to have an unmedicated birth, request a nurse who has had an unmedicated birth or is skilled at supporting them.

Fears and Worries

42. I know that millions of women have had babies and blah blah blah, but I keep thinking I'll be the rare lady who can't do it. How can I unlock my confidence and courage around my birthing abilities?

I don't think any woman — at her core — can fully fathom a baby coming out of her (unless she's already had a baby). We can conceptualize it, but the reality of it seems unfathomable. Even when we nod in childbirth prep classes and feel we're absorbing the information, it can feel impossible to get completely on board with the belief that a baby can exit our vagina, or that muscles and flesh can be expertly cut into so the baby can be retrieved. When we're sitting at home — vagina, uterus, and abdominal muscles intact — it feels inconceivable that at some point the body will go through a wild transformation to allow the miracle creature within us to emerge.

The thing is, you don't have to believe any of it is possible for it to be true. You're off the hook for not fully buying into the fact that you can do it, because whether you believe it or not, you can do it and will do it. Whether "doing it" looks like having an unmedicated birth, Pitocin and an epidural, or a C-section matters not. All of it requires courage that *will show up* when the time comes.

It's also important to remember that many other pregnant women can relate to how you're feeling — a lot more than you realize. The very natural fears and doubts you're experiencing are so much less isolating when you realize you're part of a sisterhood that shares those fears and doubts. If you don't feel chipper about the whole birthing thing, you're not broken. You're in good company.

However, having an enhanced belief in your ability to birth your baby can make the time between now and the moment you feel like you need to have a bowel movement but actually just need to have a baby a lot more enjoyable. So let's get to some practical ideas for how to do that.

What to do

Try this:

- **Find your people.** Reach out to pregnant women you know, or meet new ones by joining a prenatal exercise group or another type of gathering that attracts pregnant ladies. When you find a few candidates you connect with, invite them on a mama-date and share your feelings about birth. Many of them will likely respond with similar sentiments and support, helping you feel less alone and more understood. If they don't, they're not your people. But keep looking. They're out there.

- **Take a childbirth prep class.** Investing in this type of instruction can chip away at doubts about your birthing ability by teaching you how the body births a baby, without filling you with fear. It should also provide a bevy of techniques for pain and fear release and relaxation enhancement. Even if you don't fully buy into the techniques, practice them, as your doubts likely come more from your deep-seated skepticism about your ability to birth than from insufficiencies in the methods. By forcing yourself to practice all of them at least once and continuing to practice the ones that resonate, you'll build a powerful tool kit for birth. This tool kit will be utilized during birth whether you realize it or not.

  As a doula, I'm often amazed to see the "tool kit techniques" that come up from the ether of my client's subconscious during birth. I often hear, "I didn't even decide to use that technique, it just happened." This can occur only if your mind is filled with tools for pain relief and relaxation. Collect the tools, then trust that the ones that need to come to you will.

- **Treat yourself to a birth doula.** Set yourself up for even more birthing confidence by hiring a doula who makes you feel safe and supported. A good doula comes equipped with in-depth knowledge of many of the tips and tricks you're learning in your classes and books, and they can help you use the tools that will be most effective for your unique needs during each phase of labor and delivery.

  If you're concerned about cost, know that new doulas often provide their services pro bono to gain experience. You can also look into a volunteer doula program. There's a list of organizations that connect women with free or low-cost doula services in the "Recommended Resources" section of this book. You can also reach out to a doula in your community and ask them to refer you to a local organization, or specific doula, that provides affordable care.

- **Listen to this:** To fortify your confidence-enhancing preparation, utilize this guided meditation, which helps you visualize yourself having a happy and healthy birth experience: yourserenelife.wordpress.com /enhancing-birth-confidence/. In addition, download this birth affirmations recording: yourserenelife.wordpress.com/feng-shui-mommy -birth-affirmations-download-link/.

43. I'm a huge control freak and can't stand the thought of not knowing when I'll go into labor, what it will feel like, and how long it will take. How do I deal with all the unknowns?

I'm a card-carrying member of the Control Freak Club. So not surprisingly, the unknowns of labor were one of the most difficult parts of pregnancy for me. I found it infuriating that even though millions of women have given birth, no one could tell me exactly what to expect. But alas, with the exception of women having a planned cesarean, there's not a single lady who can know with certainty when she'll go into labor, what it will feel like, and how long it will take.

Regarding the "When will I go into labor?" component of this question, it's important to note that due dates are far from an exact science. Only about 5 percent of moms go into labor on their due date, most first-time moms don't deliver until around ten days after their due date, and while some believe ladies who have already had babies will go into labor sooner, there's no science to back that up. We just don't know. While oxytocin is the hormone that stimulates contractions, what causes the release of that hormone is still a mystery. I hear you if you're still like, "Okay, I get it. But come on, there must be *something* I can do to get things going?!" There's an effective natural induction method I'll cover below that may help you go into labor.

Now let's look at the whole "What will it feel like?" thing. While contractions often feel like an intense blend of period and diarrhea cramps, I can almost guarantee the intensity is like nothing you've ever experienced.

And every woman experiences that intensity differently. For example, some experience it as rolling orgasms (jelly!), and others experience it as a call from the body to jump out the window. We don't know exactly how the body and mind will process the intensity. Moms who have already done the damn thing don't even know what it will feel like with the next one, as childbirth is often different each time. But take heart, I'll get to the part about how to prepare for this.

And finally, we have no stinking idea how many contractions we'll have to have before that head pops out. Aargh. When it seems like you have to summon every fiber of your strength to get through each contraction, it can feel deflating to not know how many more you'll have to breathe through. If you ask women how long their labor took, you'll get answers that range from a couple hours to a few days.

So yup. It can feel like a crapshoot, especially for women who (like me) use control as a security blanket. Birth throws that blanket out the window, leaving us cold and confused if we don't know how to work through it. But luckily for us control freaks, there are ways through this fog of not-knowingness.

What to do

Well first, about that due date...

- **Think of your due date as a time of month, instead of one day.** For example, a due date of May 15 becomes "mid-May." This perspective shift helps release an obsession with a day that will likely come and go without a baby.

  When my due date came and went, I panicked, thinking there was something wrong and that my baby wasn't coming out because he probably definitely hated me. I was a wreck. I didn't yet understand that due dates are far from an exact science, as fetuses grow at different rates, and the due date is predicted by adding 280 days to the first day of the woman's last period, even though the length of women's cycles varies. Because of this, only about 4 to 5 percent of women go into labor on their due date. So do as I didn't, and break up with your due date, as this can dissolve the anxiety and sense of failure often attached to its passing.

- **Make an induction plan.** If the last tip had you asking, "But won't my care provider still be thinking about my due date?" you're correct. Many care providers start dropping the I-word (*induction*) after your due date passes. If you're not interested in induction, minimize your stress by creating a plan with your care provider, well in advance, about what you'll do if you go past your due date. As you make the plan, stick to your guns, remembering you're their client, not their patient. They can't force you into a decision you're uncomfortable with. If you feel like they're badgering you during this conversation, consider switching care providers.

  The plan many of my clients make with their care providers is to go to the hospital for nonstress tests (monitoring) if their baby hasn't arrived by forty-one weeks. If the monitoring never shows fetal distress, they keep on keeping on until baby decides to arrive.

  Natural Induction Tip: If you go past your due date and feel anxious about getting things going, consider acupuncture, as it can be one of the most effective natural ways to induce. Just make sure you find an acupuncturist well trained in the art of induction, and you let your care provider know about it.

And now, here's what to do about not knowing what birth will feel like:

- **Prepare.** Take childbirth prep classes, practice the pain-relieving techniques you learn in those classes, read the books, and watch encouraging birth videos. Every time you put in this practice, tell yourself that what you're doing will make the contractions more manageable — because it will. The breathing techniques, the pressure points, the tub, the essential oils, the positions — they all serve to get you through one contraction at a time. While they don't eliminate discomfort, they will make it easier to manage.
- **Research epidurals.** If you're still fearful about the unknown pain after you prepare, research epidurals. That way, if that's something you end up wanting, you'll be confident you're making a well-informed decision. This book provides epidural insights that can get you started.
- **Make peace with the unknowns.** To infuse your pregnancy with more acceptance for all the unknowns, listen to this guided meditation: yourserenelife.wordpress.com/unknowns-of-childbirth/.

The main thing I want you to remember, no matter how you choose to get through the sensations of childbirth, is that you *will* get through them. They will not kill you, and they will absolutely help you realize your superhero strength.

To deal with the frustration of not knowing how many contractions you'll have to get through, try these ideas:

- **Think of each contraction as its own event.** Instead of concentrating on the unknown number of contractions you'll have, focus only on one contraction at a time. As a new contraction begins to roll through you, tell yourself that all you have to do is get through that one contraction. When it's done, put your full attention on resting. Then reset, and do it again.

- **Remember that each contraction brings you one step closer to your baby.** Even if you've barely dilated over a four-hour period, those contractions are still doing something, getting you nearer the enchanting moment of meeting your babe. So welcome each contraction, even if that sounds like crazy talk.

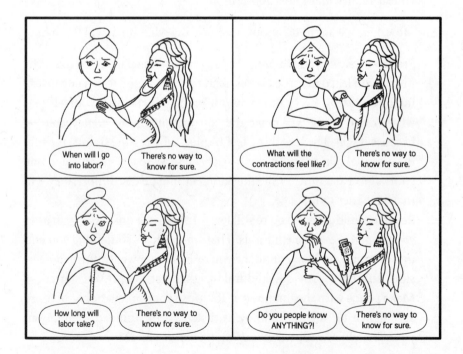

- **Don't get too wrapped up in your cervix dilation number.** While this number is a decent indicator of how far along you are, it doesn't really help us know how much longer you have to go. For example, I once supported a mom who got to ten centimeters in three hours, then had five more hours of labor before baby was born. Another woman was at four centimeters for two days, then dilated to ten centimeters in forty-five minutes and had her baby an hour later.

44. Why am I so afraid I'll die during childbirth?

You probably feel that way because a culture of fear has permeated childbirth. It bloomed when childbirth actually was a dangerous endeavor — when women weren't able to get quality care if a special circumstance came up, when doctors didn't know they needed to wash their hands between treating patients. Those women had good reason to fear death. But many of the risks those women faced are gone, and modern medical advances have made childbirth an incredibly safe experience. There is now effective protocol for even the most dangerous circumstances. And the great thing is, most women don't even need to receive medical care during childbirth; they just need a trained care provider observing them in case intervention is needed.

So now that we're covered for worst-case scenarios, we can relax into childbirth, right? We can let go of the fear of death. But that's easier said than done. Our conscious minds can know that death is a highly unlikely outcome of childbirth, but the subconscious mind still holds on to the belief. There are a few reasons for that. Media is one of them. Think about every depiction of childbirth you've seen in mainstream media. I can almost guarantee those images consisted of angry women screaming in pain. Each time you saw one of these images, a seed of fear was planted.

And then there are the scary birth stories. Some women wear their traumatic birth story like a badge of honor and love to tell pregnant women, "Childbirth will be the most painful experience you'll ever go through." I've even heard some say, "It's so painful you'll want to die."

In addition to these inaccurate, harmful messages, a fear of death during childbirth can be triggered by our mind trying to wrap itself around the process of a human coming out of our body. Many women in my classes have reported a fear that their body will "rip open" during childbirth, or that their heart will give out because of the strain. Even though these are not things that will happen, women still believe it on some level, despite all the evidence to the contrary. Much of this fear comes from the unknown. They've never had a baby, and the mind takes them to the scariest place it can imagine. Or maybe they've had a baby and the birth was traumatic. Even though they survived the experience, a part of them believes the second time around will be even more traumatic.

When this fear is at its most intense, it has a name: tokophobia. According to an article published in *Industrial Psychiatry Journal*, tokophobia — a morbid, pathological fear of childbirth — can lead to avoidance of birth and sometimes results in a woman requesting a cesarean section. The authors report a number of circumstances that could trigger tokophobia:

- **Hearing traumatic birth stories:** This is a big one. When women we trust go on and on about traumatic birth experiences, we start to think, "If it happened to them, it could happen to me." And sometimes, we take it to the next level, thinking, "But I probably won't be as lucky as they were. I'll probably be the one that dies because of those complications." But the likelihood of that is really, *really* rare.

- **Concerns about the competency of medical professionals:** Fear is an understandable by-product of not trusting that hospital staff or midwives can keep you safe. If you're convinced you won't be properly cared for if you require medical intervention, it's likely that you have experienced some form of negligence regarding medical care, or heard stories of those who have. Whatever the reasons, the "What to do" section will provide ideas for working through this.

- **Low self-esteem:** If we don't think highly of ourselves, it's hard to believe our mind and body can withstand the rigors of childbirth. (But it can!) This wavering belief in our ability to birth can water those aforementioned seeds of fear.

The good news is you don't have to just grin and bear this often-debilitating fear, regardless of where it's coming from. There are ways to face it, then move past it.

What to do

One of the most crucial steps to overcoming this fear is realizing it's not a sign of what's to come. Even if your mind believes on the deepest level that your birth will not have a good outcome, it doesn't make it so. Keep reminding yourself that the fear is a false construct of your mind, built by outdated information and stories that are part of someone else's false constructs or need to impress. And above all, know that you can overcome the fear. Know that the fear doesn't own you. Know that you are stronger than the fear. The following steps will help you believe that:

- **Find a care provider you feel safe with.** Few things are as reassuring as hearing a care provider you trust tell you that they'll keep you safe during childbirth. They can explain the protocol for all the situations you're afraid of, and they can share uplifting stories of births they've attended.

   The key here is that you trust them. If that trust isn't there, their reassurance won't mean much. So interview care providers until you find one who makes you feel safe. While it's common to have to interview a few before finding the right one, you might also discover that you don't trust any of them, regardless of how many candidates you interview. If this is the case, you might need to work with a mental health specialist to unpack and examine your unique trust issues with medical care providers.

- **Write about what you're afraid of.** An interesting thing about fear is that when we name it, it loses some of its power. So write down why you think you'll die during childbirth. Can you pinpoint where that comes from? Are other fears about pregnancy or childbirth fueling your fear of death? Write it all, letting the words flow until you find clarity. Then, make a list of the primary fears and discuss them with your care provider and/or a mental health specialist.

- **Carefully select the prenatal testing you'll undergo.** The testing that can be utilized during pregnancy is a double-edged sword. On one side, the testing can offer reassurance if it confirms everything is fine. On the other side is anxiety that can be triggered while waiting for test results, in addition to the fears that arise if results are abnormal. Because of this, it's crucial to be selective about the testing you agree to.

Speak with your care provider about what is available, and what they recommend, then carefully determine what tests are ideal for your unique situation and comfort level.

- **Avoid scary birth stories.** If someone tries to tell you their birth story, stop them and say, "I would love to hear your story if it's not traumatic and won't scare me. If you think it will, I would like you to wait to share until after I have my baby." In addition, if you come across an article, television show, or other media source that portrays birth in a scary light, skip it. You don't need to be an expert on worst-case scenarios; that's why you have a doctor or midwife.

- **Reach out to loved ones.** The aforementioned study published in *Industrial Psychiatry Journal* found that there was a 50 percent reduction in elective C-sections when women experiencing severe fear of labor and delivery told trusted friends and family members how they were feeling and asked for support.

- **Hire a doula.** Because feeling heard and supported is such a big part of unraveling your fear of death during childbirth, seeking the support of a doula can offer significant relief. To make sure you find the right person, ask friends for referrals, and keep interviewing candidates until you find the one who is a giant yes for you. You can also get a feel for how they'll support you through your fear by bringing it up during your initial meeting. How they respond will be indicative of how they'll support you through it during birth.

- **Count to ninety when you feel the fear.** Any emotion takes ninety seconds to pass through you if you don't stop it. So when you feel that fear of death gurgle up, think, "Oh, look at that. There's that fear. I'm not going to ignore it. I'm going to sit with it." Then set a timer for ninety seconds, and feel the fear until the timer beeps. Anytime you feel the emotions attached to the fear come back, repeat this exercise.

- **Create an arsenal of relaxation techniques.** In addition to the ninety-second fear release, collect practices that soothe you. For example, you could take deep breaths, envisioning calm, trust, and comfort flowing in as you inhale, and fear, tension, and dread flowing out as you exhale. You could also repeat a mantra, such as, "I'm releasing this fear because it doesn't own me. It is not real. I choose love and trust instead." Or you can simply repeat, "I am safe." As an added resource, download this guided meditation that was specifically crafted for releasing the fear of death during childbirth: yourserenelife.wordpress.com/fear-of-dying/.

- **Birth in the location that makes you feel safest.** If the idea of birthing in a hospital freaks you out, consider birthing at home or in a birth center. But if you can't imagine feeling safe anywhere but a hospital, go to the hospital. And it doesn't matter what your partner, mom, friend, childbirth educator, or whoever thinks you should do. Do what makes *you* feel most secure.

45. I'm paralyzed by the thought of birthing in a hospital. But I'm also uncomfortable with a home birth. What should I do?

I would like to say that the answer is as simple as choosing a birth center (and it might be!). But there's probably more to this question because it's really about fear, and choosing a birth center won't dissolve the underlying fears you may have. So let's start by exploring why some women are afraid of hospital births.

For many of us, the hospital is associated with injury and illness. It's the place you go when something is wrong and you need to be poked and prodded. That's enough to make anyone nervous. In addition, almost every depiction most people have seen of birth was from mainstream media: panicked women being rushed into a hospital, hooked up to machines and an IV, and then screaming at their partner (comedies), or almost dying (dramas). Those are the messages our minds have received about hospital birth. For some women, these images translate into, "I have to birth in a hospital because it's the only safe place." For others, they trigger the fight-flight-or-freeze response, making the hospital a suboptimal place for them to birth.

And now for the fear of home birth. Going back to the messages we've received from mainstream media, the rare home births shown in prominent shows or movies almost always end in an emergency transfer to a hospital, and the mother regretting her decision to try a home birth. In addition, many people have the misconception that a home birth is dangerous and irresponsible. But the reality is, if a certified midwife who has confirmed you're a good candidate for a home birth is caring for you, this environment is almost always incredibly safe. An article published in *Journal of Midwifery & Women's Health* reported that planned home births for low-risk women result in low rates of interventions, without an increase in adverse outcomes for mothers and babies. The key term in that finding is *low risk* — if you have special circumstances that could require medical care to keep you and baby safe, a hospital birth is likely the best choice. But if you and baby are all good, a home birth is a viable option.

Taking all this into consideration, it's easy to see why many women have a tricky time deciding where to birth. However, there is a way through.

What to do

The following exercises and considerations can help you discover what you're actually afraid of, process the resulting information in a way that helps you make a birthing-location decision you feel good about, and acquire tools to reinforce comfort in your decision:

- **Break down your fears.** Figuring out the makeup of our fears often makes them more manageable.
  - To do this, write *Hospital* and *Home Birth* on the top of a page. Then, under each, write everything about that birthing environment you're afraid of. Get specific. For example, under *Hospital* you might write, "The IV. The sterile smell. Infection. A mean nurse. The impersonal energy. Pressure to have invasive interventions." For *Home Birth* you might list, "Not being able to get quick care if surgery is needed. The midwife not knowing what to do in an emergency situation. Having to clean up the mess. The guilt if anything goes wrong."
  - Next, talk to a doctor you trust about your list of fears about a hospital birth. Have them give you the skinny on the object of each of your fears. For example, you can ask what's the likelihood that it will occur, and if there's anything you can do to prevent it.
  - Then, talk to a home birth midwife about your list of home-birthing fears.
  - After you've had these discussions, sit with the information as you flow through the following suggestions.

- **Consider a birth center delivery.** After you've explored your fears, visit a few birth centers. In each one, tune in to how the environment and care providers make you feel. Does it seem like a happy medium? Does it make you lean toward a hospital or home birth? Or are fresh fears coming up?

  If big doubts still come up, the base of your fears might be more about the process of birth than the environment where you'll be birthing. In this case, review question 44, about the fear of death during childbirth. This question breaks down the deeper fears of childbirth and provides tools for working through them. After you've worked these tools, you'll likely have more clarity about the birthing environment that's right for you.

- **Interview OB-GYNs and midwives.** A big factor in how comfortable women are in a birth environment is how safe they feel with their care provider. So I recommend meeting a handful of OBs and midwives (both birth center and home birth midwives) to see if you find someone who makes you feel heard and protected. This relationship will likely inform where you want to give birth.

- **Listen to this meditation.** The meditation recording at the following link helps you process the information you've gathered by walking you through visualizations of what it might be like to birth in each space: yourserenelife.wordpress.com/ideal-birth-space/.

- **Watch reassuring birth videos.** If you Google the terms "HypnoBirthing home birth videos," "positive home birth videos," and "Hypno-Birthing hospital birth videos," you'll find numerous videos showing home birth and hospital birth in a gentle, positive light. It's easy for me to tell you how safe birth can be in both settings, but actually seeing women soundly birthing in these environments can go a long way in convincing you.

  In addition, look up the video *Birth as We Know It — Educational Version* on YouTube, as it also shows peaceful births. (Some of the births are a bit unorthodox, but many are really powerful — there's even an orgasmic birth!)

- **Know that it's okay if you're not totally comfortable in your birthing environment of choice.** Regardless of where you choose to give birth, there will likely still be some nervousness when you're in that space, as it's where you'll be going through an intense life change. If you've gone through all the steps above and thoughtfully chosen the birth space that feels best, these nerves likely have more to do with what will happen in that environment than the environment itself. Avoid letting your trepidation spin into intense anxiety by continually reminding yourself that it's okay to feel nervous — I can almost guarantee that every birthing woman who came before you felt the same way. And remember that nervousness can absolutely live in harmony with excitement and courage.

- **Brainstorm how you can turn your birth environment into a sanctuary.** See "Essential Tips for the Journey" on page 302 for more information.

46. I've experienced sexual trauma and am terrified at the thought of giving birth vaginally. Is it horrible that I want to ask for a cesarean birth?

It's not horrible at all. You should have whatever type of birth you think you'd be most comfortable with. The combination of giving your body up to another human during pregnancy, being touched in a clinical manner in the same areas the abuse likely took place, and potentially feeling a loss of control in medical settings can equal a birth experience ripe with triggers and anxiety. It can also bring up fear of receiving treatment from a male doctor, nurse, or ultrasound tech. It's a complex path to navigate.

Adding to this complexity is the lack of energy many women have for managing their anxiety during pregnancy and childbirth. Because the coping skills developed after surviving sexual trauma often require significant strength to implement, the energy that pregnancy and childbirth siphon away can leave a woman feeling vulnerable to triggers and all the resulting emotions and physical responses. One survivor I worked with said pregnancy made her feel like she was on an out-of-control roller coaster of joy, fear, sadness, excitement, anxiety, and anger — until she took the steps listed below.

What to do

Take it one step at a time. Even women who haven't experienced sexual trauma can find pregnancy and childbirth overwhelming. When you're managing the added weight of being a survivor, the process can feel defeating. But if you focus on one empowered action at a time, you can navigate your way to a space of calm and trust that can carry you through a positive birth experience. Here are some ideas to get you started:

- **Rest.** This is always important, but it's especially so when navigating the added anxiety of past sexual trauma. See "Essential Tips for the Journey" on page 302 for more information.
- **Find a care provider you trust implicitly, then share your story.** After you've interviewed various care providers and have found one who makes you feel safe, tell them whatever aspects of your story you're comfortable sharing. (It may take many visits before you trust them enough to share this information.) They should then offer clear ideas on how they'll adapt their care to honor your needs. They should also be open to hearing how you want to be cared for. It's important that this feel like a collaborative relationship, and not one where they're the authority figure and you're the passive recipient of what they deem "right" for your body. They should involve you in every decision, continually reassuring you that you're in the position of control — they're just there for guidance and to provide the support you deem necessary. If they don't make you feel this way, I urge you to find a new care provider.
- **Request female care providers.** If you think being touched by men will trigger you, add to your birth preferences that you would like to be cared for only by women, and discuss this preference with your primary care provider. While this might not always be possible (for example, there might only be a male anesthesiologist available if you're getting an epidural), identifying this preference gives you a better chance of creating an environment that facilitates optimal comfort.
- **Ask for comprehensive communication from care providers.** Survivors I've supported felt anxious during prenatal visits and childbirth because they never knew when they would be touched. Some were so uncomfortable with surprise touch that they dissociated from their bodies and felt unconnected to their pregnancy and birth experiences. You can prevent this by telling all your care providers (e.g., doctor or midwife, ultrasound techs, nurses, assistant midwives, etc.) that you

need them to inform you before touching you, and to fully explain what they're doing and why.

- **Speak up when you feel uncomfortable.** Even when you make it clear you want thorough communication about required touch and you want that touch to be gentle, you might still get a care provider who isn't respectful of your requests. If that happens, don't be afraid to speak up, and if possible, ask for a different care provider.

    You might also have the experience of someone fully honoring your needs, yet still making you feel uncomfortable. If this happens, you have every right to ask them to cease touching you until you feel comfortable resuming.

- **Make it clear that it's imperative you don't lose your voice during the birth experience.** I've attended the births of survivors who had care providers who made them feel safe...until labor and delivery. These care providers assured the women that they wouldn't be pressured into decisions they weren't comfortable with and they would be treated with the same level of respect they'd received during pregnancy. But then labor began, and the promises dissolved. This resulted in the women feeling like they were no longer in control of their birth — like they were being silenced. This doesn't have to happen to you. See "Essential Tips for the Journey" on page 302 for more information on how to maintain your voice during birth.

    The importance of speaking up throughout childbirth is reinforced by an article published in *BMC Pregnancy and Childbirth* that found (not surprisingly) that the most effective guide on how to support a survivor of sexual abuse through childbirth is the birthing woman herself.

- **Ask yourself whether a vaginal or a cesarean birth seems more triggering.** Ask your care provider or childbirth preparation educator to walk you through what you can typically expect during a vaginal and a cesarean birth. As you hear about the components of each experience, take note of what raises your red flags. For example, I worked with a survivor who didn't like the idea of having an oxygen mask on her face during a C-section, while another was terrified of the idea of a vaginal tear. While it's impossible to know exactly how you'll handle a vaginal or cesarean birth, this mental mapping can help you determine what type of birth could be best for your unique needs.

- **Consider hiring a doula.** Regardless of the type of birth you select, a doula provides an additional layer of support that can soothe many of your fears and anxieties before, during, and after birth. If you'd like a doula, do as you did with care providers and interview many candidates until you find one you trust enough to share your story with. From there, be clear about the type of support you want, and what you anticipate being difficult. For example, if you've selected a C-section but are nervous about feeling out of control while under the influence of opioids, brainstorm ways your doula can create a safe container for you.
- **Think about the birth positions that might trigger you.** Certain positions can bring up memories of abuse, which is why it's important to learn the most common birth positions, and let your care providers know if there are any you do not want to be in.
- **Think about phrases that might trigger you.** Much like the birth positions, there might be phrases you associate with abuse. For example, if phrases like "Just relax" or "Don't worry, it will be over soon" have negative connotations for you, tell your care providers not to use them, and add these requests to your birth preferences.
- **Read Penny Simkin's book *When Survivors Give Birth*.** This extraordinary book dives into the complexities of giving birth while managing the PTSD caused by sexual trauma.
- **Select a childbirth preparation class that provides tools for managing fear and anxiety.** While many classes provide excellent tools for pain relief, few go deep into how to manage the fear and anxiety that can arise during the journey to and through childbirth. In my biased opinion, the HypnoBirthing and Birthing from Within modalities provide the most effective techniques for this emotional support. You can supplement these classes with my online course on Udemy, "Childbirth Preparation: A Complete Guide for Pregnant Women," which provides over fifteen relaxation recordings and an entire section on fear release. It can be found here: udemy.com/course/childbirth-preparation-a-complete-guide-for-pregnant-women.
- **Create a list of your go-to relaxation tools.** If you're triggered during birth, it will be helpful to have a list of calming techniques. To create this list, practice the techniques offered in your childbirth preparation

class, and note which ones are most effective. Provide this list to your birth companions, and explain how they can lead you through the techniques.

- **Help your birth companions pull you out of dissociation.** Dissociation — feeling disconnected from your body and the here and now — is something many survivors experience. It's a common coping mechanism, and it could occur during birth if you're retraumatized. However, your birth companions can pull you out of it with a few simple techniques.

  First, it's important for your birth companions to understand the signals of dissociation. For example, your eyes might "glaze over," or you could start moving or responding in a spaced-out manner. Essentially, you start to act really different — like you've checked out. Discuss this with your birth companions before birth, and ask the person you feel safest with to do the following if they think you've dissociated:

  - Ask everyone to leave the room.
  - Hold eye contact with you. If your eyes are closed, they can snap their fingers or say your name in a strong voice. They can then instruct you to open your eyes if you don't open them during the initial prompts.
  - Figure out a phrase you want them to use to help you acknowledge what's happening. For example, they could say, "It seems like you went somewhere else for a while. You're safe to come back to the room."
  - Once you seem to be coming back into your body, they can ask you where you are and what you're doing. They can also ask you to explain what your five senses are experiencing.
  - Finally, they can strengthen your connection to your body and the present moment by giving you an essential oil to smell, placing a cool compress on your forehead, or pressing their hands down on your shoulders.

- **Take heart that you could have a new relationship with your body after childbirth.** While it's not a given for all survivors, many report having a transformed relationship with their body after birthing their baby. The experience might help you to see your body in a new light (it's a vessel for new life!) and connect with it in ways that evoke feelings of pride, gentleness, and nurturing. Birth certainly won't erase the atrocities you experienced, but the experience can allow you to have a fresh beginning with your body.

Note: If you feel that pregnancy and preparing for childbirth could bring up intense emotions and memories, consider working with a trauma therapist.

47. What will happen if my baby needs serious medical attention after birth?

If that happens, you should continually remind yourself that it's not your fault. For a variety of reasons completely outside our control, baby's medical status can become fragile during pregnancy or birth. While sadness and fear will likely be woven into the experience, regret doesn't have to be a constant in this unexpected journey. And it shouldn't. Because in many ways, all regret does is suck you out of the present moment — and this is a present moment that requires all your energy and attention to make informed decisions and to care for your baby and yourself. Regret makes you ruminate over past circumstances that can't be changed. And sure, when everything settles down, you can review the series of events that led you here, and see if there's anything you'd change if you become pregnant again. But for now, give yourself permission to be kind to yourself. This also applies to your partner. It's natural to want to blame someone when something goes wrong, but often, that only alienates your support system. Just keep choosing forgiveness and kindness — at least in your interactions with yourself and others.

Anger will almost undoubtedly be part of your early experience as well, and that's okay. It will probably feel completely unfair that your family is having to navigate something so painful and unexpected. And it is. You deserved to give birth to a perfectly healthy baby, and it sucks that you were dealt a different hand. Let all this anger flow through and out to create space for strength. (See below for an idea of how to do that.) Because when we're constantly trying to suppress negative emotions, it's hard to find our way into courage and trust that we will make it through. But you will. Even though this might feel like an insurmountable situation, you will make it through.

What to do

While much of what you'll do during this time depends on the unique circumstances of your baby's health needs, here are some universal strategies for getting through a health crisis with your baby:

- **Keep bringing yourself back to the present.** When our child's health is in jeopardy, the mind tends to bounce back and forth between the past and the future — thoughts of the past, filled with unproductive regrets, and thoughts of the future, soaked in worst-case scenarios. Neither serves us. The most productive place for you is the present moment, where all you need to do is process and manage what is right in front of you. When your mind starts wandering to unproductive realms, pay attention to your five senses. Notice what you can see, smell, hear, taste, and touch, and let it pull you back into the now.
- **Keep a running list of questions.** When your newborn has a health condition, the questions and the storm of new information can be overwhelming. Keep track of it all by writing down your questions the moment you think of them. Then, take notes as the questions are answered. If anything is unclear, don't be afraid to ask for clarification. *Newborn Intensive Care: What Every Parent Needs to Know* by Jeanette Zaichkin also provides helpful insights on this topic.
- **Request thorough communication.** If your baby is in the NICU, you probably won't be able to be with them 24/7, which could make you antsy for information. Ensure that you stay informed of baby's health status by being adamant that the health care team regularly updates you.
- **Be treated in the same facility as your baby.** If your baby needs to be transferred to a new hospital and you're still in need of postpartum care, ask if you can be transferred to the same facility.
- **Ask to be part of baby's care.** While much of the care baby needs will likely require specialized training, there will be tasks like bathing, cleaning, and of course bonding that you can participate in. Work out a schedule with the care team so you know when to be present for these activities.
- **Create a physical anchor.** When we're crippled by fear, it can feel like we've left our body. This can be paralyzing. When you notice you're

floating into fear, ground yourself by utilizing a physical anchor. For example, you can hug yourself, push down on your shoulders, or press your palms into your eyes. When you use your anchor of choice, couple it with an affirmation, something along the lines of "It's safe to come back into my body."

- **Don't blame yourself.** Every time you try to blame yourself for what's happening, mentally step out of yourself and firmly but gently say, "STOP." After giving that stop message, treat yourself as you would a child who is broken up over something that isn't their fault. You wouldn't encourage them to be harder on themselves — you would nurture and reassure them. Do that for yourself.

- **Take time every day to let out your emotions.** Get into a private space for an hour (or for however long you have to be alone) every day and let yourself go. Scream, rage, cry, beat your fist on a pillow — let it out. Releasing these emotions can provide the clarity and calm to get you through the most difficult days of this journey. You can also journal during this time, letting out all the thoughts you don't feel comfortable sharing with others.

  If you find it helpful to have a sounding board, ask a friend or family member if they'd be willing to be this for you. Tell them straight-up that you're looking not for advice but for someone to be an active listener. I would stay away from asking your partner to do this, as they're too close to the situation. While you'll definitely be a support for one another, it's ideal for each of you to have someone else to vent to.

- **Go for a walk.** Being in a medical facility for prolonged periods can be stifling, making it hard to think clearly. Refresh your mind, body, and emotions by going outside at least once a day and walking around the block, or to a local park. Amp up the benefits of the walk by listening to soothing music or a guided meditation.

- **Nurture your basic needs.** Drinking water, regularly eating nutritious food, and sleeping help ensure that your health doesn't sustain too much damage through this challenging time. My client Sarah had a premature baby who had to be in the NICU for four weeks. She said she felt like she had to martyr herself during that time. She said the thought "My baby is suffering, so I should suffer" constantly cycled through her mind. This resulted in her depriving herself of nourishing meals, quality sleep, and regular showers. Looking back, she regrets this attitude, saying, "By doing that I made myself so physically weak and uncomfortable, which made it harder to deal with my emotions, make decisions, and even spend time with my baby. Anytime I was with her in the NICU, I would just break down."

While you probably won't feel like doing anything but worry about your baby, forcing yourself to take care of those basic needs can fortify your ability to be there for them. You don't deserve to suffer more than you already are.

- **Join a support group.** Having a child with unexpected health needs can feel very isolating — like no one else could possibly relate to your pain. But seeking the camaraderie of a support group for parents navigating similar situations can help you feel less alone, and talking with other parents provides an outlet for processing what your family is going through. Members of these groups are often wonderful resources as well, providing tips on the best care providers, helpful treatments for various conditions, and how to work with your insurance provider. Your baby's doctor can likely provide recommendations for local support groups. The March of Dimes (especially its "Share Your Story" initiative) and the National Perinatal Association also offer helpful resources.

C-sections and VBACs

48. What's a cesarean birth really like?

It's intense in ways that are similar to and also completely different than a vaginal birth. Some say a C-section is the "easy way out," but I don't agree. While the physical sensations during the surgery are typically mild, significant mental and emotional stamina is often required. And the recovery is much more involved than what's experienced by women who had a vaginal birth. I say all this because if you end up needing a C-section, I want you to know you haven't "cheapened" your birth experience or failed to "prove your strength" through a vaginal birth. You've gone through an incredible process that requires immense courage.

Here's what to expect from and keep in mind during a cesarean birth:

- **Scheduling:** If you and your care provider decide a planned C-section is the ideal option because of a special circumstance, like your baby being in a breech position or another special circumstance, the surgery will be scheduled sometime around your due date.
- **The unplanned C-section:** If you're in the middle of having a vaginal birth, but something puts you or baby at risk, your care provider might recommend a C-section. If it's not an emergency, ask them to thoroughly explain the reasoning behind their recommendation, so you can make a well-informed decision.
- **Consent:** You have to provide legal consent before the surgery.
- **Safety:** Know that the team performing your cesarean birth is composed of trained professionals who will keep you and your baby safe. Allow yourself to enter the experience with an energy of trust, as you'll be in skilled hands.
- **Support during surgery:** In nonemergency situations, your birth companion should be allowed to stay with you during the surgery. If they're squeamish, consider asking another friend, family member, or doula (if you've hired one) to accompany you, as you don't want the medical staff having to attend to anyone but you and baby.
- **Pain and numbing medication:** Before surgery, an anesthesiologist reviews your medical history and pain management options. They'll

likely recommend an epidural or spinal block to numb the lower half of your body. You'll be awake during the surgery, but you shouldn't feel anything from your waist down, with the potential exception of some pressure.

In some emergency situations — or if you have a condition that would contraindicate an epidural, like a blood clotting disorder — you may receive general anesthesia, but that's rare.

- **Further prep:** After the epidural is placed, your bladder is drained with a catheter, and an IV is started to administer fluids and any additional medication you may need. You might also receive an antacid to neutralize your stomach acid, and antibiotics to prevent infection after the procedure.
- **The screen:** To prevent you from witnessing the surgery, a screen is raised at your waist. You can request that the screen be partially lowered when your baby is lifted out. (You'll find more cesarean birth preferences in the following pages.)
- **The surgery:** When the anesthesia has fully numbed you, antiseptic is applied to your lower abdomen, and the surgeon makes a small horizontal cut above your pubic bone. They then cut through the underlying tissue — manually separating your abdominal muscles — until they reach your uterus. A horizontal incision is then made in the lower portion of your uterus, and the doctor retrieves your baby and the placenta. This typically takes fifteen to twenty minutes. You might be given Pitocin after the surgery to help prevent hemorrhaging and to ensure the uterus contracts back down to its original size.
- **Bonding:** If you and baby are in good health, you'll likely be able to hold them after delivery, while you're still lying on the operating table.
- **The stitches:** As you're falling in love with baby, the surgeon applies absorbable stitches to your uterus, and stitches or staples to your abdomen. The incision is usually so low a bikini bottom can cover the scar.

After the C-section is complete, you start the recovery process, which is different for every woman. The recovery is covered in the next question.

What to do

Create cesarean birth preferences. A common source of resistance to a C-section is lack of control, as women often feel that because the birth is literally in the hands of the surgeons, they'll lose their sense of empowerment. But this doesn't have to happen. In the absence of an emergency, many hospitals are open to moms having a voice in how their C-section unfolds, typically in the form of cesarean birth preferences. I find that creating these preferences — even if you feel certain you won't need a C-section — helps dissolve fear of the unexpected because you're preparing for all possibilities.

Some cesarean preferences that can help you reclaim feelings of control and empowerment and ensure a gentle C-section are offered below. These preferences are just samples — you should take out any that don't feel important, and add any that do. I also recommend bringing them to a prenatal appointment about six weeks before your due date to discuss with your care provider and to find out if any of the preferences go against hospital protocol. If so, you could choose to give up some preferences, or find a hospital that supports gentle C-sections.

Sample Cesarean Preferences

We request:

- **To have my arms free during the operation.** Being strapped down can induce panic. Request that your arms remain unbound so you can hold baby as soon as possible after delivery.
- **To have a nasal cannula instead of a face mask for oxygen.** Oxygen face masks make some women feel claustrophobic.
- **To have medical staff refrain from personal conversations.** Hearing the nurse's thoughts on a new dating app is unlikely to fill you with positive anticipation for meeting your baby. So request that all people in the operating room swap personal conversations with encouraging words for you — or at least limit their comments to the task at hand.

- **To have medical staff talk to me, instead of about me, as much as possible.** This can help you feel like you're part of the process, instead of "just another patient" cycling through the operating room.
- **To have music or other recording of my choice playing.** The sounds you hear during the C-section can set the tone for the experience, so ask for the ability to play songs or a guided meditation of your liking. You should also be able to bring headphones if you want a private listening experience. Use the following link to download a guided meditation created for cesarean births: yourserenelife.wordpress.com/gentle -csection/.
- **To have the screen lowered as baby is lifted out.** Seeing your baby's arrival is a powerful experience, especially for moms who cannot physically feel the emergence.
- **To have delayed cord clamping.** This helps reduce the chance of baby developing an iron deficiency, because it allows the iron- and hemoglobin-rich blood in the cord and placenta to get to baby before the cord is clamped and cut. The cord usually stops pulsating within a few minutes after delivery.
- **To have skin-to-skin contact directly after baby is born.** The release of oxytocin that occurs when you hold your baby on your bare chest supports bonding and eventual breastfeeding (if that's something you're choosing to do).
- **To have monitors placed so they won't impede bonding.** Dealing with a tangle of tubes and wires when trying to hold your baby isn't fun.
- **To have baby stay with parents at all times, unless a medical complication makes that impossible.** It's ideal for a newborn to be with one of their parents as much as possible.
- **To have a vaginal swab applied to baby (also known as "vaginal seeding").** Stay with me on this one. When a baby is born vaginally, they're exposed to a range of microbes that help reduce the risk for inflammatory illnesses, heart disease, infections, and other not-fun circumstances. A baby born via

C-section can potentially receive the benefits of these microbiomes when the care provider collects a vaginal swab and wipes it on baby's skin. It can also be wiped on your nipples before breastfeeding. Discuss this preference with your doctor or midwife, as the research is ongoing and controversial. To learn more, check out the article "The Microbiome Seeding Debate — Let's Frame It around Women-Centered Care" in the journal *Reproductive Health*.

49. What's C-section recovery really like?

After you've summoned your courage and had the C-section, it's time to recover. This journey often takes four to six weeks and requires ample patience and rest. Here are some of the steps and issues you might experience during recovery:

- **Transfer to a recovery room:** Once the surgeons have okayed you to leave the operating room, you're taken to a recovery room and monitored for a few hours. It could take many hours for the numbing medication to wear off enough for you to walk. The catheter stays in place until you can walk to the bathroom.
- **Feeding:** If baby isn't in need of medical care, you should be able to begin breast- or bottle-feeding soon after you've settled into the recovery room. You can also request to start breastfeeding in the operating room. Regarding food for you, you'll probably be cleared to eat a light meal about eight hours after surgery.
- **Blood clot prevention:** To help prevent blood clots from forming in your legs, a nurse will help you walk as soon as you're able.
- **Cramping:** It's normal to feel cramping as the uterus shrinks back to size, in addition to some pain at the incision site. Your care provider will work with you to find the best pain management solution.
- **Continual monitoring:** You'll be monitored closely during your hospital stay (usually four to six days) to ensure you don't develop an infection or have excessive bleeding. Vaginal bleeding is common for four to six weeks, but it's heaviest in the days following delivery.

- **Post-op instructions for driving and exercise:** When you're discharged from the hospital, they'll instruct you to not drive for four to six weeks and to just say no to exercise (no heavy lifting!) for six to eight weeks.
- **Continued soreness:** It's common to feel sore for at least a week or two after the C-section. Your care provider can provide pain relief options.
- **Need for open communication:** If at any point during your recovery you feel like something's off (for example, you have a significant amount of bleeding, extreme pain, or a fever), tell your care provider. Don't worry about bothering them. They'd much rather you be too cautious than not reach out when you need medical attention.
- **Long-term recovery:** You may experience lingering urinary incontinence due to weakened pelvic floor muscles. (Who said a C-section wasn't fun?!) This is totally normal and can be remedied with the help of a pelvic floor specialist. Ask your care provider for a referral.

As you heal from a C-section, you may feel disappointed you didn't have a vaginal birth — especially if you prepared for one. While it can be healthy to mourn that loss (it's okay to be bummed!), I also urge you to remember what I mentioned before — a C-section requires an exceptional amount of courage, and you deserve to honor yourself for that courage. Don't allow anyone (including yourself) to tell you that you "didn't give birth" because a surgeon was the one to physically help your baby emerge. You spent an amazing amount of time growing the baby, then completely surrendered your body to the type of birth your baby needed to have. That is extraordinary. You are extraordinary.

What to do

Keep reminding yourself of your awesomeness, while also enhancing your physical comfort by putting together a C-section Healing Kit that includes the following items:

- **Stool softener:** Pooping after a C-section ain't no joke.
- **OTC pain medication,** like ibuprofen and acetaminophen.
- **Breastfeeding pillow:** This takes pressure off your abdomen when you're feeding or just holding baby.

- **C-section undies:** These supportive, high-waisted underwear often include a silicone panel to speed scar recovery.
- **Scar balm:** This healing balm can reduce the appearance of scars and minimize itchiness. It also does wonders for stretch marks.
- **Heavy-duty maternity pads:** Beyond capturing the blood, these bulky beauties help you feel solidarity with your diaper-wearing baby.
- **Loose, breastfeeding-friendly clothing:** Essentially, stay away from anything with a waistband lower than your underboob area and stick to breathable, super comfy materials.
- **Prenatal vitamins:** Your body will likely be depleted after going through major surgery, managing an onslaught of medications, and dealing with big shifts in hormones. These vitamins help you get through it.
- *The First Forty Days: The Essential Art of Nourishing the New Mother* **by Amely Greeven, Heng Ou, and Marisa Belger:** In addition to those prenatal vitamins, this book helps you nurture your postpartum self.
- **Postpartum belly wrap:** While it hasn't been proven that these things actually work, many women swear they sped their recovery and made their abdomen feel less vulnerable.
- **Your favorite healthy snacks:** While you will hopefully have someone on hand to make you healthy meals, it can still be nice to stock up on easy, nutritious nosh you can store near your recovery area.
- **Reusable metal water bottle**
- **Electrolyte replenisher:** Slip this powder into that water bottle to ensure you're maintaining optimal hydration.
- **Your couch and remote control**

Note: I didn't include nipple salve in this list because I've found that expressing a bit of breastmilk, dabbing it on sore nipples, and letting it dry works better than any store-bought product.

50. Are VBACs really as dangerous as many assume? Why are they frowned upon in so many areas?

In short, no, a VBAC (vaginal birth after cesarean) isn't nearly as dangerous as some would have you believe. If you're having a healthy pregnancy, at least eighteen months have passed since your last C-section, you've never had a uterine rupture, and your baby is head down (vertex position), a VBAC is likely a safer option than a repeat cesarean.

According to a report published in the journal *Obstetrics & Gynecology*, a VBAC often decreases the risk of maternal mortality, the need for a hysterectomy, and complications in future pregnancies by helping women avoid major abdominal surgery, which also lowers the risk of hemorrhage and infection and shortens postpartum recovery. The American College of Obstetricians and Gynecologists also affirms that a VBAC is a safe option for many women. Despite this data, some care providers are still hesitant to support a VBAC because of concern that the mother will experience a uterine rupture. But according to the *Obstetrics & Gynecology* report, if you had a previous cesarean with a low transverse incision (very common), your risk of uterine rupture in a vaginal delivery is less than 1 percent. They also found that 60 to 80 percent of women who plan a VBAC do deliver their baby vaginally.

Even with solid information backing the safety of VBACs for women who are good candidates, a number of care providers and hospitals won't support VBACs because they think the liability risk is too high. They prefer repeat C-sections because a C-section is the most invasive option and gives them the highest degree of control, and if anything goes wrong, they can say, "We did everything we could." A survey done by the American College of Obstetricians and Gynecologists found that 30 percent of obstetricians stopped offering VBACs because of concern about liability claims or litigation. The good news is there are still plenty of care providers willing to support a VBAC, and there are plenty of ways to increase your chances of having one.

Note: Medical professionals use the term *trial of labor after cesarean (TOLAC)* to refer to planned VBAC labor while it's happening. In other words, TOLAC is the labor, and VBAC is the delivery.

What to do

Before you decide to walk the VBAC path, consider whether it's what you really want. While research supports the safety of VBAC for many women, you still need to make sure you feel comfortable having one. If you wholeheartedly want a repeat C-section, and you know that's what would make you most comfortable, there's nothing wrong with going that route. But if you're even a little bit on the fence, I recommend exploring the following suggestions, as they'll shed light on whether a VBAC is right for your unique situation:

- **Find a care provider who is an advocate of VBACs.** Some care providers say they'll let you "try" for a VBAC, but they're usually more comfortable with you having another C-section. If you really want a VBAC, you don't want that type of care provider. You want someone who has not only attended numerous successful VBACs but also wholeheartedly believes in them being the safest option for women who are good candidates. If that's you, you want the care provider you select to be 100 percent behind your decision. You want them to be your champion and do everything possible to help you get that VBAC, while of course, keeping your safety as the number one priority.
- **Get a copy of the surgical reports from your C-section.** These reports tell you the type of incision and repair used on your uterus, why you received a C-section, and if there were any complications. This informs your care provider if you're a good candidate for a VBAC.
- **Equip yourself with knowledge.** Because many people don't have an accurate understanding of the safety of VBACs, you might encounter naysayers when you share this birth preference. First of all, you don't have to talk about this plan with anyone but your partner and care provider. But if you do want to discuss it with others, arm yourself with the following fun facts that will help you educate the uninformed:
  - For a healthy woman having a healthy pregnancy, a VBAC is usually safer than a repeat C-section, as it decreases the risk of maternal mortality, the need for a hysterectomy, and complications in future pregnancies. It also lowers the risk of hemorrhage and infection, and shortens postpartum recovery.
  - The risk of uterine rupture during a VBAC is less than 1 percent.
  - Sixty to 80 percent of women who plan a VBAC do end up delivering their baby vaginally.
- **Utilize the International Cesarean Awareness Network (ICAN).** This is a nonprofit aimed at reducing preventable C-sections through

education and advocacy for VBACs. Their local chapters connect you with women in your community who have had or are hoping to have VBACs, and they can help you understand the VBAC policies of hospitals in your area and share information about the care providers that support them.

In addition, if you feel you're being forced into a cesarean, you can call the ICAN hotline at 1-800-686-4226. As they go through the menu, you'll hear the prompt, "If you feel you are being forced into a cesarean, press 3." When you press 3, you'll then be asked to press 2 if you're currently in labor. If you press 2 you'll be transferred to an ICAN representative, who very likely has legal or medical training; they can walk you through how to advocate for yourself and prevent an unneeded repeat cesarean.

- **Utilize VBAC affirmations.** If other people's fears of VBACs start getting to you, reinforce your resolve by filling your mind with these positive messages:
  - My C-section scar heals more and more every day.
  - My C-section scar is incredibly strong and will not rupture.

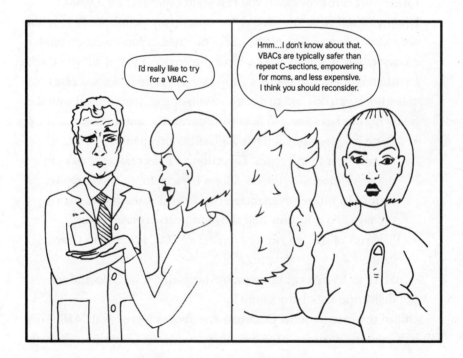

- My body will do exactly what it needs to do to have a safe vaginal birth.
- I will have a healthy and happy VBAC.
- I trust my decision to have a VBAC. I am doing the best thing for my baby and myself.
- I will be lovingly supported through my VBAC.
- **Listen to this guided meditation.** Visualize yourself moving through a positive VBAC experience by listening to the meditation at this link: yourserenelife.wordpress.com/vbac/.

51. I want to have a VBAC but can't find a care provider in my area who will attend one. What should I do?

One of my past doula clients — we'll call her Jamie — interviewed fifteen care providers in her search for one who supported VBACs. After two months of searching, she discovered there wasn't a doctor in a fifty-mile radius of her home willing to attend a VBAC. During that time she was shamed by almost every care provider she interviewed, being told she cared more about her ego than her baby's life, was uneducated and irresponsible, and would likely fail at having a VBAC. "I'm totally disgusted and disheartened," she told me after one of the worst encounters. "All these doctors care about is not being sued."

She then decided she wanted the VBAC enough to drive two hours to the nearest city to be cared for by a group of pro-VBAC midwives at a university hospital. The midwives and doctors she met with at this hospital, after confirming she was an excellent candidate for a VBAC, shared with her the latest information about how much safer VBACs were than repeat C-sections for women in Jamie's position. Almost all the data they provided contradicted what she had been told by the "fear-based gang," as she called the local doctors she'd met.

Jamie's labor came on strong and fast. She made it to the hospital thirty minutes before she was fully dilated. To lower her high blood pressure, she was given a walking epidural and quickly slipped into a state of serenity — she couldn't stop smiling and telling everyone how empowered and excited she felt. Jamie then started to push. And push. And push. After four hours of pushing the baby hadn't come out, but Jamie and the baby were in good health. I overheard a nurse say to the midwife, "If we were at the last hospital I worked, they would have forced a C-section on her hours ago." But that didn't happen. They kept gently supporting Jamie, ensuring her the baby was coming, albeit slowly. And then the baby arrived, healthy and screaming.

When I talked with Jamie a few weeks after her birth, she said, "I'm really happy I had the VBAC, but I think I would still be happy if I had to have a C-section. I felt so supported, heard, and respected by everyone at that hospital that I know they would've recommended a C-section only if it was really needed. I felt like I could trust them, and that made me okay with the idea of a C-section."

This is the essence of what many women are looking for when seeking a care provider for their VBAC. They're usually not looking for someone who will go to *any length* to get them a VBAC. They of course want someone who understands the value of a VBAC and is willing to support it when a woman is in a safe position to have one, but above all, they want someone they trust — someone who supports them in their choices and is one of their staunchest advocates. Being cared for by someone like that often allows women to loosen their grip on the desire for birth to unfold in the exact way they'd envisioned, and instead trust that it will play out in the way it's supposed to.

What to do

Begin the process of finding quality VBAC support by reaching out to friends in your area who've had a VBAC and asking for their care provider's information. You can also go to the ICAN website (www.ican-online .org/find-a-chapter-2) to find the nearest chapter, which can provide quality information on VBAC policies and pro-VBAC care providers in your area.

If you live in a smaller town that doesn't have pro-VBAC care providers, research doctors and midwives in the nearest city. You'll probably have the best luck with those who deliver at hospitals affiliated with universities, as they often have the most up-to-date information about VBACs, the risks of repeat C-sections, and how they can best support a woman through a VBAC. Finally, create a list of care providers you would like to interview. Before you meet with each candidate, call ahead to confirm they'll attend a VBAC, as you don't want to waste your time.

To conduct illuminating interviews, ask the questions below. They're intended not just to elicit information but also to provide you with the opportunity to read the care provider's body language, tone of voice, and overall vibe as they answer your queries. These nonverbal signs might be more telling evidence of whether they're a good fit for you than what they actually say.

- **Do you feel comfortable with VBACs?** The most honest component of the care provider's answer to this question will likely live in their initial reaction. If they immediately seem enthusiastic, that's a good sign. If they seem ambivalent but say they "might be willing" to support you in a VBAC "if all goes well," be wary of their timidity.
- **How many VBACs have you attended? What were the outcomes?** You want the care provider to have attended many successful VBACs. If they've attended VBACs but most ended in C-sections, take this as a potential sign that they're actually most comfortable with repeat C-sections.
- **What is your cesarean birth rate?** You want this number to be low.
- **What is the general VBAC philosophy of the hospital I would deliver in?** If for whatever reason your VBAC-supportive care provider isn't able to attend your birth, you want the hospital you'll be delivering in to be supportive of VBACs and to have a low C-section rate.
- **Am I a good candidate for a VBAC?** I placed this question after the previous ones because it's important to gain a sense of the care provider's philosophy on VBACs before having them assess whether you would be a good candidate. If it seems clear they don't fully support VBACs, this may skew their assessment of your candidacy.

  Legitimate reasons a woman would *not* be a good candidate for a VBAC are a twin pregnancy, a breech baby, placenta previa, and fetal distress. Take comfort in knowing that according to the American Pregnancy Association, 90 percent of women who have had a cesarean birth are candidates for a VBAC.
- **How confident are you that I'll have a successful VBAC?** While there's no way for a care provider to guarantee you'll have a VBAC, your experience will be more positive if they express confidence in your body's ability to move through a VBAC and in their ability to ensure your safety.

By asking these questions you're being a strong advocate for yourself and baby, while also ensuring your care provider is one of your greatest advocates.

52. Is a cesarean birth the only option if my baby is breech?

No, you have numerous options. But before we dive into those, know that it's common for babies to turn out of breech position up to week thirty-six of gestation. It's certainly still possible after that, but it's less likely, as baby is getting bigger, leaving less room for the turn.

If you are nearing week thirty-six of gestation and are feeling nervous about baby turning, the first step in encouraging them to turn is using the gentle turn techniques outlined in the "What to do" section below. From there, I discuss a more intense turning technique, called external cephalic version (ECV), and then help you explore what it would look like to vaginally deliver a breech baby. And finally, we'll look at the process of coming to terms with a cesarean birth, if that ends up being the best path for you.

What to do

Try the following techniques, after getting the go-ahead from your care provider:

- **Gentle turning methods:** If you're past thirty-four weeks' gestation, you can try natural techniques for turning baby into the vertex (head-down) position. Many of these methods are based on the belief that if your uterus is relaxed and your pelvis is optimally positioned, there's more space for baby to get into the ideal position. And because their head is the heaviest part of their body, gravity helps them rotate if there's room. These natural techniques are listed in the sidebar below.

Gentle Breech Turning Methods

- **Guided meditation:** I've created a recording to support you in relaxing your uterus while envisioning baby turning into the ideal position; you can download it at the following link:

yourserenelife.wordpress.com/breech-baby/. Beyond focusing on the physical act of creating more room in the uterus through relaxation, the essence of this meditation is to energetically connect with your baby and encourage them to turn. This is a helpful track to listen to as you engage in the following baby-turning techniques.

- **Moxibustion:** In this exercise, a witch rubs unicorn poop, eye of newt, and breastmilk on your belly. Just kidding. But the real thing might seem a little out there. Derived from Chinese medicine, moxibustion consists of a licensed acupuncturist burning mugwort close to each of your pinkie toes (the bladder 67 acupuncture point). The idea is that the stimulation of heat by these points encourages the release of estrogen and prostaglandins, which in turn stimulate mild contractions that encourage the baby to turn, without causing preterm labor. Moxibustion is usually most effective when used in conjunction with acupuncture and positions used to turn a breech baby (after you receive the moxibustion).

- **Acupuncture:** In addition to moxibustion, an acupuncturist can apply needles to points that will promote relaxation in your uterus and create an overall sense of calm.

- **Child's pose:** Encourage your baby's feet or bum to lift out of your pelvis and flip to the upper portion of your uterus by settling into child's pose. To do this, kneel on a soft, stable surface with your toes together, and knees hip-width apart. Then, lean forward and settle your forearms on the surface in front of your knees, and rest your head on your hands. From here, focus on getting your butt into the air. If you become light-headed or uncomfortable, ease out of the position.

- **On-all-fours belly dancing:** Give baby gentle encouragement to make the turn by getting on your hands and knees on a soft surface (e.g., your bed or pillows on the floor) and gyrating your hips like you were belly dancing. You can make this less boring by popping on a show or music that makes you want to gyrate. And be forewarned that this hands-and-knees hip swirl has been known to make baby-making partners randy.

- **Pelvic tilt:** Get back on that soft surface, lie on your back with your knees bent and feet planted on the floor, then lift your hips into the air. This is the bridge pose used in yoga. But we're going to make it easier by having a friend or family member stack pillows under your hips until you're able to rest in this position. Hang out here for ten to twenty minutes, listen to the guided meditation I keep touting, and repeat the process at least once a day.
- **The Webster technique:** Performed by a chiropractor, this technique helps realign the pelvis to provide more room for baby to get into the vertex position. Ask your care provider for a referral for a local chiropractor who is skilled in this technique.
- **Music:** While this is based on an old wives' tale, it's worth a try. Grab a portable speaker or some earbuds, turn on a funky jam, and place the speaker or earbuds against your pelvis. The idea is that baby will be curious about the music and turn their head toward the speaker to investigate. At the very least, this provides an opportunity to develop baby's good taste in music.
- **Spinning Babies Aware practice:** Check out the following link to look for a Spinning Babies practitioner in your area: spinningbabies.com/parents/find-a-practitioner. The Spinning Babies organization trains medical care providers and body-workers to help pregnant women utilize many of the techniques mentioned above. A practitioner can also guide you through a series of helpful daily activities, found here: spinningbabies.com/pregnancy-birth/daily-activities. In addition, you can take a class with a Spinning Babies Parents Educator, who you can find here: spinningbabies.com/parents /find-a-parent-educator.

- **ECV:** If you're not able to turn baby with gentler techniques by week thirty-six or thirty-seven of gestation, ask your care provider if you're a candidate for an ECV. In this not-too-fun-but-sometimes-effective technique, a trained practitioner will press on the outside of your abdomen, trying to turn baby's head down. It usually takes just a few minutes, but it doesn't always work.

  Factors that increase your chance of a successful ECV include having given birth before and the care provider being able to easily feel baby's head. Reasons you wouldn't be able to have an ECV include placenta abruption, severe pre-eclampsia, or signs of fetal distress. In addition, some care providers won't perform an ECV if you have low amniotic fluid levels or the cord is wrapped around baby's neck.

  While ECV is usually an uncomfortable procedure, it's worth a try, as it has fairly good success rates. A study published in *Obstetric Anesthesia Digest* reported that 33 percent of first-time mothers and 61 percent of mothers who have given birth before will have a successful ECV. And there are ways to potentially increase those success rates. An article published in the *Cochrane Database of Systematic Reviews* reported that the following treatments may improve the outcome of an ECV, but that further research is recommended.
  - Relaxing the womb with drugs like beta stimulants and calcium channel blockers
  - Stimulating the baby with sound through the mother's abdomen (see "Music" above)
  - Increasing the fluid surrounding the baby
  - Injecting an epidural or spinal analgesia to promote relaxation
  - Giving the mother opioid drugs to help her relax
  - Using guided meditation, which you might have heard about once or twice in this book
- **Breech delivery:** If the ECV doesn't work, you can start the search for a doctor who attends breech births. While these doctors do exist, they're becoming harder to find, as many medical schools no longer teach doctors how to deliver a breech baby. Your best bet is to contact a university hospital and ask if they have care providers who support vaginal delivery of breech babies. You may need to contact numerous

hospitals before finding someone. And sadly, the search may reveal that no one in your area attends breech deliveries. If you want to discuss breech deliveries with a doctor famous for his work in this area of obstetrics, and possibly receive a referral, reach out to Stuart Fischbein, MD, OB-GYN, through birthinginstincts.com.

If you find a doctor with the expertise and willingness to attend a breech birth, have a conversation with them about the risks and how they would support you through worst-case scenarios. After reviewing your medical records, they can also tell you whether you're a good candidate for a breech birth. Circumstances that could make you a good candidate include the following:

- You've given birth vaginally to one or more babies who were around the same size as the baby now in utero.
- Your baby is in frank breech position, which means their butt is down, instead of feet first. It's also ideal if their head is angled forward, chin to chest.
- You don't go into labor before week thirty-seven of gestation.

- **Coming to terms with a C-section:** With all that said, you might find that a C-section is the option you feel most comfortable with, and there is nothing wrong with that. Not feeling determined to have a vaginal breech delivery does not mean you're "giving up"; it just means you're following the path that feels intuitively right for you. And that path is different for each woman.

Part of your unique experience might also include disappointment over not having the vaginal birth you'd hoped for. You can feel frustrated by the turn of events, while still trusting that you're having the birth you're meant to have.

Labor Drugs

53. I keep hearing that everyone ends up getting an epidural. I want an unmedicated birth, but should I just give up hope?

No way! While women who had unmedicated births used to be like unicorns in places like the United States, birth norms are changing. Childbirth preparation classes and books that teach the power of the mind-body connection, fear release, and how to wield our innate ability to find calm in the face of intensity are helping women who want to have an unmedicated birth to have one. And if you don't really want one, or if you change your mind about wanting one in the middle of labor, there's absolutely nothing wrong with that. It's also important to know that really, really wanting one doesn't guarantee you'll have one. You have no way to completely know how your birth will go. However, dedicated preparation will give you a much better chance of having that unmedicated birth.

Let me tell you about Stella. She raved about unmedicated birth but wasn't planning on taking any classes or practicing any pain relief techniques. She wanted to wing it. She ended up with an epidural. Of course, she might have needed an epidural even if she *had* thrown herself into preparation, but she came to me afterward saying, "I felt totally unprepared. I had nothing when the big contractions came. I felt like they were eating me."

When Stella became pregnant two years later, she signed up for my HypnoBirthing class, my online course "Childbirth Preparation: A Complete Guide for Pregnant Women" (available on Udemy), and a Birthing from Within class. She also loaded up on books. Stella became a dedicated student of unmedicated birth. She was so curious and so passionate about practice.

A week before her due date, she told me, "While I still want an unmedicated birth, I don't think I have to have one to be happy with my birth. I feel really satisfied by all the prep I've done — it's made my pregnancy more enjoyable. And the best part is, the classes have helped me feel so empowered and confident in my unique journey that I don't feel like I have anything to prove. I don't need the 'unmedicated medal' I'm pretty sure I was striving for the first time around."

Stella had an unmedicated birth. But I believed her when she said she would have been satisfied either way.

I share all that to emphasize that while an unmedicated birth is absolutely possible and it's not a foregone conclusion you'll have an epidural, much of the wonder of wanting an unmedicated birth lives in the preparation. With that in mind, consider the ways to prepare listed below.

What to do

Find a type of preparation you jive with, making sure it's a method that provides tools for an unmedicated birth. HypnoBirthing and Birthing from Within are my favorite options. After you find your class…

- **Practice the techniques.** In addition to practicing the breathing, massage, and movement techniques as often as possible (I recommend practicing a minimum of one tool every day), put significant focus on the mental and emotional support your class provides. Many of the biggest barriers between a woman and an unmedicated birth are in the mind. Working the practices that help you replace negative, fearful beliefs about birth with hopeful, inspiring messages can remove those barriers. One of my favorite parts of the mental and emotional work found in many (good) classes is that they spill over into the rest of life. For example, after doing the HypnoBirthing fear-release practices, I felt like I had gone through intensive therapy.

- **Let it go.** After you've done the preparation and go into labor, let it all go, trusting that your birth will unfold in the way it's supposed to. And as I mentioned before, that might not be an unmedicated birth, but that in no way means you failed or didn't prepare enough. It just means that for whatever reason, your birth needed to take an unexpected path.

  Remember, if that's how it shakes out, those folks who were sure you'd get an epidural don't get to say, "I told you so." No way. *No one* has the right to make you feel shame about your birth experience. You deserve to feel pride in your body's ability to move through birth — even if birth involved Pitocin and an epidural, or a C-section. Your body still went through so much and should be worshipped as the powerhouse it is.

54. What is my care provider not telling me about Pitocin and epidurals?

Potentially, a lot. Because significant research is being done on these drugs, some care providers hesitate to share all the details because the data is always emerging and evolving. But there are also care providers who hold back information that has been well proven, in favor of supporting their agenda.

One mama I was the doula for (let's call her Sasha) was told by the ultrasound tech at her doctor's office that she had low amniotic fluid levels. When Sasha was retested at the hospital, she was told her fluid levels were normal. The on-call doctor said she and baby were healthy and good to go home. But when Sasha's doctor arrived, he disagreed and insisted she be induced with Pitocin immediately. She asked why. He said, "Because your baby could die if you don't induce." Stunned, Sasha asked if Pitocin came with risks. "No," he said. "The risks only come with not inducing." She turned down the Pitocin, but he had scared her and she didn't feel comfortable going home.

Sasha allowed this doctor to give her three rounds of Cervidil — a medication used to soften the cervix — over three days, but she stood her ground about not receiving Pitocin. Despite her and the baby's continued health, the doctor kept suggesting she was putting her baby's life at risk by not inducing. He wore her down, and she accepted the Pitocin. But it didn't work. After twelve hours on it, Sasha had only dilated to four centimeters and was exhausted. The doctor insisted she get an epidural so she could sleep. The epidural gave her a headache so intense she could not sleep. When the doctor insisted on a C-section, Sasha fired him and hired a midwife with privileges, or permission to treat, at that hospital. The midwife gave her medication for the headache, and she was finally able to rest. I knew this midwife, and she pulled me into the hallway to share all the information about Pitocin and epidurals that the doctor had failed to provide. This is the summary of what she shared:

Regarding both drugs...

• **You'll be stuck in bed.** Once Pitocin or an epidural is started, you will need constant monitoring and will be connected to an IV, meaning it will be tough to move around.

- **You're not allowed to eat.** Because of concern over aspiration during an emergency C-section (which isn't actually a risk if general anesthesia isn't used), most hospitals won't let you eat after receiving Pitocin or an epidural. While many mamas don't have much of an appetite while on these drugs, this moratorium on food can lead to exhaustion if you have to be on them for an extended period.
- **It might not work.** If you're already having contractions, the Pitocin will likely make them stronger. But if you're showing no signs of labor, Pitocin may do very little. And while an epidural almost always provides the desired effect of significant numbing from the waist down, it's possible (although unlikely) that you receive little to no relief from it.
- **There's an increased chance of cesarean birth.** There's something called a "cascade of intervention," which implies that each intervention could lead to the need for another intervention. One of the ultimate interventions during childbirth is a C-section. While plenty of women who receive Pitocin and/or an epidural have a vaginal birth, both of these labor drugs might increase your chance of needing a C-section.

Regarding Pitocin...

- **Contractions might be so unbearably strong you need an epidural.** Many women who do not want an epidural find that it's a necessity after receiving Pitocin, as it can cause extremely strong (and painful) contractions.
- **Fetal distress could occur.** If Pitocin creates contractions so strong and close together that your body and baby don't have time to rest, the baby may not receive enough oxygen, which could lead to distress and the potential need for an emergency C-section.

Regarding an epidural...

- **You'll likely need a catheter.** Because you won't be able to walk to the bathroom, a catheter is almost always inserted after the epidural has taken effect.
- **It could lead to a need for Pitocin.** Sometimes, an epidural slows down contractions so much that Pitocin is needed to keep labor going.
- **It could extend labor.** According to a study published in the journal

Obstetrics & Gynecology, women with epidurals typically have to push for nearly two and a half hours more than women without epidurals.

- **Instrumental birth is more likely.** Because it can be trickier for a mom with an epidural to push baby out (or breathe baby down), epidural use means a higher chance that forceps or vacuum extraction will be used to deliver baby.

- **You might have a drop in blood pressure.** This could also make baby's heart rate drop. However, the IV fluids you're given before the epidural is placed reduce this risk.

- **Fever could occur.** A study done by Harvard Medical School found that women who receive an epidural are more likely to develop a fever that could lead to the baby having poor muscle tone, a low APGAR score, seizures in the newborn period, and the need for resuscitation and evaluation for sepsis. The study also noted that high maternal fever has been linked to brain injuries like cerebral palsy.

- **You might get itchy.** The opioids in the epidural may make you itchy, which can often be alleviated by changing the medication or giving you an itch-relieving medication.

- **Nausea or vomiting is possible.** This is another potential side effect of the opioids in the epidural.

- **There might be breastfeeding complications.** Because an epidural blocks oxytocin — the hormone that helps milk come in and facilitates bonding — it could cause breastfeeding challenges. In addition, a mom and baby impacted by an epidural are more likely to be drowsy after delivery, which could make breastfeeding more difficult.

- **A spinal headache might be triggered.** A rare phenomenon, a spinal headache is caused by an accidental puncture being made in the bag of fluid surrounding the brain and spinal cord when the epidural is placed. If spinal fluid leaks out, an intense headache ensues — it can last for weeks.

- **Nerve damage is possible.** Another rare side effect is nerve damage caused by the epidural needle. If a blood vessel is damaged while the epidural is being placed (also uncommon), blood may collect and press on the nerve. This is one reason why women with a blood clotting disorder and those taking blood thinning medication may not be able to receive an epidural.

- **An epidural abscess is possible.** In rare cases, women develop an epidural abscess, which is an infection of the central nervous system caused by bacteria entering the epidural space. According to the book *Spinal Epidural Abscess*, only 1.2 in 10,000 women experience this.

Those are the potential outcomes of Pitocin and epidurals that are widely recognized — the possible side effects your care provider should share with you. But what about the potential outcomes they won't share? The outcomes that haven't been conclusively proven, but are interesting to consider? Following are possible risks with labor drugs still being researched, as of 2020:

- **There is a possible increased chance of baby developing autism.** Limited research has found that babies of women who had Pitocin and an epidural during labor were 2.77 times more likely to exhibit an autism phenotype. Because not all babies of women who received labor drugs in these studies went on to develop autism spectrum disorder, it's believed the drugs must interact with other factors to cause autism. These other potential factors are being studied.
- **There is a possible link between Pitocin and bipolar disorder.** A study published in the *Journal of Affective Disorders* found that babies exposed to Pitocin during birth had 2.4 times increased odds for developing bipolar disorder than babies not exposed to Pitocin. They also found a potential connection between Pitocin and cognitive impairment in childhood.

While this is compelling research to keep an eye on, I don't believe it's a reason to turn down labor drugs if they're really needed. Both studies acknowledged that continued research is needed.

So what happened to Sasha? She had her baby, after crazy-high amounts of Pitocin were used to force her body into labor, and the epidural was kept in for over twelve hours so she could handle the abnormally strong contractions. She had a vaginal birth but was exhausted and dissatisfied with her birth experience. She and baby both had an infection, which a nurse suspected was caused by all the vaginal exams Sasha received over four days in the hospital. When we processed the birth experience, Sasha said she never would have said yes to the labor drugs if the doctor had provided all the information.

On the flip side, I've been to many births where Pitocin and epidurals were used after the mother received all the up-to-date information and made an informed decision she felt good about. But the key here is *receiving all the up-to-date information*. While this section provides a jumping-off point for arming yourself with information, ongoing research means this information is ever changing. There's a lot you can do to make sure you're getting as much current data as possible.

What to do

Ask a lot of questions before saying yes to any intervention, and don't let anyone brush away your concerns or questions. Demand thorough answers.

Here are questions to help ensure you're well informed about your unique situation and options:

- **Is this an emergency?** If the situation is actually an emergency, the care provider should be able to succinctly state why it's an emergency, and what the wisest course of action is. This is the primary reason we have care providers at birth — in case of an emergency.
- **Is there an evidence-based medical reason you're recommending this intervention? If so, explain it to me.** Some care providers recommend an intervention based solely on their personal experiences, and not on evidence-based research. This is fine if they're up-front about it, but you can better understand where the recommendation is coming from by including the term *evidence-based* in your question.
- **Is this intervention really necessary? What are the alternatives?** An article published in the *Journal of Perinatal Education* reported that when these two questions are asked, the rate of unnecessary intervention significantly drops. It's believed this occurs because these questions inspire meaningful discussion that allows the mother to make a well-informed decision.
- **Can you give me time alone with my birth companion so we can discuss this?** This one's in the form of a question just to be polite. If it's not an emergency, the caregiver should absolutely give you privacy to make a decision with your birth companion.

After you've received all the information, make a decision that feels right for *you*. Maybe your questioning revealed that an epidural, Pitocin, or both could actually minimize your chance of needing a C-section. Or maybe you determine the potential benefits of receiving the labor drugs aren't worth the risk. It's not a black-or-white choice — the decision to accept or reject these drugs is never "right" or "wrong."

55. Is there any chance an epidural could paralyze me?

Yes, but it's *really* unlikely. A study published in the *British Journal of Anaesthesia* reported the estimated risk of permanent harm following a spinal anesthetic or epidural as less than 1 in 20,000. This risk is often considerably lower for women in labor, as they tend to be healthier than those people receiving an epidural because of illness or injury.

The rare times paralysis has occurred, it was because of direct injury to the spinal cord; a spinal hematoma, which is an accumulation of blood in the epidural space; or an epidural abscess, an infection between the outer covering of the brain and spinal cord. However, even these are circumstances that don't always lead to paralysis.

What to do

If possible, don't let fear over this minuscule risk stop you from receiving an epidural if you really need one. It's more likely you'll be struck by lightning than experience paralysis from an epidural.

In addition, be sure to tell the anesthesiologist if you have a blood clotting disorder or have been on blood thinners. This should all be in your chart, but it's still wise to mention it.

If you feel an epidural is the right choice for you but you're afraid of paralysis, ask the anesthesiologist to reassure you. Hopefully, they'll be able to outline how experienced they are and what an excellent track record they have, and to explain that with modern-day training and tools, paralysis doesn't need to be a concern.

They should also tell you which sensations to expect, and which to report, as the epidural is being placed. Many women experience stinging, burning, pressure, a sensation of coolness, or all of these in their back as the numbing medication is applied and the needle is inserted. It's not supposed to be too intense. (The worst part is having to hold still while you have contractions.) But if you have any of the following sensations, you should tell the anesthesiologist immediately:

- Sudden loss of sensation in one or both legs
- Sharp, shooting pain
- Uncontrollable shaking in your legs
- Intense hot flash
- Anything else that feels "off"

Relaxation tool: Download this guided meditation and listen to it as the epidural is being placed, or anytime throughout labor, to reduce anxiety and enhance calm: yourserenelife.wordpress.com/epidural -meditation/.

Sex and the Vagina

56. I want to have an orgasmic birth. Is it possible?

Yes, ma'am, it's possible! But that might not mean having an actual orgasm. Only about 6 percent of women have orgasms during birth, and much of that is due to genetics — those ladies aren't Aphrodite, they're just lucky. According to a study in the journal *Biology Letters*, genes account for 34 to 45 percent of a woman's ability to climax. However, it's near impossible to know if you have orgasm-inclined genes. What you do know is how easy it is for you to have an orgasm. If you're a climax machine, maybe your genes are helping you out, or maybe you just have your finger on the pulse of what turns you on. Whatever the reason, if it's fairly easy for you to orgasm, you have a better chance of orgasming during labor. That doesn't mean all hope is lost if you really have to work to get that pleasure-explosion — the "What to do" section will help you up your chance of floating in a sea of orgasms (or at least a little lake) during birth.

Beyond genetics, what's the deal with orgasms showing up amid an experience many tout as exceptionally painful? First of all, two of the regions in the brain that are active during orgasm — the anterior cingulated cortex and the insula — are also active during painful sensations (Oh hi there, contractions). In addition, orgasm and childbirth both produce strong surges of blood, oxytocin, and endorphins and stimulate the birth passage, cervix, clitoris, and vagina. So there you go — *orgasm* and *childbirth* aren't the antonyms many believe them to be.

But now I want to shake up this question. I want to propose we shift the term *orgasm* to *orgasmic*. Because even if you're not rolling in orgasms as you're getting that baby out, you can still have a birth filled with euphoria, empowerment, transformation, joy, connection, and love: essentially, an orgasmic birth. Think about it — although we all love our orgasms, can't you think of hundreds of instances in life where you weren't orgasming but still felt incredible? You can bring that goodness into birth.

What to do

Set yourself up for orgasms during birth, and/or an orgasmic birth, by releasing preconceived notions about pain, shame around sexuality, and doubt about your ability to birth.

- **Prepare.** Most women who have orgasmic births prepare thoroughly, often taking at least one childbirth prep class, reading the book *Orgasmic Birth* by Elizabeth Davis and Debra Pascali-Bonaro, and watching the documentary *Orgasmic Birth: The Best Kept Secret*. They then practice many of the techniques learned from these resources on a daily basis, specifically fear-release practices. As my grandma would say, they didn't go into birth all willy-nilly.
- **Hold a belief in an orgasmic birth.** Going into labor with the belief that an orgasmic birth is possible can transform your experience and make it more likely to lead to an orgasmic birth. As I mentioned, this orgasmic birth might not be filled with orgasms, but it will be composed of a trust that birth isn't all about pain; can be infused with moments of deep connection with your body, baby, and partner; and can unleash a power and confidence that will make you feel like a total goddess. This type of birth is just as good (or at least almost as good) as a birth sprinkled with orgasms.
- **Examine your beliefs about sexuality.** Did you grow up with a belief that sex and masturbation are taboo? If so, you're not alone, and it's not too late to reprogram. You can begin shifting your perceptions of sex and masturbation by first examining what your beliefs are, and where they came from. Are they things you actually believe on the deepest level? Or are they ideas planted by someone else?

  Next, connect with your sexuality in a new way by partaking in the art of masturbation, and taking note of what turns you on. What type of pressure and speed does it for you? Where do you like to be touched? Share your findings with your partner. Then, talk with them about getting more creative during sex by playing around with positions, dirty talk, eye contact, or anything else that piques your arousal. And finally, do the things you've just talked about.

To support this sexual reprogramming and awakening, listen to this guided meditation: yourserenelife.wordpress.com/orgasmic-birth/.

- **Edit key birth words.** Remove fearful, constrictive terminology from your childbirth lexicon by making a few substitutions. Begin by swapping the term *contractions* (it sounds so restrictive!) with the word *surge*, as it sends more fluid, pleasurable messages from the mind to the body. And instead of saying or thinking the word *pain* when you're having a surge, name the actual sensations you're feeling. For example, "I feel a pulling up in my abdomen, a tightening in my back, and pressure in my vagina." These swaps give you a better chance of tapping into the ecstasy that can live in childbirth.

- **Consider a birth center or home birth, or create a soothing hospital room.** Because it's easier to have an orgasm, or feel orgasmic, in a space that feels homey, soothing, and private, choosing to birth in a birth center or at home will likely increase your chance of having an orgasmic birth.

  However, if the idea of birthing in a hospital comforts you, you might experience anxiety if you birthed anywhere else. If that's you, think about how to transform your hospital room into a birth sanctuary. For example, you could bring battery-powered candles, a soft robe and cozy socks, a silk pillowcase, a portable speaker and playlist of relaxing music, an essential oil diffuser and your favorite oils, honey sticks, and anything else that comforts one of your five senses. In addition, hiring a doula can add an incredible layer of support to a birth in any location, but especially in a hospital.

- **Ask for complete privacy.** You're unlikely to have an orgasm while your midwife and her assistant whisper about birth stuff in the corner or a nurse checks your vitals. Up your chance of feeling free enough to let waves of pleasure wash through you by asking anyone you don't feel comfortable moaning in front of to leave the room.

- **Stimulate your clitoris.** Clitoral stimulation is one of the surest paths to an orgasm, and it can make you less sensitive to painful stimulation — it's like a medication-free epidural. But many women are hesitant to masturbate during birth because they feel strange mixing this sexual act with bringing their baby into the world. There are two ways to get around this.

One, go into the bathroom for ultimate privacy, or as I just mentioned, ask everyone to leave the room, with the exception of your partner, if you're comfortable with them being there or even helping you.

Two, if the sexual component of masturbation is tripping you up, change the way you think about it. Think of it as just another pain-relieving tool you're using for childbirth. It's not masturbation, it's a "pain-soothing vaginal massage." And if you really want to up your chances of reaching that sweet O, do as many women before you have done and use a vibrator.

- **Moan.** When you feel yourself at the tipping point between pain and pleasure, let out long, low moans to release painful energy and call in euphoria.
- **Rub your nipples, and make out with your partner.** These sensual acts awaken arousal and release oxytocin, which can speed up your birth by triggering more effective surges.
- **Breathe.** As you feel a surge coming on, take in a long, deep inhalation through your nose, allowing your lower and upper abdomen to fully expand. When you reach full capacity, exhale through your nose at the same slow pace. As the surge intensifies, you'll likely hit a "wall of resistance." When this happens, your mind will try to trick you into thinking that continuing to breathe in and expand your abdomen will cause an explosion of pain. But the opposite is true. Continuing to inhale and expand will bust past that wall and help you access the relief that can lead to pleasure.
- **Remember that pain isn't the enemy.** Many have the misconception that an orgasmic birth is free of pain. But often an orgasmic birth consists of repeatedly coming to a tipping point between pain and pleasure, and swaying between both until you make the decision and take the actions to tip fully into pleasure. And sometimes you'll tip into pain, and that's okay. Pain isn't a bad sign during childbirth; it doesn't mean you're doing anything wrong — it's an organic part of the journey. When you can surrender to it, instead of resisting or fearing it, it often transforms. Almost every woman who has had an orgasmic birth will tell you that she danced with both pain and pleasure, and it made for a fuller experience.

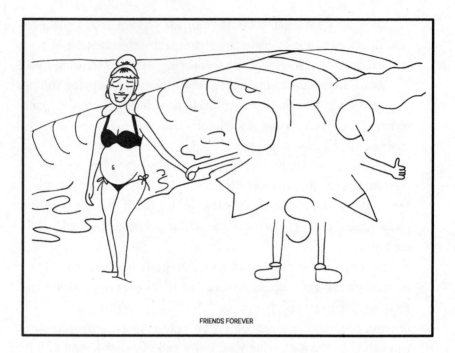

FRIENDS FOREVER

- **Connect to an orgasmic energy orbit.** Envision a never-ending supply of warm, golden energy spiraling down from the stars, becoming more and more concentrated as it swirls through your body. This energy is most potent as it moves through your uterus, out your cervix, and finally washes over your vagina and clitoris. Feel this energy activating your endorphins as it moves down. Train your mind and body to easily tap into this orgasmic energy by practicing this visualization every morning and evening.
- **Submerge yourself in warm water as much as possible.** The relief that warm water provides allows your muscles to relax and become more susceptible to orgasmic sensations. If you don't have access to a tub during birth, sit in the shower.

57. Is a vaginal tear as scary as it sounds?

No. My perineum tore during birth, and I had no idea until they started stitching me up. And I didn't have an epidural. But I get why women are horrified by the idea of a tear in one of the most sensitive parts of their body. It sounds awful. The thing is, the combination of a buildup of endorphins, the numbness caused by the pressure of baby's head, and the Goddess-like determination to get the baby out makes many women oblivious to a vaginal tear, regardless of whether or not they have an epidural.

To provide further insight about vaginal tears, here are answers to the most common questions I get about this topic:

- **How likely is a tear?** It's common for a first-time mom to tear, but again, you probably won't even notice it until after birth. The recommendations in the "What to do" section can help reduce the likelihood of a severe tear.
- **How big are the tears?** While tears range in size, they're usually much smaller than we imagine. First-degree tears are only a few centimeters, while a fourth-degree tear (the most intense) is rarely longer than an inch.
- **How are tears repaired?** Minor tears usually don't need any repair beyond time and rest, while more extensive tears require absorbable stitches. The area will be numbed before the application of the stitches. In rare cases, anesthesia is used.
- **What is the recovery like?** It's not too bad — you just feel really sore for seven to ten days. Depending on severity, tears take anywhere from a few days to a few weeks to fully heal. The "What to do" section provides recovery tips.

What to do

To help the emergence of baby be a gentler experience for your perineum, thus minimizing your chance of a severe tear, follow all the suggestions in the "What to do" section from question 63 (the one about pushing). I would especially focus on the perineal tissue massage — make it your part-time job starting around week thirty-four or thirty-five of gestation. It's one of the best things you can do to make your perineum more elastic and less susceptible to tearing.

If you feel the fear of a tear might hinder your ability to birth with calm and confidence, listen to this fear-release guided meditation: your serenelife.wordpress.com/fear-of-tearing/. I also recommend envisioning your perineum as a rose that gently and easily opens. You can also watch time-lapse videos of flowers opening, focusing on how easily their soft petals unfurl — there's no strain in their bloom. As you do this, remember that your perineum was also designed to soften and expand when it's time to bloom.

In regard to what to do after a tear, here are a few strategies for soothing discomfort and promoting healing:

- **Kegels:** Attempting Kegels (even if you can't feel them) promotes circulation, which can speed recovery.
- **Sitz bath:** Soaking your perineum in warm water can ease pain and itching. You can also ask your care provider if there are medications or additives you can put in the water to aid healing. If you'd rather not bother with sanitizing your bathtub, purchase a sitz bath kit that fits in the toilet and allows you to dunk your perineum. As an added bonus, a sitz bath also works wonders on hemorrhoids! Yay!
- **Witch hazel pads:** These medicated pad liners — soaked in witch hazel extract — are the vagina's best friend, offering instant cooling relief when slipped in the underwear.
- **Anesthetic spray:** In addition to the witch hazel pads, ask your care provider to recommend an anesthetic spray to numb the perineum.
- **Fiber:** Your first bowel movement after childbirth might be nerve wracking. I felt certain I would bust my stitches and poop out my innards — but I didn't, and you won't either. However, the essential act of clearing your bowels could be uncomfortable if you're passing hard stools. Soften up that poo by eating fiber-rich foods and drinking lots of water. You can also ask your care provider if they recommend using a stool softener the first few days after birth.

58. Will my vagina look like minced meat after a vaginal delivery?

I'll not mince words (hee-hee) — most vaginas look pretty beat up after vaginal childbirth. With all the stretching and potential tearing, the vagina won't be easy on the eyes for a while. But the good news is, it won't stay that way. Tears heal, and stretched skin (slowly) bounces back. The one thing that might be permanent is a darkening of your vulva, as it could experience a shift in pigmentation. So while your petunia will never look exactly like it did pre-childbirth, it will go back to a semblance of its former self after six to twelve months.

Something else to expect from the first few days of life after birth is that you will have heavy discharge. There will be lots of blood, mucus, and tissue coming out of you, requiring you to don a diaper-like pad. While the load will likely lessen within a week, you'll probably need pads for four to six weeks.

What to do

If you're squeamish, or if you experience more pain when focusing on a sore area of your body, don't stick a mirror down there for a while. However, if you want to marvel at everything your courageous vagina went through, take a look — it's pretty fascinating. And don't be embarrassed by its appearance. The two of you went through a lot, and you're allowed time to heal. Tummies are squishy, stretch marks are prominent, and vaginas aren't pretty in that fourth trimester — and that's okay. Be patient with your body, and grateful it helped you grow and birth new life.

Regarding how you can minimize tearing and make your perineum more elastic, check out the "What to do" section from question 63.

Skin and Appearance

59. Will it be weird if I want to be totally nude during labor?

Not at all. For some women, having clothes on during birth can feel distracting and restrictive. Taking it all off can leave your mind clear to focus on breathing, moving, or doing any other relaxation techniques that help you move through contractions. And no one supporting you during birth will think twice about you being naked. Doctors, nurses, midwives, and doulas are totally used to all states of undress when supporting a laboring mom.

To ensure you stay comfortable with your nudity during birth, be really clear about who is and who isn't allowed in your birthing space. For example, if you don't want your father-in-law dropping in when you're doing naked hip swirls, let everyone know that no one is allowed in the birth space unless they get explicit permission from you.

What to do

Keep reminding yourself that there's *nothing wrong* with being buck naked during birth. Then consider the following:

- **Put it in your preferences.** Add the following line to your birth preferences: "I request complete privacy during birth. In addition to the necessary medical care providers, only the following people are allowed in the birth space [insert names]."
- **Tell your partner.** It can be helpful to give your partner a heads-up about your desire to be nude, especially if you think they'll be uncomfortable with it. But don't let them dictate what you do and don't wear during labor. You can give them the courtesy of a discussion, but you get the final say in what you wear.
- **Bring "just in case" birth clothes.** It doesn't hurt to have a nursing bra, robe, and loose, comfortable clothing on hand in case you feel like being clothed during certain phases of labor.

60. I'm getting really focused on what I'll look like during and after labor. I'm especially concerned about looking bad in photos. Should I bother with doing my hair and makeup when labor starts?

Before I get into the specifics of this question, I want you to consider that your decisions regarding your looks during labor should be totally based on your feelings about yourself, and not on how you think others might judge you. Anyone around you during birth will be so in awe of what you're doing they won't give a hoot what you look like. You'll look like a goddess to all who lay eyes on you, even if your hair is a mess and you're covered in sweat.

With that said, I definitely wouldn't bother with makeup (no matter how much you love it), as it will probably end up running down your face when you sweat, get into water, or cry. Regarding your hair, I can almost guarantee it will also get mussed up during labor. But because the undoing of the hairdo won't cause anything to run down your face or sting your eyes, there's no harm in doing your hair beforehand, especially if it ups your confidence and provides a distraction during early labor.

Something I *would* do during early labor is take a shower — if you have the time. And I would go all in with that shower: wash your hair, shave your legs, exfoliate your butt. Do whatever you need to do to feel super fresh. I did *not* do this before I went to the hospital to birth Hudson, and I remember many moments of feeling grimy. No one seemed to notice my griminess (nor would I have cared if they did), but I didn't like the feeling — it was distracting. If you're wondering why I didn't just take a shower while in labor, the answer is that I had to use every drop of my mental and physical facilities to move through each contraction — there was nothing left for shampooing.

What to do

As mentioned, let's skip the makeup, only do the hair if you really, really want to, and say yes to a shower. Regarding photos, if you've hired a birth photographer or would like your partner or doula to take photos, and you are concerned about what you'll look like in the photos, there are a few things you can do to prepare:

- **Become one with raw images.** Consider that you might enjoy having photos that capture the unfiltered realness of your birth experience, wild hair and all. Of course, if that's not your thing, no worries. Just be your brand of beauty.
- **Ask your photographer to check in before taking a photo.** Setting this parameter lets you decide in the moment whether the taking of the photos will make you too aware of how you look, distracting you from the task at hand. Or you might decide that you don't care how you look and are happy to have them capture some of these once-in-a-lifetime moments as is.
- **Request touch-ups.** If the photographer is someone you feel really comfortable with, ask them to touch you up before they start snapping. For example, they can push the hair off your forehead, readjust your robe, or move the barf bag out of the frame.
- **Bring beauty basics.** When you get to the blissful period when baby is in your arms, you might want makeup applied before taking the shots that'll be texted and posted. You might also want a hair touch-up. If you think this is something you'll desire, pack a bathroom bag with a hand mirror, hairbrush, and your makeup essentials (e.g., some concealer, blush, and mascara), so your birth companion can easily retrieve the goods while you bond with baby.

Fluids and Other Bodily Emissions

61. I know everyone asks about pooping during birth, but let's be real; will the care providers pull a face behind my back if I poop?

While no one enjoys wiping poop off another human, your poop is the least of your care providers' worries. They just want you and baby to be healthy. And they've likely seen so much poop during deliveries they won't have much of a feeling about you doing it. They'll just silently jump into "poop protocol" and swipe it away before you realize what happened. Every mom I've seen poop during birth had no idea they'd done so — they were more concerned with other situations, like pushing a human out of their vagina.

Something else to consider is that when people talk about pooping during birth, they're not referring to a full bowel movement. They're talking about little bits and pieces popping out. "Rabbit turds" is what a midwife I know lovingly calls birth poops. (Yes, I got into this business for the glamour.)

What to do

Talk with your care provider about that aforementioned poop protocol. They'll be able to assure you that pooping is nothing to be worried about, and that the people caring for you won't be offended if that's part of your story. They can also tell you how they typically handle this incredibly common occurrence. In addition, these steps can help you feel more confident:

- **Don't do an enema.** This could cause unneeded discomfort and doesn't make much of a difference during childbirth. The beliefs that an enema could shorten labor or decrease the risk of infection have been debunked.
- **Stay on top of your fiber and fluid intake as you near that due date.** Constipation is always uncomfortable, but it can be especially unsavory when you're in labor. Drinking plenty of water and eating avocados, lentils, chickpeas, raspberries, and other fiber-rich foods will keep things moving, helping to ensure you don't have a backlog when it's baby time. (If you really want a treat, whip out those prunes.)

- **Visit the bathroom at least once an hour during labor.** Even if you don't feel like you need to go, spending time on the toilet gives your body the freedom to purge any urine or fecal matter you might not know you need to release. And this release enhances comfort.

Tinkle Tip: If you have trouble peeing, put a few drops of peppermint oil in the toilet bowl, place your bare feet on a cool surface, and dip your hand in a cup of cold water. (Who said those prank scenes in summer camp movies weren't teaching us valuable life lessons?)

General

62. I'm very reserved and cringe at the idea of screaming or cursing, or having strangers see my vagina, butt, and breasts during birth. Will this impede my ability to labor?

It's unlikely that your sense of modesty will impede labor, primarily because even the most modest mamas will tell you their modesty almost entirely dissolved when they were in labor. But even if that doesn't happen, you'll still be fine because you have control of who's in the room with you, and how covered you are. While many believe this is a given for birth at home or in a birth center, somehow they don't feel they have power over who is in the room at the hospital. But you absolutely do. You can make it clear in your birth preferences that you don't want hospital staff in the room when you're laboring, with the exception of the nurses needing to monitor you every hour or so and an occasional visit from your doctor. In regard to delivery, you can request that only absolutely necessary hospital staff be present.

You also have control over the nonmedical staff who are with you. You don't have to say yes to that friend or family member who really wants to be at your birth if you don't think you'd be comfortable with them present. You don't even have to have your partner there if you think their presence will throw you off. (For more on this, see question 38.)

Essentially, you have every right to go into labor with your modesty intact — you don't have to change. But again, birth might change you any-ways, especially if you have an unmedicated birth, as the intensity of the sensations will likely eliminate your concerns about nakedness, cussing, and so on. If you get an epidural, you'll be more aware of your modesty, but you'll also have more energy and focus to advocate for your wishes for privacy and coverage. And if you have a C-section, nothing but your abdomen and upper bikini line area will be exposed.

What to do

Home in on the elements that make you uncomfortable. For example, are you hesitant to have your vagina exposed? Do you not want your breasts shown? Are you nervous that you won't be able to control what you say, or how you sound? Does the idea of your partner seeing birth fluids come out of you make you nervous? Write down everything that's making you uneasy, then try the following:

- **Put your needs in your birth preferences.** In this document, you can ask to be assigned only female care providers (whenever possible), and that no medical or midwifery students be allowed in the room. You can also request that people knock before entering your birthing space, only stick around if their presence is absolutely needed, keep your lower half covered with a sheet during vaginal exams and baby's descent, or anything else you think will make you more comfortable. And when making these preferences, don't worry about offending anyone. This is *your* birth, and you get to ask for what you want.
- **Talk with your care provider about your concerns.** Discussing your qualms with your care provider will not only help them better understand your needs, but will also give them a chance to offer fresh ideas for keeping you comfortable during childbirth.
- **Make a "Please Knock" sign.** In addition to putting this in your birth preferences, make a sign for the door of the room you'll be laboring in that says, "Please knock, and wait for permission before entering." This ensures no one surprises you when you're in a state of undress, or any kind of state you're not comfortable with certain people witnessing.
- **Pick out super comfortable clothing.** If nakedness is a concern, consider finding a really comfortable nursing bra. You could also bring a robe, and wear underwear that's not too restrictive. Just make sure these are items you don't mind getting birth juices on.
- **Wear earbuds.** Nervous about cursing, moaning, or screaming? Pop in your earbuds and play your favorite music or guided meditation, so you're less aware of what you sound like. As for the people in the room who don't have earbuds in, I can almost guarantee they won't care about profanity or any loud noises you make.
- **Determine how your birth supporters can help.** Making a plan for how your people can advocate for your desire to stay covered and maintain privacy helps ensure you don't have to do anything but focus on birth. Discuss with them beforehand what's important to you, and offer ideas for how they can best support you.

- **Request the bare minimum number of vaginal exams.** In many cases, vaginal exams aren't required during birth, so if they make you uncomfortable, opt for none, or few.
- **Have your partner stand by your head when baby is being delivered.** If you're uneasy with the idea of your partner witnessing the release of discharge and blood, a potential vaginal tear, or other components of your vagina's journey through childbirth, talk with them about staying away from that area as baby emerges. It's good to talk about this well before you go into labor, as your partner might have strong feelings about seeing your baby come out. You, of course, have the final say over who sees what during birth, but your partner's feelings might sway your decision.

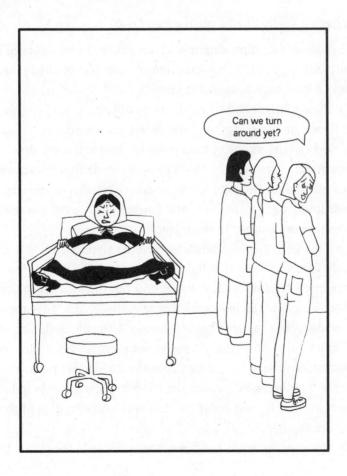

- **Ask that the room be cleared as soon as possible after baby's delivery, so you can begin breastfeeding (if you're choosing to breastfeed).** If breast exposure is a concern, remind everyone that you want only absolutely essential care providers in the room after baby is delivered. You can also drape a blanket over baby after you place them on your bare chest.
- **Remember that your care providers have seen it all.** The wonderful people who support women through birth have seen all degrees of nudity, heard birthing women scream and curse the wildest of phrases, witnessed them pooping, and observed the whole range of other raw displays that birthing evokes. Essentially, there's nothing you can do that will make them blush.

63. What's it really like to push a baby out?

It's like pushing a flaming watermelon out a fleshy hole the size of a baseball. Just kidding. Actually, this experience is completely different for each woman. I'll give you a couple of examples.

My client Chelsea had taken my HypnoBirthing class and was a devout believer in breathing her baby down (an alternative to pushing). For weeks beforehand, she practiced the birth breath every time she was having a bowel movement, and in her regular meditation practice she envisioned successfully helping her baby emerge in this gentle way. When she went into labor, the midwife and I were called to her house and she began a very long journey through labor.

Tired but determined, Chelsea worked her HypnoBirthing tools, continuously focusing on surrendering and expanding. Twenty-four hours later, the midwife said the head was almost out. Chelsea began doing her birth breathing, and ten minutes later the midwife said, "Give me one big push." And just like that, her baby was born. I was shocked. Almost every birth I've attended consisted of a big announcement when the mom was fully dilated, and everyone getting in position to help her push. A nurse or midwife would then loudly coach the mom to press her chin to her chest and push like her life depended on it. It was usually a long process. But not this time.

My birth, on the other hand, was the epitome of the classic pushing you see in the movies. My feet were in those scary-looking metal stirrups, I had a spotlight on my vagina, a nurse was nervously watching the monitors, my husband looked like he was about to faint as screams, blood, and probably some poop came out of me, and the doctor kept telling me to "Push harder! Harder! Harder!"

I did as I was told. I wailed like a banshee and worked so hard I spiked a fever. I pushed for three hours before Hudson came out. When he arrived, his hand was pressed against his face (something called *nuchal hand*), which is likely what made the pushing such a long, hard process. But I don't think that was the only reason. Even though I knew about the birth breathing technique, I hadn't really believed in the power of it, and I didn't have a doctor who supported it. But who knows, even if I had Chelsea's unwavering belief in breathing the baby down, I might still have needed to push harder harder harder, whether because of the nuchal hand or just the structure of my body.

I share these stories to make the point that the experience of pushing (or breathing) a baby out can range from gentle to super-duper intense. So much of it depends on the woman and the baby. And while how the pushing process unfolds is mostly out of your hands, there are ways you can prepare yourself for the experience, which I cover in the "What to do" section. Before we get to that, let's look at the questions about pushing I get most often.

- **What does it feel like?** For many women, pushing doesn't feel nearly as uncomfortable as they think it will, even if they don't have an epidural. Because of the pressure of baby's head on nerves in the vagina, a numbing sensation is often present during pushing. This numbing is usually accompanied by intense pressure — essentially, it feels like you're about to take the biggest poop of your life. Some women report a "ring of fire," an intense burning sensation, when baby's head is crowning. But most women I've worked with (myself included) said they never felt it. As strange as it sounds, I found pushing to be the most comfortable part of childbirth, albeit the most exhausting.
- **What can make it harder?** A baby in the posterior, or "sunny-side up," position is one of the most common situations that can make their emergence trickier. In this position, baby's face is pointing toward the

front of your body, which can make it challenging for them to get past your pubic bone. It doesn't make vaginal birth impossible, just harder. There are tips for repositioning a posterior baby in the "What to do" section. You'll also find a link for the video "How to Reposition a Posterior, or Sunny Side Up, Baby" in the book's "Recommended Resources" section.

Numerous other circumstances can complicate pushing — here are the ones you can actually do something about:

- **Lying on your back:** This position doesn't utilize gravity and can narrow the birth canal. Being on all fours, lying on your side, or squatting are all preferable for most women. If you have an epidural, ask if you can lie on your side while pushing.

- **An epidural:** As an epidural can make it difficult to feel and coordinate the birthing muscles, pushing when you have one can be tricky, but not impossible. I've witnessed many midwives tell moms with an epidural who had fully dilated to *not* push, and let contractions do the work instead. In many of these cases, the mom didn't have to push until baby was almost out. Some call this delayed-pushing technique *laboring down*. You can also ask if the epidural can be turned down when you're ready to push, so some sensation returns.

- **A tired uterus:** If you've had an incredibly long labor, your uterus might get tired, and tired uterine muscles can complicate baby's descent because they may not be able to contract as effectively as needed to push baby out. Some care providers recommend Pitocin if they suspect the strength of contractions is waning, as it can give the uterus a much-needed pick-me-up.

- **How long does it take?** Unfortunately, there's no answer for this one. Some women push for ten minutes and the baby is out, and others push for hours and still need the support of forceps or vacuum. Following the tips in the "What to do" section can increase your chance of shortening your push time.

- **What is it like for baby?** While it's impossible to know what baby is thinking during this process (I suspect it's something along the lines of "WTF is happening?"), monitors tell us that many babies experience

a dip in heart rate every time their mom engages in heavy-duty pushing, as there's usually a drop in oxygen during this time. The heart
rate usually bounces back up when the contraction and push are complete. This is another reason why the gentler pushing methods can
be beneficial — they don't require mom hold her breath. However, if
there is a special circumstance requiring that baby come out as soon
as possible, the more intense pushing could be worth it. Your care provider can help you determine what is safest for you and baby.

What to do

While there's no way to know what type of pushing will be most effective
for your body and baby, or how you'll process that experience, these techniques will help you go into the event as prepared as possible.

- **Do the perineal tissue massage.** This massage will prepare your per-
  ineum for baby's head.
  - First, coat your pointer and middle finger, or your thumb,
    with an unscented, organic oil.
  - Then insert the fingers two inches into the vaginal opening, and
    move them in a U-shape along the inner edge of the perineum.
  - I recommend applying more pressure when you reach the
    tautest skin (area between the vagina and anus), as this is the
    skin most likely to tear during birth.
  - As you push to the point of discomfort, utilize pain-relieving
    techniques like deep breathing and facial relaxation. This
    makes the perineum become more elastic, and helps mentally
    prepare you for the vaginal stretching during crowning.

  I recommend doing this nightly for about ten minutes, starting at
  around week thirty-four or thirty-five of gestation.
- **Get baby in the optimal position.** Cephalic presentation (the best position for baby to be in) is when baby is head down, facing your back,
  with their chin tucked to their chest. Your care provider can help you
  determine if baby is in this position.

  If they're not facing your back, here are a few things you can do
  to give them the space to get into this position, which they'll usually
  instinctually do if they're physically able.

- Get into the yoga position called "child's pose" and really stick your butt into the air. You can also gently sway your hips. Stay in this position for at least five minutes (unless you feel woozy), and practice once a day.
- Get on your hands and knees and gyrate your hips.
- As often as possible, sit in a position where your pelvis and belly are tilted forward. The easiest way to do this is to sit on a wedge cushion. If you're sitting on a birth ball, make sure your knees are lower than your pelvis.
- Sleep on your side instead of your back.
- Avoid sitting in bucket seats, or leaning back into the sofa.
- You can also try the techniques provided in question 52, about options for a breech baby.

- **Prepare your pelvic structure.** A deep squat (with the support of a spotter) or the yoga poses "child's pose" and "cat-cow pose" can all help relax and lengthen your pelvic floor muscles.
- **Practice birth breathing while pooping.** Because the "birth breath" stimulates the natural expulsive reflex, it can help you poop *and* get a baby out with minimal pushing. Many mamas don't believe this until they experience its effectiveness while having a bowel movement. So...
  - While sitting on the toilet, take in a quick and strong inhalation through your nose.
  - As you slowly exhale, feel the power of the breath being pushed down the back of your throat, through the uterus, and out your vaginal opening.
  - While you exhale, you'll organically create a low sound and gentle vibration in your throat. You'll also feel your expulsive muscles bearing down.
  - Repeat until you expel that poo!
- **Ask your care provider how they typically guide women through baby's emergence.** Gaining an understanding of the instructions your care providers usually provide through this phase of birth helps you determine whether their process resonates with you. If it doesn't, talk to them about how you'd prefer to navigate pushing.
- **Think of how you want to be guided through pushing, or breathing baby down, and add it to your birth preferences.** After you've

determined if you'd like to try birth breathing or want to go with more traditional pushing, add it to your birth preferences. I also recommend listing how you'd like to be guided through this experience. For example, women I work with often use the phrase, "I request calm prompts from only one person. No loud 'cheerleading' please."

- **Utilize the "laboring down" technique.** In laboring down, you allow the uterus to push baby out with only contractions, and not your pushing efforts, after you've fully dilated. This can conserve energy, reduce your chance of tearing, and provide a gentler experience for baby. Many women I've supported use this technique until they can no longer suppress the urge to push.
- **Choose a position that takes weight off the tailbone.** Standing, kneeling, squatting, being on all fours, or lying on your side allow more expansion in the pelvis, potentially leading to an easier emergence for baby. Changing positions can also help if pushing progress seems to stall.
- **Apply a warm compress and oil.** Help the perineum soften and expand (which minimizes tearing) by asking your care provider to place a warm washcloth on your perineum, in addition to massaging it with oil.
- **Go limp between contractions.** Contractions and pushing can take *a lot* of energy. Allow yourself to recharge between push sessions by closing your eyes, going totally rag doll, and taking slow easy breaths. You can also ask that no one talk to you unless absolutely necessary.
- **Consider having a mirror held between your legs.** Seeing the top of baby's head between your legs can be an incredibly motivating visual. If you're into this idea, bring a hand mirror to your birth, and ask someone to hold it between your legs when baby is crowning.

64. Will I be judged if I want to eat my placenta? And is it worth it?

Maybe, to both questions. I believe that anyone who judges you for your birthing or parenting decisions isn't worth your time. Sure, people close to you have every right to not understand your decision, but they don't have a right to make you feel shame for the decision. And what's the deal with some people having such a strong reaction to those wanting to ingest their placenta? Well…

Many believe that consuming the placenta is a dangerous, "hippie dippy" thing to do. They're not entirely wrong. It can be dangerous in certain circumstances, and I know lots of hippies who are all about noshing on that placenta. But I believe what's really behind these conceptions is that the idea of someone eating their placenta brings up visions of dicing up the organ and tossing it in the frying pan, or even throwing a few raw chunks in a smoothie. While that's been known to happen, it's not what placenta consumption usually looks like. Most women get the placenta encapsulated and take a few of the pills each day.

Before I get into the specifics of ingesting the placenta, know that it's a controversial topic because very little research has been done on it. And the studies that have been done were limited, providing inconclusive results. Because of this, I think it's important to talk to your care provider before making this decision. Then do what feels best to *you*.

To increase your knowledge of what it means to consume your placenta, let's look at some facts:

- **How is it encapsulated?** The placenta is washed, steamed (sometimes with herbs), dehydrated, and ground, and then the powder is encapsulated.
- **How could eating it help?** Anecdotal evidence has suggested that ingesting the placenta can do the following:
  - Increase energy
  - Balance hormones
  - Prevent anemia through restoration of iron levels (However, it's been found that most placenta pills contain a very modest amount of iron.)
  - Lower chances of developing postpartum depression

  Some believe these benefits are caused by the placebo effect. As a big believer in the mind-body connection, I don't think there's anything wrong with that. But I've also heard from women who felt that their placenta pills *dampened* their mood and energy. In addition, there are potential risks to consider.
- **What are reasons I might *not* want to eat the placenta?**
  - **Group B strep:** If you have group B strep (GBS), there's a possibility it could infect the placenta. The infection could

then be passed to the baby through breastmilk after you ingest the pills. I've known plenty of women who tested positive for GBS, encapsulated their placenta, and had no issues with their baby being infected, but it's important you're aware of the risk before making the decision.

- **Infection:** In addition to GBS, it's possible for the placenta to be contaminated by other intrauterine infections. There's also the potential for contamination during the encapsulation process, if it's not handled properly.

- **Hormones:** Estrogen in the placenta pills could increase the risk of blood clots. And the presence of progesterone could impede prolactin, which is responsible for milk production. Estrogen can also suppress prolactin.

What to do

Talk with your care provider. If they simply tell you not to encapsulate, ask them why. Ask questions until you get a clear view of where they're coming from. If you feel that what they're sharing is primarily based on personal beliefs instead of more solid evidence, consider talking with a few placenta encapsulating specialists to receive a more well-rounded perspective. After gathering information from numerous sources, sit with the decision until you're clear on what you feel most comfortable with.

If you choose to move forward with placenta encapsulation, here are questions to ask the specialist:

- Did you receive formal training and certification? What did that consist of? Do you engage in continuing education?
- How many placentas have you encapsulated?
- What are the risks of placenta encapsulation? Have your clients ever had adverse effects?
- Are there certain STDs or infections that would rule me out as a candidate for encapsulation?
- How do you handle and store the placenta before you're ready to encapsulate?
- Where do you encapsulate? What are the sanitation procedures for your equipment and workspace?

- Would you be willing to encapsulate in my kitchen if that's what I'm most comfortable with?
- How do you make sure my placenta isn't mixed up with someone else's?
- How do you encapsulate the placenta?
- What temperature do you use to steam the placenta? Is it high enough to kill potential blood-borne pathogens?
- What do you encapsulate the powder in?
- Will you be immediately available to pick up my placenta? If not, how should I store it until you arrive?
- How soon will you deliver my pills?
- Will you provide a dosage recommendation?

When you start taking the pills, pay attention to how they make you feel. If you start feeling down or notice a drop in milk supply, consider not taking the pills for a few days to see if the negative symptoms go away. Because there isn't much quality evidence about this, each woman taking these pills is essentially acting as a guinea pig, which ends up great for some, and not so much for others. Each body seems to respond a bit differently.

65. What if part of my placenta doesn't come out of my uterus? What will my care provider do?

If part of your placenta doesn't vacate your uterus within around thirty minutes after baby is born (something called a *retained placenta*), it will be evicted. As a full or partial retained placenta could cause hemorrhage (excessive bleeding) or infection, your care provider will utilize various methods until the entire organ has been birthed or removed. But you don't have to be too worried about this, as it's pretty rare. According to an article in the *International Journal of Women's Health*, a retained placenta occurs in only 1 to 3 percent of deliveries.

There are three types of retained placenta:

1. **Placenta adherens** occurs when contractions are too weak to push the placenta out and it remains loosely attached to the uterus. This is the most common type of retained placenta.
2. **Trapped placenta** is when the cervix begins to close before the placenta has been expelled.

3. **Placenta accreta** occurs when the placenta attaches to the muscular walls of the uterus, instead of the lining of the walls. This is sometimes diagnosed before birth and usually results in the care provider recommending a C-section.

You care provider will check your placenta after its birth to confirm that it's fully intact. If they suspect part of it is missing, they may perform an ultrasound to confirm. From there, they'll take steps to remove the remaining pieces. However, it's possible for a care provider to miss that a portion of the placenta is still in the uterus. In that situation, you might experience a fever, excessive bleeding, constant pain, or stinky discharge.

How does my care provider get it out? One of the first things they'll likely do is administer medication that encourages the uterus to continue contracting. (This is often done pre-emptively.) Breastfeeding can also trigger contractions. You might also be told to urinate, as a full bladder can impede the placenta's expulsion.

If these methods don't work, they may have to move on to manual removal, or surgery. In the case of manual removal, the care provider administers anesthesia and/or analgesia, reaches their hand into your uterus, and "sweeps." Essentially, they feel around and remove lingering placenta. This doesn't feel great — but it usually works. Surgeries to remove the placenta include dilation and curettage (aka D&C), hysteroscopy, and laparoscopy. A hysterectomy is needed in rare cases. Antibiotics are given after the treatment to reduce risk of infection.

What to do

While there's not much you can do to avoid the rare occurrence of a retained placenta, there are a few ways to be proactive:

*   **Avoid prolonged use of Pitocin.** According to the article in *International Journal of Women's Health*, prolonged use of Pitocin could increase the risk of a retained placenta. So use Pitocin only if it's absolutely necessary — not just because a care provider thinks it would be cool to speed things up.
*   **Pay attention to your postpartum symptoms.** If your care provider believes the full placenta was birthed but you experience fever,

excessive bleeding, constant pain, or stinky discharge, or you just feel that something is off, let your care provider know so they can confirm you don't have pieces of retained placenta.

- **Know how to stay calm if you experience a retained placenta.** Stick a few of these retained-placenta relaxation tools in your back pocket for the unlikelihood of this happening to you:
  - If you're told you have a retained placenta, immediately start taking deep breaths, helping to prevent panic from taking over.
  - Have someone on hand to hold the baby, as pain medication may need to be administered. However, continue focusing solely on your baby until a recommendation is made and you make a decision. This can help your mind from spiraling into a place of fear.
  - Keep reminding yourself that you're being taken care of by trained professionals. While it's not fun to have a retained placenta, they'll take care of you, and you'll be fine.
  - If a manual removal or surgery is needed, close your eyes and envision your body filled with and surrounded by a warm, golden light that's keeping you calm and safe.

Mothering

You have your baby in your arms, and everything is perfect now. Right?...Wait — no? Well, you're not alone. I naively thought the birth of my son would mark the end of physical strangeness and emotional chaos...but it was only the beginning. The blood loss, hair loss, hemorrhoids, vaginal tears, hard-as-rocks boobs, sleep deprivation, and wild, all-consuming love for a stranger are so intense — and it happens so fast. Then we start to get the side-eye and "suggestions" from friends and family wanting us to parent the way they parented, whether they're conscious of this desire or not. It's a lot.

While so much about early motherhood is enchanting, there are also many hard things we should get out in the open. Because when we don't talk about the not-so-enchanting elements of this experience, we become susceptible to shame, guilt, and a desire to retreat.

My hope is that you'll become more comfortable acknowledging, and moving through, the murkier aspects of motherhood. I hope that you'll get used to talking about, seeking support for, and not hating yourself for any part of the experience that's holding you back from joy, fulfillment, or a solid connection with your child. And if you get in a flow with this supportive system of reflection and action now, while your baby is a baby, it will become second nature as you navigate the Wild West of the other phases of parenthood.

Relationships

66. My friends are a huge part of my life, but none of them have kids. I'm starting to feel really isolated. What should I do?

Let me paint you a picture. Lady gets pregnant with Baby. Lady's friends are super excited for her and want to support her. They throw a baby shower. They do most of the same things they've always done, only Lady's wine is replaced by mocktails. Everyone is confident their friendship will seamlessly flow into Lady's life with Baby, but no one talks about what that will look like. And then Lady has Baby. The friends show up to ooh and aah, then everyone leaves. Friends want to invite Lady to this and that, but they don't want to pressure her or make her feel bummed she's missing out, so the invites dry up. Friends want to call, but they don't want to bother Lady. "Maybe she's trying to nurse? Or sleep? I should probably just let her call me when she's ready." Lady is elbow-deep in diapers and exhaustion and at first doesn't notice the radio silence. But then the fog of the fourth trimester begins to fade, and she notices. She notices that she feels isolated. She wants to call Friends, but doesn't. She thinks she'll just bore them with mom-talk.

This is a classic case of Postpartum Friendship Dissolution. As you probably noticed, much of it is birthed from lack of communication.

While your relationships with your buddies will definitely change, they don't have to end. Your life circumstances have been shaken up and turned upside down, but you're still you — the you that loves your friends, and vice versa. There has to be a way to save those friendships. But how? How do you sidestep Postpartum Friendship Dissolution and walk the path of Postpartum Friendship Evolution?

What to do

Talk to your friends, one at a time, about how you're feeling. (If you're reading this while pregnant, talk to them before you have the baby, so you can all prepare for the changes.) These conversations aren't meant to cause guilt for either party — they're opportunities for you to be vulnerable and to cocreate a plan for how the relationship will look moving forward. After you let them know you value their friendship and need more of them in your life, the two of you can brainstorm ways you can connect. For example…

- Maybe your friend loves talking on the phone, and you can schedule calls for times you'll be on a walk with baby.
- Or maybe this friend lives nearby and is often free to join you for those walks.
- Maybe this is the friend you used to see live music with or take dance classes with. While it will likely be hard to meet up for your activity of choice as often as you used to, you could commit to doing it once a month — or whatever works best for your schedules.

After you've created the plan, forewarn your friend that you won't be as reliable as you were before baby. Motherhood is predictably unpredict-able, potentially causing you to cancel plans at the last minute because of a sick child, or an AWOL babysitter. Being forthright with this information will hopefully prevent your friend from being annoyed that you're not able to show up for the friendship in the same way you used to.

In addition, ask them to reach out if they haven't heard from you in a while. As a foggy-brained new parent, it can feel near impossible to remember how many days you've been wearing those pajama bottoms, much less when you last contacted your friends. Remind them that radio silence doesn't mean you don't care; it just means you're overwhelmed.

Here are some additional considerations when navigating friendships as a new mom:

- **Be thoughtful of conversation topics.** While your non-mom friends probably won't mind hearing a bit about motherhood, they won't be able to relate to it and will likely tire of the topic if it's not kept to a minimum. Ensure your time with friends is filled with connection by asking each one about their life, and bringing up topics you used to love gabbing about. If you're worried you're incapable of thinking of anything but mom-topics, keep a running list of conversation starters you think would be interesting to your friend. For example, if the two of you love celebrity gossip, write down juicy tidbits you can bring up. If you're politics fanatics, list hot topics you want to get their opinion on. You won't always have to put this much effort into talking points, but while you're trying to find your footing on the balance beam of parenthood and friendship, this forethought will pay off.

Note: If your friend is not child-free by choice, it might be best to steer clear of all talk of baby, unless they ask. Hearing about you living the life they desperately want could be devastating, and it could drive a wedge in the friendship. For more on this, see question 7.

- **Know that you might need to let go of some friends.** Not all friendships will stand the test of motherhood. While it might be painful to let those friends drift away, you can honor them by sitting with the idea that they were meant to be in your life for a certain period of time, and now it's time to part. This parting will likely be made easier by the fact that your time is now seriously limited, and you have to be selective about who you spend time with.

  After I had Hudson, only three of my prebaby friends were still standing. These were the friends who weren't offended if I forgot to call or text back, or didn't reach out for months at a time. These were the friends who would try to make a meetup happen if I randomly had a free hour and reached out to them last minute. These were the friends who would come to Hudson's birthday parties, even when they were the only ones without kids. They understood the constraints of my new circumstances and didn't fault me for them. They were free of drama (at least the not-fun kind) and always there when I needed them.

- **Find new friends.** One of the most natural parts of parenthood is making new friends. The playgroups, time at the park or library, and other baby-centered gatherings all create organic opportunities for fostering fresh friendships. And many of these connections will feel refreshing as you can gab about the trials and triumphs of parenthood without feeling self-conscious.

While these new relationships will likely be easier to maintain and should absolutely be nurtured and enjoyed, you should still use the suggestions above to hold on to at least a few of your pre-parenthood friends. Those are the folks you probably feel most comfortable being your unfiltered self around, which is a dynamic that can feel like gold as you navigate the unsure footing of early motherhood.

67. My partner seems resentful of my relationship with our baby. I don't want my romantic relationship to suffer, but I also think my partner should understand how important it is for me to bond with our baby. What should I do?

"I laughed at him when he told me he was jealous of my connection with the baby," Madison said. "I seriously thought he was joking. I had blood leaking out of the pad attached to my disposable underwear, our baby was latched on to one nipple, and milk was leaking out the other. When I realized he wasn't joking, I yelled at him. I was so mad. Then he started crying, and I walked away." Madison, a past doula client, called me the day after this went down with her husband. Insulted by how he was feeling, she got a little pissed when I suggested we try to see things from his side. I don't blame her; I would've also been miffed if someone tried to make me see my husband's point of view if he even insinuated that anything was hard for him when our son was a newborn. However, staying in the space of anger and defensiveness only blocks us from strengthening our relationship with the person who's supposed to be our biggest supporter in early parenthood.

This is such a tricky situation because many of the emotions being triggered in you and your partner are likely coming from subconscious programming. For example, your partner's inbuilt fears of abandonment or inadequacy could be sparked when you begin to devote time to baby that used to be reserved for them. And then there's your emotions: if the primal instinct to care for your infant feels threatened, you could easily lose empathy for your partner's emotions.

In addition to those subconscious responses, the resentment your partner feels about your relationship with baby could stem from circumstances that developed during pregnancy. For example, your partner probably wasn't able to experience the same level of connection you might have fostered with the baby when pregnant — and that might have been hard on them. And now you're nine months ahead of them when it comes to bonding with the baby. In addition, if you decide to breastfeed, there's another significant bonding activity your partner can't participate in. It's understandable that they might feel left out. But of course, you've done nothing wrong by growing your child and choosing to breastfeed. Like I said, it's tricky.

Both of you might find it near impossible to fully understand where the other is coming from, as each person's point of view will feel so completely "right" to them. But strangely, that's a great place to start — realizing you're both just doing and expressing what feels true for you. Neither of you intends to hurt the other (I assume). From the base of that understanding you can start to build resolution.

What to do

Work through the following strategies while constantly reminding yourself that this isn't a "win or lose" situation. There's not one party that gets to be the righteous victor. The only "winning" comes when you both develop some empathy about what the other is feeling, and you start working together instead of apart.

- **Talk it out.** Create the ideal environment for a productive conversation by setting a communication ground rule: you each get the opportunity to share without interruption. As hard as it is, don't let yourself get bogged down in rebuttals and thoughts about that thing you feel like you really, *really* have to say right this second. Because then you don't hear anything your partner says, because you're just trying to remember that thing you wanted to say. Let that inclination go in favor of truly hearing what your partner is trying to express. If something really needs to be said, you'll remember it when your turn comes.

  Then, when your partner lets you know they're done sharing, resist the urge to immediately jump into what you disagree with. Instead, first repeat the key messages you feel they're trying to express. They can then let you know if you interpreted them correctly, or if there's something important you misperceived. This will help them feel heard and give you an opportunity to objectively review what they shared. Then, take a beat before getting into how you feel, as the pause can help you get into a thoughtful space, instead of a defensive one.

  This process might feel super frustrating at first, and it can be really hard to stick with, but by doing your best to follow it you'll set yourself up for a productive conversation that doesn't spiral into hurt feelings and a fractured relationship.
- **Create more opportunities for your partner to bond with baby.** A

great way to help your partner release jealously over your relationship with baby is to help them foster their own relationship with baby. Once they get to see what all the fuss is about, they'll be less inclined to judge you for wanting to spend all your time with that adorable little nugget. You can support this bonding by giving them alone time with baby. This is important because when you're near, baby will likely only have eyes for you. They can start with small activities like short walks, bottle feedings, and diaper changes. It's simple stuff that can make a big difference.

- **Accept your partner's help, even if they don't do things your way.** I've talked to numerous partners (my husband included) who felt like they were more of a nuisance than a help after their baby was born. I get this. Us mamas usually develop routines and preferred methods for caring for our babies pretty early on. When our partner tries to take on some of those responsibilities but doesn't do it in the way we've labeled as "best," it can be easy to feel like it's more efficient for us to just take care of all the baby business. But as hard as it is to cede control over a task you're probably the master of, giving your partner more responsibility when it comes to baby will help them feel like a part of the team, instead of an outsider peering in.

- **Remember that your partner is also going through big emotional and physical shifts.** While you definitely win the award for navigating the biggest changes, your partner is also working through sleep deprivation, an identity upheaval, and a slew of other shake-ups that are likely enhancing their feelings of confusion over where they stand, and their need to talk to you about it. Under "normal" circumstances they might have more perspective about what's going on and might even be able to move past it without discussion — but in the raw state they're in, the shift in your relationship could feel like the end of the world. I say all of this to give you a frame of reference for where your partner is coming from. Remember that neither of you is doing anything wrong; you are both doing the best you can to navigate your brave new world.

- **Notice if you start pulling away from your baby.** If your partner's jealousy is severe enough that it's impacting your bond with baby, consider seeking professional support to work out the most effective and safest way to move forward. While it's normal for your partner to feel resistance to the changes in your relationship, you shouldn't be made to feel like you have to choose between them or your baby.

68. My partner and I fight all the time about how to care for our baby. It's exhausting. What should we do?

How to care for tiny, defenseless offspring can stir up major beef between parents — even parents who didn't think they even had strong opinions about how to care for a baby. What some of us don't realize is that we're carrying all sorts of baggage into parenthood. Either we consciously or subconsciously believe that the way our parents parented is the way to go, or we want to do things the exact opposite of the way our parents did it, or we are somewhere in between. And of course, life experience sprinkles more baggage into the mix. If the baggage your partner brings to parenting conflicts with your own, major disagreements can arise. And these disagreements can get really heated, as you're both fighting for what you think is best for your baby — a precious person you've likely fallen head over heels for. The stakes can feel unreasonably high. Ceding to the will of your partner might seem like an unimaginable scenario, much more so than when you're arguing about less-precious topics.

Here's an example: From day one, my mother-in-law has stood firm in the belief that babies should sleep in a crib, ideally in their own room. She is the leader of team "Let Them Cry It Out." Because my husband treasures his parents, who have raised six kids, he believes they know what's best in most realms of parenting. I also treasure my parents, who are not cry-it-out advocates and slept with my brother and me when we were infants, putting us either in their bed or in a crib in their room.

None of this initially seemed to be a problem. For the first few weeks of our son's life, my husband didn't argue when I decided to bed-share. Things were going great. Our son happily fed and snoozed by my side, we were all getting adequate sleep, and we were adhering to all the safety guidelines for bed-sharing. But then Eric's mom started peppering us with questions about where the baby was sleeping. And next came the assertions that if he didn't get used to sleeping on his own, he would be in our bed until college. The result: my previously "let the baby sleep wherever you want him to sleep" husband was suddenly pushing me to change the sleep plan.

I immediately bristled. Not only was this arrangement the only one that allowed Hudson and me to sleep more than three hours a night and facilitated ample nighttime feedings, but also it felt intuitively right to me. The thought of being pushed to not have my baby beside me at night triggered all my Mama Bear instincts. Intense arguing ensued. We would *go at it*. And honestly, we never really reached a resolution. It was a parenting stalemate. I just kept doing what felt right, and he stopped challenging me as much. This particular argument would flare up every now and again, but other baby-care issues eventually took its place.

I've retrospectively discovered the suggestions in the "What to do" section, and I hope to use them with our second baby. For now, I hope I can help you do better than I did.

You see, you and your partner aren't arguing because your relationship is broken, or because one of you is a bad parent. You're arguing because you both feel like it's your duty to protect the well-being of your offspring and you might believe your partner has a seriously misguided parenting point of view. Without intentional strategies and a mega-dose of active listening and understanding, it might be tricky to pull out of the cycle of baby-care arguments. So putting in the work to implement these positive changes is worth it, because ultimately, finding peace with your significant other and figuring out ways to parent as a team will likely benefit your baby more than any decision in all the topics you're fighting about.

What to do

Just yell, "Mama knows best!" when your partner questions your parenting....Sigh. If only it were that easy. Because it's not, try these strategies instead:

- **Get other people out of the mix.** Regardless of how wise your parents, in-laws, siblings, friends, or whoever are about parenting, they shouldn't get a say in how you care for your baby. I would get furious when I felt like my husband was parroting parenting views I knew he'd gotten from his mom. And I'm sure he felt the same. We both wanted to communicate with our partner, not with a proxy for our mothers-in-law. You can kick those people out of your conversations by mutually agreeing to ask your parents (or whoever is in your ear) to stop providing parenting opinions unless you ask for them. Let them know you respect their point of view but need to go at it without their input.

- **Get the right person in the mix.** While I just told you to get other people out of your baby-care decisions, the one exception could be a pediatrician you both resonate with. This neutral party can ideally provide information that guides your parenting decisions and resolves discord. But the key here is that your partner goes with you to these appointments, as they'll likely be more open to the guidance if it's received firsthand. This will also give them the chance to ask illuminating questions.

- **Determine the root of your parenting opinions.** It can be wild to discover what our true beliefs are after unraveling ourselves from the parenting influences of our past. To start that unraveling, ask yourself the following questions about any belief you and your partner are in conflict about:

  - Is this a parenting method I came to believe in because it's what my parents, siblings, or other loved ones did and insist on as the way to go?

  - Did I do extensive research that led me to believe this was the right choice for my family?

  - Does this instinctually feel right? Or does it feel wrong, but the idea of finding a new way feels scary and unknown?

  Keep digging into the layers of the belief until you discover where it came from. From there, you can determine if this is a belief that truly feels like the best choice for your family, or begin building a new belief based on fresh experiences and research.

- **Write each other letters.** As you probably know, it can be really hard to get your point across, or absorb your partner's point of view, when you're in a heated argument. You can bypass that distracting, unwanted heat by both composing letters about how you're feeling, explaining your beliefs about the baby-care situation in question.

  This letter allows you to really explore where you're coming from and communicate in a way that's fueled by a desire to help your partner understand you, rather than to make them agree that you're right and they're wrong. In turn, reading your partner's letter can open your mind and heart to where they're coming from, and help you move forward with the decision-making process with enhanced understanding for the "other side."

Agree to not discuss the letters until you've both had time to process them and can talk without strong emotions distracting from the main objective: finding a solution that's best for your baby.

- **Try out your partner's baby-care wishes on a trial basis.** If the baby-care strategy your partner is suggesting is not something you believe would be damaging to your child, you could agree to try it their way for a few days. For example, if they're all for cloth diapers and you're a disposable devotee, you might agree to give cloth diapers a go for a week. At the end of that trial you might still loathe cloth diapers, but your partner will at least feel like you heard them and gave their preference a whirl. And maybe some of these trials could transform a few of your parenting views. At the very least they'll bring more harmony and respect into your relationship.

- **Create a safe word.** Help prevent your arguments from getting into damaging territory by creating a safe word or phrase. This is a word or phrase that can be used when one of you realizes the conversation has taken a turn for the worse and is no longer productive.

  Because Eric and I usually argue in the evening, our phrase is, "We need to go to bed" — and not in a sexy way. This phrase helps us realize fatigue and short fuses are making us mean and irrational. It doesn't always stop the argument, but it at least makes us check ourselves.

- **Research together.** When you can't find common ground on a certain baby-care issue, research solutions together. Skim the same parenting books, peruse articles and studies about the baby-care topic, speak with your pediatrician, or engage in any other activity that allows you to absorb the same information. This joint research gets you on the same page (or at least in the same chapter), so you can find a solution without too much arguing.

- **Write down your joint parenting philosophy.** Once you've worked through most of your disputes about baby care, work together to create a shared parenting philosophy. As you create it, consider questions like these:

+ What type of parents do we want to be?
+ What values are important to us?
+ How do we want to nurture our baby?
+ What type of emotional climate do we want to create in our family?
+ How do we want to handle disputes and discipline when our baby is older?
+ What do we hope to get out of parenting?
+ In what ways do we hope parenting helps us change and grow?
+ What aspects of our childhoods do we want to infuse into our child's life?
+ What aspects of our childhoods do we want to leave behind?

Keep riffing, exploring, and taking notes until you've created a document that can inform your parenting decisions moving forward. And of course, this document can be adapted as your family evolves.

69. My partner is showing signs they're going to leave. Should I address these concerns, or try to ignore the situation? Can I do this alone if they do leave?

I first want to acknowledge that regardless of whether or not your partner actually leaves, the fact that you're feeling this way must be so hard. Parenting a newborn is stressful enough when all is well between the parents, but when you're worried about your baby-raising partner skipping town, you're forced to grapple with a mess of emotions no new mother should have to deal with. For example, you might feel scared, angry, sad, and a range of other emotions that could come with the major uncertainty you're facing. Some might tell you to "just try to be strong, push the concerns aside, and power forward," but I think bottling these emotions and ignoring your concerns just delays resolution. One of the strongest things you can do is feel the emotions and express those concerns. And don't worry about *trying* to be strong, because you already are — your strength is a bright light at your core that can never be extinguished, no matter who enters or exits your life.

Regarding the path of parenting alone, you can absolutely walk it if you must. While it might feel like your world would end if your partner left, it wouldn't break you. You are just as capable as the millions of single mothers out there, and you would find your footing even if it feels like the hardest thing you could ever do. I'm hands-down more impressed with the single mothers of the world than the Olympians, Academy Award winners, and Nobel laureates, because these women are constantly summoning their courage, resilience, and dedication. They don't get to clock out or take a sabbatical. They're all in, all the time. That might sound overwhelming, but *you can do it* if that's how life unfolds.

What to do

Take small steps to figure out what's going on, and build up your confidence and autonomy, which will be valuable even if your partner stays. Here are some ideas to get you started:

- **Address your fear.** Instead of stewing in fear over whether your partner is planning to leave, tell them what you're thinking. You'll likely be met with one of two reactions. One: they're shocked you've been thinking that and make moves to help you feel better. Two: they squirm because you've hit on something they've been considering. Either way, you've stepped out of the unknown and got the conversation started.

  If they're not planning on leaving but something about them is still making you uneasy, you can begin addressing their behavior and what you'd like them to change. If they are thinking of leaving, you can dive into why they're feeling that way, if it's something that can be resolved, and if you even want to resolve it.

  As tempting as it can be to live in limbo, asking the question that's probably been driving you crazy can untangle those knots in your stomach and give you something real to work with.

- **Consider whether you want them to stay.** It might seem unfathomable that life could be better without your partner, but it's worth considering. Once you move aside from the very natural fear of being alone, how do you feel about your relationship? Does your partner nurture your emotional, mental, and physical well-being? Or do they threaten or ignore it? Do you feel safe and cared for when they're with you? Or tense? Are you relieved when they're out of the house for a few hours? Continue exploring your interpretations of the relationship until you get a hold on how you really feel about it. This deeper understanding can guide your feelings and actions moving forward.

- **Seek counseling.** If you determine that you're dedicated to keeping your partner in your life, and they're willing to put in the work to mend the relationship, discuss the possibility of seeing a couple's counselor. This objective support can give both of you an outlet for your emotions and healing strategies tailored to your unique situation. While some associate counseling with high costs, many mental health specialists accept insurance or provide pro bono services through family support centers.

- **Make a loose plan for what you'll do if they leave.** Many major changes seem insurmountable until we break them down into smaller steps. So to help yourself realize that you will make it through if your partner leaves, make a list of all the challenges that will erupt after they leave. For example, "Less income to pay rent. No one but me to watch the baby. A fear of being the only adult in the house at night. A loss of companionship." Then start listing potential solutions to the changes. For example, "Find a new living situation. Ask friends and family members for help with childcare. Install a security system to enhance my sense of safety, or ask a family member to move in. Reconnect with my friends." While this list won't magically dissolve your challenges, it will at least show you that there's a way forward.

- **Shift your focus to yourself.** When we believe that much of our safety and happiness is based on our romantic partner, it's easy to be terrified of the idea of them leaving. It can be crazy making to put so much stock in the actions of a person you can't control.

  Take back your sense of power and calm by shifting your focus from making sure your partner will stay to nurturing yourself — committing to actions that make you feel more whole and capable of caring for yourself and baby. Understandably, this is much easier when not navigating the fatigue, hormonal upheaval, and uncertainty of life with a newborn. But taking small actions like going on a morning walk with baby, drinking more water, making a list of career goals you'd like to pursue when you've gotten through the haze of early motherhood, calling a friend or family member who lifts you up, and doing anything else that makes you feel good, and isn't based on your partner's actions, can make a powerful difference.

The key to getting these small actions to actually help is that you're doing them to support yourself, not to change into a person you think your partner will be more likely to stay with. Do it for *you*, the person you'll always be in a relationship with.

70. I resent my baby for getting all the attention, and I feel invisible. How can I start feeling like I matter?

Isn't it a wild emotional shift to go from getting ample help and compliments when the baby is inside you, to suddenly being seen as their leaky accessory after going through all the work of getting them out? And sure, there are folks who ask about the birth and tell you how great you look (bless them), but really, most people are all about the baby. This can be nice at times, as you may score much-needed downtime while others coo and ooh over the baby, but then there are the times when you crave to be seen as more than a mother — as more than the lady carrying around that adorable creation everyone wants to hold. You crave conversation about that book you're writing, or that cat-grooming workshop you went to… or whatever your thing is. You want to be honored for being the powerhouse who grew and birthed a baby while also having all of these other amazing qualities. You're not selfish for feeling this way.

For the first six months of Hudson's life I felt completely invisible. When people came up to us, their eyes would immediately lock onto him. If they engaged me in conversation, their eyes would stay on him, and the topic would almost always be his eating, pooping, or weight-gaining habits. I felt like I was his personal assistant. Or PR rep.

A big part of my frustration was that these interactions were a physical manifestation of what was going on in my own head. Almost every thought I had, every action I took, involved Hudson. I could barely remember what made me an individual. While I loved him deeply, I also felt twinges of resentment that he had robbed me of my individuality. Luckily, these feelings began to fade as he grew and became less dependent on me. And of course, because motherhood is crazy like this, him needing me less made me have moments where I missed him needing me all the time. Geesh.

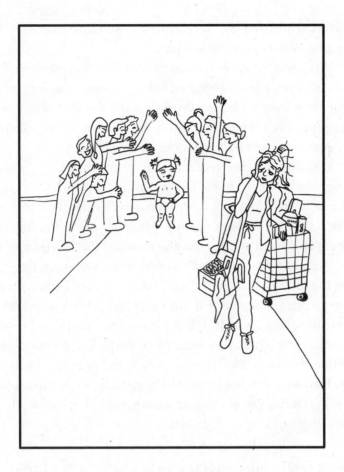

What to do

Remember that in the early days of motherhood it's so normal for your life and identity to feel fully wrapped up in baby. However, you can create a lifeline to your unique self by making a list:

1. **Create a list of all the things that make you feel like you.** This list can contain anything, from something as simple as taking a shower or organizing the closet to tasks as complex as creating a graphic novel or starting that business you've been dreaming of.

2. **Put the items on the list into three categories.** The first category will contain the actions that are absolute essentials and should be prioritized immediately (for example, taking a shower every day, and going on a walk three times a week). These are the things you'll bring to your

support system and say, "Let's figure out who can watch baby during these times so I can do these things."

The second category will consist of actions that are incredibly important to you but can be put on hold for six months, as month six is often when baby is a tad less dependent and able to be with others for longer periods. My top two items in this category were meditating for fifteen minutes and writing for one hour, every day.

Finally, move the remaining actions on your list into category three, which consists of the things that will come back into your life after baby's first birthday. By this time, you'll likely be in your groove with motherhood, sleeping fairly regularly, and feeling comfortable setting up consistent childcare. This is around the time I started teaching HypnoBirthing classes and amped up my writing career.

3. **Use the list.** Pull out your categorized list whenever you're forgetting who you are or wondering if you'll ever get back to that person. After a day of feeling invisible, this list helps you breathe and remember that there will come a time when life settles back into a more balanced rhythm. And no, life will never go back to feeling exactly like it did before baby was born, but it will start being more layered and consisting of people seeing you as a unique woman, not just the person that baby is clinging to. Things will get better.

71. I find it really boring to take care of a baby all day. Does that make me a bad mom? Is there a way to make it more entertaining?

Girl, I feel you. When Hudson was a baby I felt like I was on a hamster wheel of feeding, butt cleaning, spit-up dodging, cooking, not showering, and walking around in circles saying, "Shh." I felt like my life had been drained of creative, thought-provoking stimulation. I was mega-bored hanging with a person who didn't talk and cared only about my boobs. And I was pretty sure I was missing crucial mothering pieces.

It's no wonder we feel like there's something wrong with our boredom when we're constantly told how magical it should be to interact, bond, and help baby learn about the world. These are all essential tasks that plant seeds for the emergence of independent, vibrant humans. So shouldn't we feel inspired and excited by them? I suppose some women are, but I wasn't.

If you relate, let me start by saying how super-duper normal you are for feeling this way. You're not an evil Grinch incapable of connecting with your child. You're an adult who craves activities that challenge your mind and awaken your creativity. At first glance, caring for a baby does none of these things, and often it just makes us feel incompetent and frustrated. But when we dive deeper into the nuances of baby care, there is something to be done about baby-care boredom.

What to do

Toy around with these ideas:

- **Incorporate your interests into baby care.** For example, it's important to talk to baby so they're exposed to language, but who said you have to talk to them about mundane topics or read to them from cardboard books? Give your babe language exposure by reading aloud from a magazine or that book you've wanted to read. And music — scrap the Mozart (unless that's your jam!), strap baby to your chest, and get a workout by shaking your butt to nineties hip-hop while making funny faces at baby.
- **Think of innovative ways to make baby tasks more interesting.** Do this by listing your daily baby-care activities on one side of a sheet of paper and writing your interests and talents on the other half. Then, start brainstorming how you can fuse the lists, mixing and matching your interests and talents with baby-care obligations.

  For me, diaper changes became more compelling when I used the time to challenge my writer's brain to come up with new lyrics to favorite songs. Breastfeeding was made way less boring by putting a TV tray and my laptop by my nursing chair and writing weird poetry while Hudson ate. And I made sure I still interacted with him by asking questions about how I should get around tricky prose.
- **Remember that you don't have to parent the way others do.** Bringing your unique self into motherhood is one of the best ways you can quell boredom and foster an authentic bond with your baby — it will help them get to know the real you. And if your way doesn't look

anything like the way of your sister or the ladies in your mom group, that's okay. We all get to forge our own path.

While life with baby will eventually become less boring, regardless of what you do, liven up your mama-baby relationship *now* by injecting motherhood with the stuff that makes your mind do a happy dance.

72. I don't feel connected to my baby. I don't even like to look at them. Am I a monster?

You're not a monster. Not even a little bit. You're one of the many women facing postpartum blues or postpartum depression. According to a study published in *Morbidity and Mortality Weekly Report*, one in nine women experience symptoms of postpartum depression. But some believe the number is actually much higher, as many mothers don't feel comfortable talking about their depressive symptoms.

While it's easy to convince yourself that the lack of connection with your baby is a sign you're lacking some essential "good mother" chip, it probably just means that wonky hormones, plus the ingredients of exhaustion and extreme change, are impacting your ability to bond. However, just because the causes of what you're experiencing aren't dark and sinister doesn't mean you're not feeling like this is the end of the world. Many of us are given the consistent message — especially during pregnancy — that the bond between a mother and child is unbreakable. That it's the greatest love story we'll ever experience. When that's not our reality, it can feel life shattering.

Something important to remember as you navigate this likely heart-breaking experience is that it's *temporary*. While any form of anxiety or depression can easily trick us into thinking we'll never feel better, that's rarely the case.

If you're sad and unable to develop a bond in the two weeks following baby's birth, you might be facing the common phenomenon of postpartum blues, which is believed to be caused by a combination of your hormone levels plunging and a struggle to adapt to the abrupt changes of motherhood. If the feelings of sadness and disconnection don't lift after two weeks, you might be experiencing postpartum depression.

It's also important to realize that you're not scarring your child, or your future bond with them, by not feeling connected *now*. The mother-child bond develops over a lifetime, and it will happen for you, even if you first have to navigate medical and emotional support. And it's wise to seek that support. Sadly, about 60 percent of women with symptoms of depression do not receive a clinical diagnosis, and 50 percent of women with a diagnosis do not receive treatment. As added incentive to seek support, consider this: studies have shown that while postpartum depression can have short-term impacts on infants, there are rarely long-term emotional effects if the mother receives treatment early on.

What to do

Get help, as you should not have to navigate this pain alone. While I totally get the resistance to being open about your depression (I waited two years before I asked for help!), I can almost guarantee that your care provider won't judge you. They'll probably be relieved you were brave enough to speak up. And I want to remind you again that postpartum blues or depression is not a fatal character flaw; it's a very common by-product of going through the intense physical and mental shifts of pregnancy, childbirth, and early motherhood. It doesn't mean you're a bad mother, or that you'll never bond with your baby. Asking for help is actually one of the best things you can do for your baby.

Here are a few support-steps you'll likely need to take:

- **See your primary care provider.** The first stop on the path to moving past postpartum blues or depression is your care provider. They can help evaluate what's going on and refer you to a mental health specialist. They might also prescribe medication, like an antidepressant. For many women, medication is a key player in getting out of the grips of postpartum depression.
- **Be consistent with counseling.** After you find a mental health specialist you resonate with, commit to showing up. When I was depressed, I canceled on my therapist all the time because I felt too listless to leave the house. Needless to say, I didn't get much out of the relationship. Years later I faced another bout of depression and forced myself to see

my therapist once a week. If I couldn't get out of bed, I would Face-Time her. I always felt lighter after our sessions and gleaned serious benefits from our time together — and I also needed medication.

As hard as it can be to keep showing up for counseling, it's one of the most potent ways you can nurture yourself through depression. Even if some days you're sure you have nothing to say to your therapist, you'll benefit from simply arriving at the appointment.

- **Find quality care for baby.** As you navigate this challenging time, it will be essential to ask trusted loved ones for help with your baby. Being their sole caregiver while trying to get through depression might feel impossible, which is why calling in reinforcements can ensure that you and baby get the care you deserve.

  You might resist this because you don't want to tell people about your depression. This is normal, but you'll probably be amazed by how supportive friends and family are when you trust them with your vulnerability. (And you might also be surprised to learn that some of your loved ones have been through the same thing.)

- **Continue to spend time with baby.** While being with your baby might be a painful reminder of how disconnected you feel, it's important to continue being with them, even if you have to fake affection. Because "faking it 'til you make it" might just help you develop an authentic bond with baby, and it will definitely support them in feeling bonded to you. If you don't trust yourself to adequately care for your baby on your own, ask an adult to be with you when you're spending time together.

73. I get really defensive when I receive unsolicited parenting advice. It's so bad I've been snapping at strangers and find it hard to be around friends and family members who have kids. How can I navigate this advice without creating tension?

Unsolicited advice is composed of an interesting mix of motivations and emotions, as the advice-giver is usually trying to make themselves feel important and helpful, while the advice-receiver often feels like they're being told they don't know what they're doing. For the most part, the only kind of advice that doesn't cause tension is the solicited kind. So yup, it's perfectly natural for your hackles to rise when someone starts preaching about sleep training, insists you'll kill the planet if you use disposable diapers, or shares some other opinion that primarily serves to pump up their ego. And while you have every right to be annoyed or defensive, remember that you and the advice-giver likely have two completely different perceptions of the conversation. They think the two of you are bonding over their knowledge and helpfulness, while you feel like they're judging your parenting and putting their opinions where they don't belong. Keeping that in mind can significantly reduce your defensiveness.

Something else that could be happening is that you're feeling insecure about your parenting knowledge and choices, and need space to figure out what feels best for you. People telling you what you should do can make you feel rushed to make decisions and even more insecure about your base of knowledge. If you're feeling this way, I encourage you to remember that *you're* the expert on your child. You're the guru of your family, even if you haven't consumed as much parenting literature as the other person or haven't found all the answers. (And spoiler alert: no one ever finds all the answers.) So instead of letting the advice get to you, take it as a sign that it might feel good to take some alone time to meditate on what's going on with your baby, yourself, or your family and what solution intuitively feels right. If you don't know where to start, use that alone time to research the issue and make a list of potential solutions that resonate with *you*.

It's also common to feel the urge to tell the advice-giver why certain advice wouldn't work for your family and, in the case of something like corporal punishment, why you think it's wrong. But the fact is, they don't want to hear it, and you don't want to waste your breath. You don't have to convince them their advice is misguided, or the way you're doing something is working fine, or you're confident you can come up with a solution on your own. You don't owe them any explanation, and you don't have to get sucked into a parenting debate — save your energy for something enjoyable. Here are some tips for slipping away from advice sessions with minimal effort and emotion.

What to do

Scream "No!" when someone tries to give you advice. Just kidding. Try this:

- **Keep parenting challenges to yourself when you're with chronic advice-givers.** Minimize the chance of receiving advice that might activate your defensiveness and anger by dodging parenting conversations with people prone to offering advice.
- **Compose go-to responses.** When most people give advice, the response they want is an unsarcastic version of, "Oh my gosh, thank you! I never would have thought of that. You're a genius! What would I do without your superior insights?" But you don't have to give them that. You get to think of a response that allows you to shut down the outpouring of advice without getting into an argument. I usually say something like, "Hmm. That's interesting. I'll think about it." If they continue with the advice, I'll interrupt with an, "I'm so sorry but I think my baby just pooped. I'll be right back." And then I'm not right back.

  Here are additional responses you can tinker with:

  - "[Insert the parenting choice here] is working just fine for us. No need to fix what isn't broken."
  - "It sounds like that worked great for your family. I love how there's so many unique ways to raise a child, and that every family gets to make their own decisions."
  - "I'm sure that's an ideal option for some families. We're going to keep doing what feels right for us."
  - "We tried that, but it didn't work for us. Just shows that each child is different!"
  - "I'm doing what the pediatrician advised." And it doesn't matter if this is a lie — it will likely shut down the advice or judgment, as people are often loath to go against the word of an expert.
  - "Luckily, we don't have to agree on the right way to [insert parenting topic here]. We can each do it our own way."
  - "Thanks for your concern."
  - "I'll keep that in mind. *Anyways*, tell me about that book club you joined."
- **Check in with yourself after receiving advice.** After you've gotten out of an unwanted-advice conversation, take a pause and look objectively at the advice. Do you instinctually know it won't work for your family? Does it go against your parenting philosophy? If so, fuggedaboutit. But if the advice sparked some interest, file it away for later use.

- **Remember that the advice-giver is (probably) coming from a good place.** Most people aren't trying to insult or annoy when they give advice — usually, they're genuinely trying to help. Hold on to this belief when they blast you with their counsel. While you don't have to agree, or even listen to it, remembering that they're probably not intending to insult you can help you stay calm enough to gently extract yourself from the conversation, instead of raging.
- **Avoid being the advice-giver.** I like to preach about how annoying unsolicited advice is, but I myself give it all the time. And I'm working on this. Be better than me and swallow your advice when it tiptoes to the tip of your tongue. I can almost guarantee that people would prefer your empathy or your questions about what *they* think they should do over your wisdom (as wise as it might be). And of course, if they ask for your opinion, you can let it rip.

74. I know there's a whole movement about not judging mothers, but I'm still afraid I'll be judged. How can I feel secure in my parenting decisions and manage the judgment when it comes?

There sure is a movement to stop judging mothers. And for good reason! Us poor mamas have everything from side-eye to full-on trolling thrown at us for putting even a finger out of line. But where to put "the line" is the biggest problem. What's the definition of that line? Where the heck does it live? Each parenting camp (and there are many) will give you a different answer to those questions. And all of those camps are certain their way of parenting is The Way to parent. It's a dangerous recipe for excessive judgment that sadly causes mothers to feel unsure and shamed about their parenting choices.

I wish I could tell you the movement to *let moms be* has resulted in a rosy world where all parenting trolls say, "You know what, I don't agree with you, but that's okay! I'm sure you have your reasons." But it hasn't. The judgment still exists, and not just on the internet. Family gatherings, mommy-and-me groups, preschools, parks, and all the other places where mothers and offspring congregate can be ground zero for judgment, even from people who know better and mean well. And it will probably always be that way.

So what to do? Luckily, I've developed this fairy dust that you blow in the face of anyone who starts judging your parenting, and they suddenly understand where you're coming from. Or no...maybe I haven't. But wouldn't that be cool?

What's actually cooler is the realization that the only person we need to convince to stop judging us is ourselves. When we figure out how to be solid in our unique parenting choices and realize it's not the right way, or the wrong way, but *our* way, we're free to stop caring (at least as much) about the judgments that come from external sources. It's like my mom said for the entirety of my teen years and was annoyingly right about, "What other people think and say about you has nothing to do with you." You just need to get right with you.

The main reason people judge another's parenting decision is because that decision is different from what they're doing, and they process it as that person implying that they're doing it wrong. Their judgments are essentially saying, "Nah-ah, *I'm* not doing it wrong, *you're* doing it wrong." So ultimately, the judgment comes down to that person's own stuff. I know this because I used to be a big-time judger. I wouldn't do it openly; I would do it behind people's backs like a civilized person. When I finally started looking at why I did that, I realized that every time I judged someone's parenting choice it was because that choice ignited my own insecurity. For example, I had a friend who shared how they no longer let their toddler have screen time because he got too obsessed with it. I was so triggered by this. I immediately went to my husband and was like, "There's no way they're actually doing that. They have to be lying. And if they're not lying, they're just going to make their kid obsessed with screens when they're older because they were deprived as a child." My judgments completely came from the fact that I was feeling guilty about how much screen time I let our son have. But I didn't want to give it up because it made life so much easier. I was fighting hard to feel okay about my choice, even though I didn't. As you can see, those harsh judgments were all about me and my stuff.

What to do

Keep reminding yourself that judgments aren't personal and that you can trust yourself — then try the following:

- **Above all, listen to feedback from your intuition.** You already know the best way to parent your unique child, in the unique circumstances you live in. Deep down, it's all there. But the opinions of others, books by the experts, how we were parented, and various other factors muddy the waters, making us second-guess our decisions.

  To step out of that muddiness and make decisions that feel intuitively right, get into a quiet space and ask yourself about the parenting decision you've been conflicted about. For example, "Where should my baby sleep?" When the voice of your mother or that expert or whomever starts babbling, push them away. Seek the answer that makes your insides happy. When you find the right answer for *you*, your stomach will unclench, your chest will feel light, and your heart will say, "Yes! That feels right!" And you don't have to ask permission to listen to these feelings. You can just do what feels right.

  And the cool thing with decisions is, you can always change them. If you decide cosleeping is right for your family, but then circumstances change and it no longer seems like the best option, you can edit what you're doing. And while many parenting decisions might have to be made with a partner, you'll be able to discuss the options with more clarity when you first determine what decision makes your insides happy.

  Caveat: Some of your decisions will come more from that place in your brain that's craving ease than your deep wells of wisdom — and that's okay. We will never be perfect parents. We will sometimes be like, "Yeah, I know I shouldn't let my kid watch so much *SpongeBob*, but it's saving my sanity right now, so oh well." We've all been there. Heck, I'm there while I type this.

- **If someone's disapproval triggers you, explore that.** When my mom gently insinuates that I might try something different with Hudson, I. Get. So. Angry. Irrationally angry. When I started looking at where that came from, I noticed that the angrier I got over a suggestion, the more my insides (those traitors!) thought she was right. She knows me so well. She knows when I'm not honoring my instincts. And I *hate* when she's right, because obviously we all hate when our moms are right, right?

  So if someone's judgment really ticks you off, explore whether you're being triggered because what they're suggesting is what you actually feel is best deep down, or because it just doesn't feel good to be judged. If it's the latter, remember that their response to your choices has way more to do with them than you, and go on your merry way.

- **Find soothing tools for when you're triggered.** When I feel judged I immediately get defensive. I want to lash out. Sometimes I do lash out. But when I catch myself, I keep my ego from raging by saying, "I hear you, but I really have to pee. Let's press pause on this, and I'll be right back." It sounds ridiculous, but it works like a charm. This protocol gives me the opportunity to be alone and get hold of my emotions. I'm able to step away from what was said and figure out if the person was being hostile, trying to be helpful, or just making an offhand comment they didn't intend as a judgment. Usually, I'm able to come back to the conversation with some perspective and more self-control.

  You certainly don't have to use my "I gotta pee" trick, but I encourage you to make a plan for how you'll respond when judgment causes an ego flare-up.

- **Feel free to *not* share your parenting philosophy.** If you're with someone you know won't understand your parenting choices, you have every right to not discuss them. For example, if your judgy in-laws are constantly asking why you do this or that with your child, you don't have to explain yourself. You can simply say, "It's just something that works for our family. We're not saying it's the way everyone needs to parent, but it's the way we're choosing to parent." If they harp on about what they think you should do or how kids were parented "in their day," feel free to just smile and nod while using your brainpower to figure out which Netflix show to watch tonight, or tell them your tampon is leaking and walk away.

- **Steer clear of toxic parenting spaces, online and IRL.** Certain Facebook groups, some parenting forums, get-togethers with parents you know you aren't aligned with...these are all environments where toxic judgments run amok. While of course there are exceptions, you'd be wise to avoid gatherings you believe will be saturated with strong, maybe even hurtful opinions, especially when you're still trying to figure out how you want to mother. There's nothing wrong with guarding your heart.

- **Broaden your perspective on judgment from loved ones.** The potential exception to my "stay away from toxic environments" spiel is family gatherings. While certain familial situations are definitely toxic and should be avoided, there are others that are uncomfortable just because a family member is having an awkward time being involved in your child's life.

  For example, let's say one of your child's grandparents gets to see them only twice a year. Every time you see that grandparent, they might be full of suggestions for how to parent. You would be within your right to be incredibly irritated by this. But riddle me this — what if the unsolicited advice was the family member's misguided way of feeling more connected to your child? What if they feel that sharing their "wisdom" is a gift that will enhance your family's life? If you suspect this is where a judgy family member is coming from, you might help them find other ways of feeling connected — for example, taking on some feedings or diaper changes or, in the case of older kids, having a few one-on-one outings. If this doesn't stop the "Maybe you should try..." comments, feel free to straight-up tell them that while you respect their insight, you'll let them know if it's needed.
- **Resist the urge to make your own judgments.** While placing judgment can feel so juicy in the moment, the "high" never lasts. Moral of the story: If we don't want others to judge us, we shouldn't judge them. We're all doing the best we can, and we all deserve more understanding and "you do you" from our fellow parents.

75. I have a loved one who had a miscarriage and seems to have a hard time being around my baby. How should I navigate this relationship?

Very gently, and without your defenses up. The reaction your loved one is having has nothing to do with how they feel about you or your baby, and everything to do with their emotions about their pregnancy loss. They are probably navigating immense grief, and being around someone that has the one thing they want most can feel heartbreaking. I learned this the hard way.

One of my closest friends — we'll call her Zoe — had a miscarriage when my son Hudson was two. Zoe and Hudson had an amazing bond that evaporated as soon as she lost her baby. She would tense when Hudson ran to her for a hug, and she avoided his requests to play. He was heartbroken, and I was irritated. "Can't she see that she's hurting his feelings?" I would think. I never said anything, but I'm sure I was giving off a vibe.

I didn't *get it* until I went out to lunch with her one day. Every time we neared a pregnant woman or small child, Zoe would stiffen and look away. When a woman with a stroller sat near us at the restaurant, I noticed her bite her cheek, resisting tears. She was suffering. I had been so wrapped up in how Hudson was responding to her standoffishness that I hadn't really seen her pain. From that point forward, I planned meetups that didn't involve Hudson or the high potential of running into any of her other triggers. I would go over to her house, take her out for a drink, go to a belly dancing class, or do anything that distracted her from motherhood, even if it was only for a few hours. And you can be sure I didn't bring up mom life when we were together.

After Zoe eventually gave birth to a healthy baby girl, she brought up her postmiscarriage reaction to children. "It killed me to not hang out with Hudson, and my sister's kids," she said. "But it all made me angry, and so sad I felt like I couldn't breathe. I wasn't angry at any of you; I was just mad at life, and my body, and how unfair everything felt. You and my sister were my safe places, but when your kids were around, being with either of you sucked." She told me how the situation with her sister was especially complicated because all family gatherings involved her kids. "Of course I didn't expect her to not bring her kids to, like, Easter dinner, but I kind of wish my family would've given me an out for some of those things. I just wanted permission to be sad, and disgruntled, and not show up for a while."

And there it is. She wanted permission from the people who loved her to navigate the miscarriage in whatever way she needed. She didn't want people trying to cheer her up or saying, "That will be you soon enough" when watching kids running around. She wanted people to tell her that everything she was feeling was okay, and they'd be there for her no matter how much or little she needed them. She wanted people to check in, without forcing a hangout.

While every woman handles the loss of a pregnancy in a different way, almost every woman I've known who has navigated miscarriage relates to this story, myself included. They want you to be there for them without unknowingly subjecting them to more pain. Sound tricky? It doesn't have to be.

What to do

Here's how to show up for your loved one during her journey through pain and loss, without sacrificing joy for your journey into motherhood:

- **Let her lead the way.** The person best able to provide insight into how you can support your friend is your friend. Request one-on-one time with her, and ask how you can best support her. You can throw her a major bone by letting her know up front that you're cool hanging without your baby and will do your best to not talk about motherhood, unless she brings it up. This will likely make her feel relieved, as she might have been nervous about making these requests. Letting her know that she can't offend you with her requests will make her feel safe to share and spend time with you.
- **Give her an out.** While you don't want to withhold invitations to gatherings, it's compassionate to let her know you totally get it if she doesn't feel comfortable attending. This helps her feel included, without the pressure. And while it's tempting to say something along the lines of, "You totally don't have to come, but I really hope you do," I would cut out the second half of that sentence. We mean well when letting someone know how much we'd love them to show up, but all it does is put social pressure on them. Instead, convey a message along the lines of, "If *you* want to come, please do. But I also completely understand if you don't feel up for it. Whatever you want is the best decision."
- **Regularly send a "thinking of you" text.** I have a client who experienced a miscarriage, divorce, and cancer diagnosis in the same year. "I felt a big need to go within," she said, reflecting about that year. "I told my people I needed space, and everyone listened. They listened so much that I completely stopped hearing from them. I didn't blame them, because I had pretty much told them to do that — but it made

me feel isolated. Then my cousin started sending short texts. She'd write, 'Hey! You don't need to respond but I just wanted to let you know I love you and am thinking of you.' She would send some variation of that a few times a week. I usually didn't respond, but I appreciated those notes so much. It made me feel like even though I was in a space where I needed solitude, I hadn't been forgotten."

You can be like this cousin, sending loving, no-strings-attached messages to let your friend know she's not alone, even if she wants to physically be alone. If you don't receive a response, it doesn't mean she didn't appreciate the thought. Don't give up on her; just keep letting her know you care.

Tip: Add to your thoughtful texts by occasionally having your friend's favorite treats or flowers sent to her house. You could also send a comfort box from an infant loss support program like Three Little Birds (threelittlebirdsperinatal.org) or a card from the #IHad AMiscarriage line (shop.drjessicazucker.com).

- **Don't bring up your baby unless she does.** Baby-brain tries to wipe the memory of everything but baby topics, which might be the last thing your friend wants to talk about. I used to prepare for meet-ups with friends I assumed didn't want to talk baby by making a list of interests we shared. My overpreparing tendencies would then lead me to Google those topics to come up with interesting stuff to talk about. You obviously don't have to do that, but you might prep yourself to keep anything pregnancy or parenting related from slipping out of your mouth. And of course, your friend may straight-up ask you about, or bring up, baby or parenting topics — if so, share openly, while being careful not to go overboard. Pay attention to her nonverbal cues, slyly shifting the conversation if you notice she is becoming uncomfortable. While the first few conversations with her might feel forced and awkward, you'll eventually become comfortable with the new unspoken guidelines of your relationship.

- **Let her know you're comfortable hearing about what she's going through.** Sadly, some women feel like a pariah after a miscarriage. They feel like people are tiptoeing around them, trying to ignore the death-colored elephant in the room. You can minimize this discomfort and make your friend feel safe to share by asking if she wants to talk about how she's feeling. She might not, but just knowing you're not afraid of the topic might help her feel like she's not an island no boat wants to stop at.

- **Call her baby by name.** If your friend shared the name of her baby, use it when talking with her. This helps convey that you don't think of the miscarriage as trivial, that you understand a child she was deeply connected to passed.

- **Don't feel guilty for your joy.** You have nothing to feel guilty about. You have every right to have a beautiful, healthy baby — and to be happy about that. While you don't have to talk about that beautiful baby with your friend, you do get to feel shame-free gratitude for motherhood.

76. Since giving birth to my second baby, I've been finding my first child kind of irritating. Am I a bad mom for not feeling equal favor for my children?

While most parents swear they feel the same about all their children, that's usually not true. A study published in the *Journal of Family Psychology* found that 74 percent of mothers and 70 percent of fathers reported preferential treatment toward one child. This isn't surprising, as personalities, shifting life circumstances, and a slew of other factors impact how we feel about the people in our life, meaning there will be seasons when we enjoy spending time with some people more than others — and our children aren't immune to this.

While you probably *love* all your children so much you'd die for them, that doesn't mean you equally enjoy spending time with all of them. For example, you might have an adorable baby who can't talk back, a four-year-old who worships the ground you walk on, and a teenager who primarily communicates with eye rolls. Not surprisingly, you'd probably prefer to hang with the little ones. Even if your children are close in age, you'll likely still have your "favorite." Like if the two-year-old has intense emotions that trigger you, and your baby is super mellow, you'll probably favor the baby. There is nothing wrong with any of this. You can love all your children unconditionally while not liking them equally.

Something else to consider is that your older child might be feeling especially "needy" right now. They can sense that your focus has shifted, and they want your attention. Many children, even older ones, often seek this attention by acting out of character or creating disturbances. Essentially, they create circumstances that force you to pay attention to them. And because sleep deprivation and the endless needs of a newborn make it hard to recognize the deeper meaning of these outbursts, it's easy to lash out and create even more of a divide between you and your child. This will probably resolve itself as your family settles into its new structure, but in the meantime, you can call on your partner or other adults close to your older child to spend more time with them. You can also ask these adults to take the baby for short stints so you can spend one-on-one time with your firstborn, even if it's the last thing you want to do. (No judgment!)

It's also important to remember that your favor may shift as you and your children change. As life continues molding your family, you might find that one child's irritating traits are dissolving, while your "favorite" child begins getting under your skin. And remember, that preverbal baby will eventually find their voice, and it's anyone's guess how you'll respond to what they have to say. Isn't parenthood exciting?!

What to do

Keep reminding yourself that while it's totally normal to like one child more than the other, it's still important to not engage in differential treatment (aka treating one child better than the other) and to continually ensure that all your children know how loved they are. These activities can help you do that:

- **Examine what bugs you about the child you don't like as much.** It can feel really icky to not know why you don't like one of your children as much as the other. This not-knowing can lead you to believe you're a bad mom, cold hearted, or just destined to have a tumultuous relationship with that child. I don't think any of that is true. I'll bet there are specific reasons why certain things about your child trigger you. Let's figure out what they are.

    When you find yourself inwardly (or outwardly) rolling your eyes at this child or gritting your teeth, notice that. Press pause and objectively look at what's happening. What about this moment is irritating you? Is your child responding to something in the same way your partner does, a way that you wish they didn't? Are they responding in the opposite way that you would, and that's triggering? Does their behavior remind you of someone you don't like, and that dislike is being reflected onto your child? Does their behavior remind you of flaws in yourself you want to avoid? Is your child acting needy in a moment where you feel stretched thin? Unravel the situation until you figure out what the core source of your annoyance is.

Developing this deeper understanding about your child and how you respond to them will support you with the upcoming activities, and help you realize that neither of you have a fatal flaw or are intentionally trying to irritate one another. You're both just doing your best to feel loved, seen, and heard as your family adapts to the big changes brought on by a new baby.

- **Create intentional opportunities to bond with your not-the-favorite child.** Now that you've started pinpointing why your child irks you, brainstorm activities you can do together that have the lowest potential for irritation. For example, snuggling on the couch and watching a movie, making a smoothie, or building a LEGO tower might be situations that allow you to be together without getting peeved with each other. When it's time to do activities like cleaning up, brushing teeth, getting dressed, or other tasks that typically find you and your child clashing, you could tap out and call in your partner, at least while you have a newborn. While this won't always be possible, being aware of situations that typically cause you to get frustrated with your child, having another adult take on these situations, and investing time in the activities that are usually harmonious can begin shifting your parent-child relationship.
- **Talk with your partner.** If you have a partner in this parenting thing, they can help you see your relationships with your children more clearly. They likely witness your interactions with the kids more than any other adult and can support you in identifying dynamics you're not aware of, or easing up when you're too hard on yourself. For example, they can let you know if your actions make your favoritism clear, and if you're overly harsh with the child that's bugging you. They can also help you make a plan for how the two of you can provide all the

children equal care and attention, which might look like them picking up the slack with the child who's frustrating you, making sure they don't feel neglected.

- **Help your kids feel emotionally safe.** If you sense the child you don't favor as much is picking up on your energy, remind them how much you love them and let them know what's going on — in an age-appropriate way. For example, my friend Amy has an eleven-year-old son who really irritates her. "He is me in a little boy's body," she said. "He's constantly showing me all the things I don't like about myself, and I have no patience for it." Her daughter, on the other hand, has a temperament similar to Amy's husband's. "She's so easy to be with," Amy said. "Sometimes when I'm spending time with her in the morning and her brother wakes up, I feel angry. I feel like he's going to ruin my mood before he even does anything."

Needless to say, Amy was wracked with guilt about this, especially when her son straight-up asked, "Mom, why don't you like me?" Amy was inclined to tell him all the things that would make him feel better, but she decided that would only mask the problem. Instead, she told him that because he was so much like her, he sometimes reminded her of things in herself she wanted to change. She told him it wasn't fair to take this out on him, and asked him to let her know when she was being unkind. He now says, "Mom, are you seeing you in me?" when he senses that he's bugging her.

If Amy's son had been younger, she probably wouldn't have gone into the whole "You remind me of me" thing, as he might not have been able to process that. Instead, she could have acknowledged his feelings, asked questions to get more insight into what was making him feel unliked, and then assured him that things would change.

Above all, stay aware of how you're treating each child so you can avoid hurting anyone, glean insights into how to improve these relationships, and tune in to your children so you can tell when they are in need of reassurance that you love them deeply.

77. My pet used to feel like my child, but now that I have a human child I never want my pet around because I'm nervous they'll hurt the baby. Should I find my pet a new home?

Isn't it wild how having a baby can change your perspective of almost everyone in your life? Especially your animals. It's like one minute your pet is a constant companion and best friend, and then, bam, your baby's born and that pet suddenly feels like a looming threat. This can feel jarring and heartbreaking. While you're celebrating and savoring the new love that's come into your life, you're also mourning the relationship you're losing. Because even if your pet is able to stay in your home, it's unlikely your bond will ever be the same, as you now have a new creature to dote on. On the other hand, if you determine it's safe to keep your pet, their life may become even richer as they develop their own bond with baby. Everyone can win.

Regarding your fear of your pet hurting the baby, there's no guarantee either way. But there are ways to objectively look at the situation and make a decision that's best for all involved. And luckily, it's not very often that a family needs to remove a pet from their home for baby's safety. In most cases, training, limiting and/or supervising your fur-baby's contact with your human baby, and taking other precautions can ensure your baby's safety without the need to say goodbye to your pet.

What to do

Here are some ideas to keep your baby safe while also nurturing your pet's well-being:

- **Consider whether your pet has ever been violent.** One of the best ways to determine if your pet will cause harm to your baby is to review their history. Has your pet been aggressive toward other animals or humans? How do they react to children? Is there anything about their personality or history that would lead you to believe they might cause harm to your baby? Answering these questions honestly can be an important first step in making your final decision about rehoming.
- **Hire a trainer.** A trainer can not only help your pet break bad habits but can also help you determine if they're a threat to your baby, as animal trainers are often experts in the behaviors of their animal-of-choice and know the signs that indicate an animal could be a danger to others. If the trainer believes your pet is safe to stay in your home, and you agree, you can ask them to help your pet break certain habits to

create a safer environment for baby. For example, if you have a dog that jumps on people, is used to sleeping on your bed and getting on other furniture, and normally goes into the room that is now the nursery, the trainer can help you teach them that those habits are no longer allowed. If you're reading this during pregnancy, I recommend working with a trainer before baby is born.

- **Introduce your pet to baby's scent.** As most animals have a heightened sense of smell, prepare your pet for the array of new odors baby will supply by having them smell an article of clothing that the baby has worn, before they meet the baby. Pet them as they're taking a whiff, as this can help them create positive associations with the baby's scent.

- **Don't leave your pet alone with the baby.** Make sure you're always present when your pet and baby are near one another. Both children and animals can be erratic, so you'll want to monitor all interactions until your baby is much older. In addition, begin teaching your baby that it's not okay to pull the dog or cat's tail, for example, by gently removing their hand if such an action occurs.

- **Stay aware of your pet's emotions.** Keep an eye on how your pet responds when they hear baby cry, for example, or when they're simply around baby. Is their personality unchanged? Are they acting more aggressive or skittish than usual? Do they seem depressed? Do they shake or show other signs of anxiety when baby cries? Are they indicating stress by averting their eyes or moving away when baby is around? Your observations can inform how you navigate their relationship with your baby. A trainer can also provide invaluable insight into what various behaviors indicate, and what, if anything, should be done.

    Tip: You can prepare your pet for your baby's cries and other noises by playing recordings of baby sounds when you're pregnant. It can be telling to see how they respond to the recording.

- **Organize extra care for your pet.** Because your pets will likely be dealing with emotions that range from irritation to depression as your attention shifts from them to the baby, ensure they still feel the love by asking friends or family members to spend time with them during the first few weeks postpartum. If you have a dog, find people who can take them for a walk or a romp at the dog park. If you have a cat, ask a fellow cat lover to come over and give them attention. And of course, whenever possible, remind your pets they're still important to you by carving out bits of time throughout the day to spend with them. In addition, when your pet is with you and baby, be sure to also pay attention to them so they don't feel jealous of the baby.

- **Ease into baby-pet interactions.** When you've determined it's safe to allow your pet to meet your baby, take it slow. Start by having someone hold your pet while you hold the baby, and allow the pet to slowly move toward the baby. They'll likely sniff them, and maybe give a little lick. During this initial interaction (and all the following) stay as calm as possible, as pets and babies are sensitive to our energy and will react accordingly. A tense mood makes everyone else tense. So take deep breaths, and trust that the meeting will go great.
- **Read *Good Dog, Happy Baby*.** This excellent book by dog trainer Michael Wombacher provides an effective twelve-step process for preparing your dog and family for a new baby.
- **Know that you're not a horrible person if you need to find your furbaby a new home.** As heartbreaking as it is to determine your baby really isn't safe around your pet, the decision to find them a new home will be best for all involved. Not only will you be keeping your baby safe, but you'll also be ensuring your pet doesn't spend the rest of their life being scolded and shut off from the family, and you won't have to suffer the distress of being the one to hand out that punishment. While it's devastating to say goodbye, you're ultimately doing right by all involved.

Fears and Worries

78. The thought of sudden infant death syndrome (SIDS) keeps me up at night. Why does it happen, and how can I prevent it?

I was so afraid of SIDS, I couldn't fall asleep the first night of Hudson's life. When I couldn't hear him breathing, I placed my hand under his nostrils, waiting for the small puff of warm air that would confirm he was still alive. The fear of SIDS would have kept me from sleeping all through the next few months if the bone-deep exhaustion of motherhood hadn't pulled me under. While many people talk about how amazing life is when a baby sleeps, my baby sleeping was one of my biggest sources of anxiety. And really, how could we not be terrified of SIDS? Defined as the sudden, unexplained death of an infant under the age of one, SIDS usually occurs when the baby stops breathing during sleep. Understandably, we want to figure out why it happens, and how we can prevent it.

While there's been significant research on the topic, there's still not a clear understanding of why it happens. But there are many theories, and these have led to certain safeguards we can implement to minimize the risk of this heartbreak striking our families.

The common SIDS risk factors are listed in the sidebar below. But before we get into that, I want to note that rarely does one factor cause SIDS. Often, the following elements must be present for SIDS to occur — if just one is removed, SIDS is much less likely to occur:

- **Vulnerability:** A defect or brain abnormality that impacts a baby's heart or lung function (such as the serotonin condition described below) can make them more susceptible to SIDS. Essentially, this vulnerability makes it more difficult for the body of a baby faced with an environmental complication (see below) to trigger a protective response.
- **Environmental complication:** While most babies can manage environmental complications like lying facedown on a mattress or overheating, babies who are vulnerable and are six months old or younger are less able to respond protectively and so are at higher risk for SIDS.
- **Developmental changes:** Infants six months old and younger experience rapid growth and change. These changes could temporarily

disrupt internal systems that impact breathing. This is one reason why SIDS is most common in babies between the ages of two and six months.

There's not much you can do about baby's vulnerability or age, but the "What to do" section (pages 224–26) helps you cancel out most environmental complications.

Common SIDS Risk Factors

Here are many of the most common risk factors for SIDS:

- **Issue with serotonin-producing neurons:** Properly working serotonin neurons are needed to maintain the continued functioning of the heart and lungs. Here's how it works: The brain facilitates the flow of oxygen to the heart and lungs. If someone has sleep apnea, for example, they stop breathing, and the brain gets alerted that there's not enough oxygen and too much carbon dioxide. Then the brain triggers a protective process called *autoresuscitation*, which usually consists of big gasps.

  The belief is that in some cases of SIDS this protective mechanism is not triggered. A study done by Harvard Medical School found that when serotonin-producing neurons are inhibited, the brain's ability to autoresuscitate and save the body from apnea is impeded. Continued research could lead to screening that might help detect infants at higher risk for SIDS.
- **Sleeping facedown:** According to the book *SIDS Sudden Infant and Early Childhood Death: The Past, the Present, and the Future*, the prone (facedown) position has been found to increase the risk of rebreathing expired gases, overheating, and accidental suffocation. Placing an infant on their side to sleep is also not recommended. In 1994, a campaign called "Back to Sleep" was launched, urging parents to lay babies on their back for sleep. This lowered the rate of SIDS by 50 percent.

- **Sleeping on a soft surface, or near soft objects:** A soft sleep surface or objects that could cover a baby's face (like blankets, pillows, or stuffed animals) increase the risk for accidental suffocation and overheating.
- **Rebreathing:** This consists of a baby breathing in the air they just exhaled, which causes oxygen levels to drop and carbon dioxide to rise. Putting a baby to sleep on their stomach or having a blanket or other soft material in the crib that can cover their face can result in rebreathing.
- **Overheating:** As overheating could cause respiratory issues or depress a baby's ability to wake up, it's been found to be a risk factor for SIDS.
- **Respiratory infection:** An article published in the medical journal *Hippokratia* found that a mild degree of respiratory viral infection was observed in 80 percent of SIDS cases. In addition, a study published in *Immunopharmacology and Immunotoxicology* reported that common bacterial toxins found in the respiratory tract, in association with a viral infection, could contribute to SIDS in an infant during a developmentally vulnerable period. An infection can be especially dangerous for a baby sleeping on their stomach, as this prone position could increase airway temperature and stimulate bacterial colonization and bacterial toxin production.
- **Maternal smoking and secondhand smoke:** Maternal smoking during pregnancy is considered one of the greatest risk factors for SIDS, as it can lead to premature birth and low birth weight (both risk factors for SIDS), diminish lung growth, increase the chance of developing respiratory infections, and impair the baby's ability to wake themselves. And exposure to secondhand smoke after birth could impact the baby's inflammatory response during an infection and limit their body's ability to respond to threats to the heart caused by inflammation.

- **Being born prematurely:** A study published in the journal *Pediatrics* found that many premature babies have impaired blood pressure control, meaning if they have a drop in blood pressure during sleep, their body wouldn't be able to quickly respond. In addition, premature babies often have a higher risk of developing respiratory distress, do not have strong sucking and swallowing reflexes, and have a higher risk of infection because of an underdeveloped immune system.
- **Long QT syndrome:** This heart rhythm condition can potentially cause fatal arrhythmia — when the heart beats too fast or slow or has an irregular pattern. According to a study in *Journal of Biological Research*, long QT syndrome accounts for 12 percent of SIDS cases.
- **Toxins from the mattress:** While I want to be super clear that this theory hasn't been thoroughly tested, I think it's worth sharing. A New Zealand scientist and chemist, Dr. James Sprott, believes the phosphorus, arsenic, and antimony found in some fire retardants used on crib mattresses can mix with mold created from the baby's urine, spit-up, and drool to create toxic gas. He believes the inhalation of this gas could contribute to SIDS. An additional theory is that body heat can contribute to the release of volatile organic compounds (VOCs) in mattresses.

  Again, this theory hasn't been conclusively proven, but I think it's worth it to bypass this potential risk by purchasing an organic crib mattress from a company that's Global Organic Textile Standard (GOTS) certified. If that's too pricey, you may be able to prevent the release of these gases with a mattress cover specifically designed to block toxic gases. (If you're wondering where the information about cosleeping is, go to question 97.)

As research continues, new potential causes of SIDS will likely be revealed. Your care provider can provide information about the most up-to-date SIDS research.

What to do

While there's no foolproof way to prevent SIDS, the following can help you significantly reduce your baby's risk:

- **Practice healthy habits during pregnancy.** The American Academy of Pediatrics reports that babies of women who obtain regular prenatal care, do not smoke, and abstain from regular illicit drug and alcohol use during pregnancy have a lower risk for SIDS.
- **Put baby on their back for sleep.** Even if your baby seems to be more soothed on their stomach, always put them to sleep on their back.
- **Breastfeed.** The American Academy of Pediatrics states that babies who are exclusively breastfed have a 50 percent lower risk of SIDS, as breastfeeding provides the following benefits:
  - Supports the baby's ability to arouse from sleep more easily
  - Decreases incidence of diarrhea, upper and lower respiratory infections, and other infectious diseases
  - Supports the overall immune system
  - Helps the brain systems that control breathing to mature
  - Minimizes allergies that could cause inflammation in air passageways
  - Reduces gastroesophageal reflux
  - Supports the development of the oral cavity and throat muscles, helping to keep the airway open
  - Enhances the mother's awareness of the baby
- **Ensure that the crib is empty, and use a sleepsack.** Have baby sleep on a firm mattress with a fitted sheet — there should be nothing else in the crib, not even crib bumpers. Regarding clothing, put baby in a breathable sleepsack, which is a "wearable blanket." This allows them to stay warm without using a blanket that could bunch up around their face. If the weather is so warm that you yourself are using little more than a sheet for coverage, your baby will likely be fine in a onesie or a light sleepsack.
- **Create a cool environment.** As it's important to prevent overheating, keep the thermostat between sixty-eight and seventy-two degrees Fahrenheit, have a fan on in baby's sleep area, and clothe them in the aforementioned sleepsack or onesie. In addition, it's not advised to put them to sleep in a hat, as it can trap heat.

- **Open windows when weather permits.** Fresh air helps keep the air in baby's sleep environment cool and clean, minimizing SIDS risk factors. If the weather allows and you feel it's safe, open the windows in your baby's sleep zone, being sure to insert a window guard when they become mobile.

- **Cleanse air with plants and an air purifier.** Enhance the cleanliness of the air in baby's room by using an air purifier and placing one or two air-purifying plants in areas of the room they can't reach. Plants that can cleanse the air of harmful toxins, like trichloroethylene, formaldehyde, benzene, and xylene, include the peace lily, gerbera daisy, florist's chrysanthemum, red-edged dracaena, and English ivy.

- **Use a firm, GOTS-certified organic crib mattress or a toxin-resistant mattress cover.** As the toxins in standard mattresses might increase the risk of SIDS, opt for a GOTS-certified organic crib mattress or wrap the mattress in a cover that's a "toxic gas shield."

- **Make sure baby's bed adheres to Consumer Product Safety Commission (CPSC) guidelines.** A government organization that oversees products sold in the United States, the CPSC provides recommendations for purchasing a safe infant bed; see "Safe Sleep — Cribs and Infant Products Information Center" at cpsc.gov/SafeSleep.

- **Skip swaddling.** While the research is ongoing, a study published in *Pediatrics* found that swaddling might increase the risk for SIDS, as it could hinder a baby's ability to wake up during cardiovascular stress.

- **Have baby sleep in your room for at least the first year of life.** A report by the American Academy of Pediatrics recommends that babies sleep in their parents' room for the first twelve months, as this can reduce SIDS by up to 50 percent. While there's not a definitive reason for this outcome, it's believed that a baby will arouse from sleep easier when sleeping in a room with others, and that parents are better able to monitor the baby when they're in the same room.

- **Consider a bedside sleeper.** These aptly named baby beds are essentially bassinets that can be pushed up next to your bed and readjusted so baby is level with you. Some also have a side that can fold down, allowing you to easily access baby. If you go this route, make sure you select a bed that meets CPSC safety standards. Ideally, it will have a thin and firm mattress that's no more than an inch thick. In addition, net or mesh walls are preferred, as they increase airflow.

- **Stay away from cigarette smoke.** As breathing in secondhand smoke can be incredibly harmful to infants, remove your baby from any area where someone is smoking. And because smoke can linger on furniture, carpet, and other material, it's best to not have baby in the home of a smoker, which is why it's strongly advised that any smoker who lives in the same home as an infant quit smoking. In addition, do not let anyone who smokes hold baby, as smoke can linger in hair and clothes.

- **Ensure that all babysitters and childcare facilities you utilize follow these safety guidelines.** Whenever anyone else will be caring for baby, make sure they adhere to this sleeping protocol. If baby will be at a day care, have someone there walk you through their protocol. You can also stop in during naptime to see them in action.

    The same goes for a babysitter; walk them through your sleepy-time routine, ensuring they understand its importance by having them repeat it back to you. You can also provide a simple written reminder. For example, "Put baby to sleep on their back, in their designated, empty bed, without a blanket and in a sleepsack or onesie, depending on temperature. And turn on the fan."

    If a parent or in-law seems resistant, remind them that this is not a request. While they might have done things differently when their children were infants, it's up to you how your child is put to sleep.

- **Contact your pediatrician if baby seems to have respiratory issues.** As respiratory issues can be a SIDS risk factor, contact your care provider if baby has a cough, breathing issues, or any symptom that concerns you.

79. I have horrific thoughts about awful things happening to my baby. Sometimes I imagine being the person inflicting harm. Am I crazy? Am I a danger to my baby?

I would stop breathing whenever I let myself think about something horrible happening to my baby. Leukemia. A deadly car accident. SIDS. A kitchen accident. The list goes on. The thoughts would slam into me out of nowhere. One time, I was changing Hudson's diaper and had a vision of him and Eric being in a lethal head-on collision. I froze. Diaper in midair. I was there. Feeling all the feelings I assume I would feel if that — the worst — happened. Then Hudson peed on me, and I snapped out of it. These thoughts didn't come every day, but they came often enough that I had to build walls. I refused to let my mind go there. And if it tried, I would combat it with heavy-duty distraction.

When the distractions got too exhausting and less effective, I saw a therapist. She helped me find a balance between running from the nightmares and letting them swallow me. She also helped me recognize that *feeling* like something horrible was about to happen didn't mean anything was actually going to happen. It was just a false thought triggered by the facts that my newborn was so vulnerable and I was almost entirely responsible for keeping him alive. She offered heaps of techniques, and I tried them all. The ones that worked are in the upcoming "What to do" section. But according to the therapist, what I experienced was pretty mild. Some women get so buried in nightmarish thoughts about their baby they can barely function.

One of the most frightening mental phenomena some new parents experience is thoughts of intentionally or accidentally harming, or even killing, their child — a type of something labeled "intrusive thoughts." Most report that they don't actually *want* to harm their baby but still have vivid thoughts of doing so. These thoughts can really become frightening for a parent when they're doing something like bathing their baby, driving with them, or partaking in other activities that present obvious risks. It can cause an almost constant state of paranoia, and keeping things under control can take debilitating amounts of energy. For obvious reasons, this is a mental state parents rarely tell anyone about, out of fear their baby will be taken away. But what many don't realize is that these thoughts are more common than you'd expect. A study published in *BMC Psychiatry* found that between 70 and 100 percent of new mothers report unwanted intrusive thoughts of infant-related harm, and half of all new mothers have intrusive thoughts about harming their infant on purpose. These thoughts don't make you a monster; they're just a sign you're experiencing a very treatable psychological condition. Any mental health specialist worth their salt will not even think of reporting you, as long as you can honestly acknowledge that you find the intrusive thoughts disturbing.

When these intrusive thoughts become consistent and regularly impact your ability to function, they might be a sign of postpartum obsessive compulsive disorder (OCD). This can manifest as obsessive attempts to suppress the intrusive thoughts, partaking in obsessive rituals that you are convinced will prevent harm from befalling your baby (like constantly praying or checking on them), or avoiding triggering situations like bathing the baby or driving with them. Not surprisingly, OCD has been connected to issues with serotonin regulation and elevated levels of oxytocin — both of which are hormones impacted during pregnancy and the postpartum period. Obsessions with intrusive thoughts can also be triggered by stressful situations and a rapid increase in responsibility, which are both major elements of early parenthood. Because of these factors, some mental health specialists believe slight OCD tendencies might be a normal by-product of the postpartum experience.

The rarest but most serious cause of these violent thoughts is postpartum psychosis. This condition usually consists of an inclination to harm the baby, extreme paranoia, hallucinations and delusions, sleep disturbances, and disorientation. It typically presents within a week of the baby's birth. Unlike moms with conditions like postpartum OCD, those with postpartum psychosis rarely realize that they shouldn't be having thoughts of harming their baby — they don't find the thoughts terrifying or appalling. This is a situation that requires immediate intervention.

What to do

If the thoughts you're experiencing are limiting your ability to function, get support from a perinatal mental health specialist. They will likely recommend cognitive behavioral therapy, and they might recommend medication. Follow their advice before you try any of the other suggestions listed below, as you deserve the support of a mental health specialist who can take the unique circumstances you're working with and help you craft a customized treatment plan. They can also help you normalize what you're experiencing, which can be an immense relief.

With that said, I want to acknowledge that summoning the courage to tell someone about your intrusive thoughts can be one of the most challenging things you ever do. The good news is, a condition like postpartum OCD is no longer seen as a "scarlet letter." Ongoing research is helping us understand that these conditions are not signs that someone is a dangerous miscreant, but rather they're symptoms exhibited by a perfectly normal human experiencing a treatable psychological phenomenon. There's no shame in speaking up and accepting help. And in the most extreme cases, speaking up might save the life of you or your baby. From there, consider the following:

- **Remember that the thoughts aren't "real."** One of the only good things about horrific thoughts about your baby is that they're likely a shocking contrast to your other thoughts. This contrast can make it easier to pinpoint when a thought is intrusive — aka a thought that is produced not by the real you but by the condition you're navigating (e.g., OCD, anxiety, or depression). This realization can help you separate from the thoughts and remember that they're not indications of something you will do, or even want to do, and they aren't markers of how you feel about your baby.
- **Write down what's true.** If you start getting lost in all the horrible things that could happen, home in on what's actually real by writing it down. For example, you might write, "I grew and birthed my baby — that wasn't easy; it took strength and courage. I provide a home and nourishment for my baby. I'm not broken. These thoughts aren't me. These thoughts aren't true. I love my baby. That's true." Keep writing until you feel firmly planted in your truth.
- **Bring yourself back to reality with your five senses.** Another way to pull your mind out of a swirl of worst-case what-ifs is asking, "What do I see, smell, taste, hear, and feel?" Keep listing things your senses are experiencing until the intrusive thoughts loosen their grip.
- **Remind yourself that you're not crazy.** When you have intrusive thoughts, you're experiencing a symptom, just like someone with the flu experiences the symptom of a fever. And just as the flu can strike anyone, intrusive thoughts can strike anyone. So when you have the symptom of intrusive thoughts, continually remind yourself that you're a whole, amazing person having an uncomfortable experience that will pass with the right support. And as long as you recognize that the thoughts are disturbing and are nothing you should act upon, you're doing fine, as this is an indicator that you're not experiencing postpartum psychosis. Of course, these thoughts aren't fun, and they

could be a sign of postpartum OCD, an anxiety disorder, or post-partum depression, so get that support, mama.

- **Find a support group.** In addition to seeking support from a perinatal mental health specialist, it can be helpful to find an in-person or online support group composed of women having similar thoughts. This can help you feel less alone, normalize your experience, and help you develop a deeper understanding of what you're going through. To ensure you find a quality group, ask your therapist for recommendations.

80. Sometimes I fantasize about running away. Do I need help?

When I was a new mom, I fantasized about running away to a beachside hotel and sleeping until I no longer felt like I was living underwater. I had it all planned. I would loot my savings so I could pay the hotel in cash and no one could track me through my credit card. I would leave my cell phone under my mattress with a note saying, "I'm alive, but barely, and I'll return when I'm ready." The closest I got to this was stopping at the beach parking lot on my way home from Target one day, rolling down the windows, and sleeping for thirty minutes. Most new moms, as well as veteran moms, admit similar fantasies. So we're not alone.

But just because we're not alone doesn't mean it feels good to want to run away from our lives. Something that might help you feel better is knowing most moms that have the running-away fantasy don't actually want to ditch their families forever; they're just looking for a few hours (okay, maybe a few days) where they don't have to take care of anyone's needs but their own. They want some precious time to screw their head back on. To get so deeply asleep they're facedown, drooling into a pillow in a pitch-black air-conditioned hotel room. To order room service. To remember what their dreams are. To take a shower, or a poop, without someone crying for them. I think this is a totally normal, valid fantasy.

With that said, if you feel like you want to run away because it seems you're of no value to your family, you feel too sad or anxious to care for anyone, or you've become so obsessed with thoughts of running away it becomes hard to function, you might be experiencing postpartum depression, anxiety, or OCD. In that case, a perinatal mental health specialist is the person to see. They can help you figure out what's going on and provide specialized support.

What to do

Recognize that this fantasy is not a sign that you weren't meant to be a mother; instead it's trying to guide you toward a life where your needs are honored. Here's how to listen to that guidance:

- **Let yourself feel entitled to help and alone time.** Some women think they should thank their lucky stars when someone steps in to help with their baby. Or that they need to sing their partner's praises when they offer to hold the baby while mama sleeps. While it's fine to feel thankful and express that thanks, you should also *expect* this support, and even demand it. It shouldn't be something you stumble upon as often as you find a leprechaun passing out Xanax at the end of a rainbow. You should stumble upon help and time for yourself as often as you throw a load of spit-up-stained shirts into the wash.

  What I'm saying is, when you start fantasizing about running away, make a clear plan with your partner or your go-to baby-care person about when you need them to take baby, and for how long. Some women feel that in asking their partner for this support they're asking for a favor, but no. You're not asking for a favor. You're asking your *partner* to provide something that is your right, not a privilege. So as uncomfortable as this might initially be, I encourage you to clearly let them know what you need, instead of asking if it's something they'd be willing to do. Claim your right for support.

- **Fulfill your fantasy.** Because the fantasy of playing hooky from your life is usually sparked by a need for alone time, grab it by the horns. When your baby is an infant and incredibly dependent on you, maybe the most you can hope for is a few hours out of the house. But you should take it! Use that time to get a massage; bring a blanket to the beach or a local park, lie down, and sleep in the fresh air; or take your journal or laptop to a coffee shop and write. Do that thing you really want to do but keep thinking, "Nah, I don't have enough time."

  When baby is a bit older and can survive without you for a night, consider booking a hotel room (and using it). And yes, there will probably be guilt and hesitancy and all that other mom stuff when you prepare to leave, but if you can force yourself to get to that hotel and fully focus on *you* for twenty-four hours, you'll return as You 2.0.

- **Learn from your fantasy.** Do me a favor and take a minute to envision what you would do after running away. After you take care of the basics like sleeping, eating, bathing, and maybe having a good cry, what do you see yourself doing? What are the things you would do to make yourself happy if you had no one else to care for? Let yourself go there, then write down what you see.

I did this when Hudson was a newborn, and I saw myself going on sunrise beach runs, taking long showers, sipping coffee while getting absorbed in a writing project, napping, watching some good ole reality television, and eating dessert I didn't have to share. It was pretty basic stuff. What I realized was that while I wasn't at a place where I could check off all those activities every day, I could sprinkle them in. So from that point on I committed to doing at least one activity from my fantasy list each day, and it was life changing. I now have a seven-year-old and am thrilled to say I usually do some version of everything on my fantasy list every day. And I didn't have to run away from my family to do it!

So use your fantasy, mama. Use it to inform how you start blending your fantasy world with your real world.

- **Let yourself do less.** I'll bet that when you envisioned your fantasy you saw yourself juggling way less than you are now. There's a reason for that. Moms are taught to stretch ourselves so thin we're transparent. Cook fresh, organic food. Exercise. Feed baby on demand. Never let them sit in a wet diaper for longer than 3.5 minutes. Maintain a clean, organized home. Call your mom. Keep a foot in your career. Nurture your romantic relationship. Shower. Brush hair. Have a bowel movement. Burp baby. Sleep. (Wait, no, scratch that.) Oy vey. It's just so much. But here's a wild idea. What if you let yourself just cross *some* of the stuff off the list? (At least for now, when baby is such a fresh human and so demanding.) What if you asked someone else to do the cleaning and grocery shopping? What if you let yourself do less and know that it's not giving up, but getting smart? Try it out for a week and see how it feels.
- **Tell someone where you're going.** I know a few women who went to the grocery store and ended up at a local hotel. In all cases but one, the women called their partner to let them know where they were. While those were awkward conversations, the partners at least knew

they were safe. In one situation, the mom did not inform anyone and turned her phone off. Her sister found her right before her husband called the police. Don't let that happen to you — it will just cause more stress. Play hooky if you feel you have no other choice, but make sure the person caring for your baby knows what's up.

81. I had a horrible childhood and am afraid I'll replicate that with my child, as I have no good parenting role models. Am I destined to be a bad parent?

The fact that you want to step away from the negative parenting patterns of your parents is amazing — you've already taken a huge leap away from those patterns. Many people grow up in dysfunctional households and never identify what they should try to do differently with their children. You're in an eyes-wide-open position that's filled with possibility.

I also invite you to consider that your horrible childhood can be a blessing as well as a curse when it comes to parenting your child. It's a blessing because you *get* to start from scratch, and a curse because you *have* to start from scratch. Regarding the blessing, you have a clean slate you get to fill with your own way of parenting. You get to seek out parenting philosophies that resonate with you, then use pieces of these philosophies to craft your own. It can be an exciting, enlightening process. Regarding the curse, the idea of starting from square one can feel overwhelming. You don't have positive parenting presets. You don't have memories filled with happy parenting moments to lean on. You — and your partner, if you have one — are tasked with starting from the beginning. Again, a blessing and a curse.

What to do

Stand firm in the knowing that you're in no way destined to be a bad parent. You are a wholly unique human who gets to make her own decisions. The dated belief that all women turn into their mothers is ridiculous — you get to choose who you become. You get to choose how you want to parent. The following ideas will help you get on the path that will shape you into the amazing parent you're destined to be:

- **Get specific about parenting traits you don't want to repeat.** While you realize you don't want to parent like your parents, it can be helpful to break down exactly what it is they did or didn't do that you found damaging. For example, did they ignore you, talk down to you, use corporal punishment, withhold affection, leave you home alone before you were old enough to care for yourself, shame you?

  As painful as it might be to dredge this all up, it can be liberating to explore what your parents did and how it impacted you, so you develop a clear picture of how you want to parent. And if you find this difficult to do on your own, seek out the support of a mental health specialist, especially if you experienced abuse.

- **Determine the type of parent you want to be.** Once you pinpoint the parenting methods you don't want to use, it'll be easier to determine what methods you want to try. A good place to start is figuring out what the opposite of the negative parenting methods you listed would be. For example, you might list, "actively listening, building up the child's confidence, using communication instead of physical force to discipline, being openly affectionate, never leaving the child alone (until they're old enough) or with iffy childcare, supporting the child in navigating failure without shame," and so on.

- **Research.** The parenting methods you list in the previous step will probably reveal parenting topics you want to learn more about. For example, maybe you're unsure what nonviolent communication is, are at a loss about compassionate ways to discipline, and want to discover how to be more comfortable with physical affection. Start researching the topics you're drawn to, and take note of all the ideas and methods you want to try. This will be an ongoing activity, as what works for your family will shift over the years. But every minute of research adds to your base of knowledge and enhances your dedication to being a loving parent. There's a list of helpful parenting classes and books in the "Recommended Resources" section on page 337 to get you started.

  In addition to this traditional research, you can research parents you respect. For example, if you appreciate the way your partner's sister parents, you can spend time observing what she does and doesn't do, and ask questions about her parenting philosophy. The more you're around parents who show there's a better way, the more you'll develop confidence that you can also choose a better way.

- **Don't forget about your intuition.** While I'm all about that research, I'm also a big believer in your intuition. The fact that you recognize the damaging aspects of your childhood probably means you're in tune with your emotions and gut instincts about what feels right and wrong to you. Lean on these instincts as you navigate parenting.

  For example, when your child is a toddler and they become upset for no apparent reason, you'll likely have an instinct about how you can support them. And sure, this instinct might be informed by the parenting research you've done, but it's mainly coming from your inner knowing — your ability to tune in to your child and support them in the way that works best for both of you. In some ways, the most important thing you can do as a parent is learn to trust your intuition, and take the time to listen to it when parenting decisions arise.

- **Stay aware of any impulses to emulate unwanted parenting habits passed on by your parents.** As strong as your loving intuition is, it's not perfect and will sometimes give way to subconscious habits learned from your parents. But all is not lost if that happens. It simply means you're a human who — like every other human — inherited a few of your parent's habits. The cool thing is, habits can be changed when they're noticed. So whenever you have a parenting moment that makes you feel icky, analyze it. For example, if your child is being very persistent about their need for attention, and you snap at them in the way your mother used to snap at you, clock that. You might think, "Hmm, it's interesting that I responded in that way. How can I stay more calm next time, and respond in a way I feel good about?"

  The tricky thing is, it can be hard to have this insight when we're stressed, as stress can automatically push us into ways of being and thinking we learned as a child. However, developing the habit of using stress-relieving tools like breathing or walking away from a situation until you've calmed down helps you step out of the responses your parents ingrained in you, and choose something else.

  Essentially, managing stress and keeping your eyes open to the negative influences of your parents' parenting are two of the best ways to prevent your parents' unwanted influence from bleeding into your parenting experience.

- **Be wary of your parents' current influence.** If your parents are a regular fixture in your life, stay attuned to whether your parenting habits change when they're around. For instance, I have a friend who had a painful childhood and spent years working through her issues with her parents. She eventually got to a place where she could have them in her home for visits — her children were four and eight when these visits began.

What she realized was that she changed the way she treated her children when her parents were around. She either reverted to parenting methods they had used, or went overboard with the new methods she'd learned. "It was like I left my rational mind and based my parenting on their reactions to my children," she said. "I either wanted to please them, or show them I was a better parent than they were. My kids and husband started dreading visits from them because it changed me so much."

It got so bad she had a sit-down with her parents. She told them how she felt when they were around and explained that if the visits were to continue, they had to hold their judgments and let her parent the way her children were used to. This didn't immediately solve all the issues, but it set guidelines that helped prevent her parents' influence from derailing her thoughtful parenting choices.

- **Know that you won't be a perfect parent, and that's okay.** No matter how much effort you put into being an amazing parent, you will make mistakes. Your kids will yell at you, you might yell back, some doors will be slammed, and tears will be shed. This is an inevitable part of parenting, and something no one escapes. When this happens, I encourage you to not punish yourself with guilt and shame, but instead to chalk it up to one of those good ole learning moments and move on. The less time you spend lamenting your parenting mistakes, the more time you can spend loving on your children and yourself.

82. Until my baby is vaccinated, I don't feel comfortable taking them out of the house or exposing them to anyone but my partner and me. Am I being paranoid?

I don't think you're being paranoid. But let's peel back the surface of your feelings by considering a few things. First, if your baby has a compromised immune system, it's wise to be cautious about being around too many people until they're less vulnerable. And if you're in the thick of flu season or have family members who have been battling a "bug," it's best to avoid exposure for you and baby.

If you have a healthy baby, you're likely fine to go out. This is especially true if you're breastfeeding, as breastmilk fills your baby with antibodies and other goodies that work wonders at protecting them from harm, at least for a few months. The one "going out" caveat is that you might want to avoid incredibly crowded areas, like theme parks, malls, and cruise ships, for example, as these are the types of environments that can breed the spread of infection.

With that said, consider whether your hesitancy to leave the house or have people over also has to do with your need to integrate with all the changes you're going through. Becoming a parent is one of the most massive, sudden transformations a human can go through, which makes it natural to want to pause interaction with the outside world until you get your bearings.

Whatever your reasoning, I recommend following your instincts. If you're yearning to leave the house but guilt over exposing baby to a virus is holding you back, get creative about safe ways to go out. For example, you could go on walks, so long as you have a hard line with strangers trying to touch baby, which strangely happens more than you'd expect — people see something cute and want to touch. You could also meet friends for a picnic at the park or go to an uncrowded restaurant and sit on the patio. Essentially, choose activities that allow you to be outside, without having close contact with others.

If you want people to come over but worry about invisible dangers they might carry into your home, be strict about them washing their hands as soon as they arrive and holding off on coming over if they're sick. Your pediatrician can also let you know if there are vaccinations you should confirm that others have before coming over. For example, whooping cough was a big problem when Hudson was born, so I and everyone who would be frequenting our house were vaccinated with Tdap before he was born. In addition to all that, you have every right to not allow anyone to hold the baby.

That's my long way of saying that what you're feeling is your maternal instincts giving you a strong signal that you should explore.

What to do

After contemplating where your hesitation to go out with baby or have people over is coming from, consider the following actions, as they can provide a welcome sense of security:

- **Get a recommendation from your pediatrician.** If you're raring to get out but fear keeps popping up, ask your baby's pediatrician for their suggestion. They can guide you based on your baby's unique health circumstances and any public health concerns you should be aware of.

  For example, I'm writing this during the Covid-19 outbreak; for obvious reasons, this pandemic makes it easy to decide whether to go out or not. But even when we're not in the midst of a pandemic, flu season and a flare-up of other viruses could cause the pediatrician to advise you to stay close to home for a while. Regardless of their recommendation, you'll likely have more clarity after the chat.

- **Breastfeed.** While breastfeeding isn't a substitute for vaccinations, the milk does give baby an extra layer of protection for about six months after birth. Breastmilk does this by providing antibodies that support the immune system and protect against diseases you have had or have been vaccinated for. These antibodies can bind to potential pathogens and prevent their attachment to the baby's cells. In addition, breastfeeding can enhance the baby's response to certain vaccines.

- **Get vaccinated.** Protecting yourself is one of the best ways to protect your baby. So confirm with your care provider that you're up to date on vaccinations, and ask if they recommend any new ones. Many advise pregnant women to get a Tdap vaccine and a flu shot during pregnancy.

- **Don't let others touch baby until they've washed their hands.** Because close contact, touch in particular, is one of the main ways viruses spread, require anyone who wants to hold baby, or even just touch them, to wash their hands for at least twenty seconds first. And remember, you have every right to not allow others to hold or touch baby if you're uncomfortable with it.

- **Verify the health standards of the day care facility you use.** If your baby will need day care before they're vaccinated, confirm the health standards of your preferred center by reading their health and safety inspection report. Many centers post these online, and you can also ask them for a copy. In addition, ask them about their handwashing policy, vaccination requirements and records for those old enough to receive shots, guidelines for keeping a sick child home, and anything else you feel is important. The Child Care Aware website offers excellent resources for finding quality childcare: childcareaware.org/families /choosing-quality-child-care/starting-child-care-search/.

- **Avoid crowded spaces.** As I mentioned before, crowded areas increase baby's risk for contracting a virus. While the risk is probably pretty low when an outbreak isn't occurring, if you're feeling anxious you can enhance your peace of mind by avoiding crowded spaces until baby is vaccinated. For unavoidable sites like airports, minimize baby's exposure by washing your hands as often as possible, not letting anyone touch them, and minimizing their contact with public surfaces.

- **Know that it's okay to want to stay in.** If baby's health is only a portion of your hesitancy to interact with others, and all parts of you resist the idea of going out or socializing, trust that. Honor your need for time and space.

- **Create a loose script for when people hassle you about your need for space.** Because it can be hard for others to understand your request for space — especially when they're yearning to meet that adorable baby — come up with a go-to response for when you're questioned. For example, "The pediatrician recommends we keep baby home and away from others for [insert your desired period of time here], and for baby's safety we're going to honor that." Even if the pediatrician didn't recommend this, I'm all about blaming it on them, as others are often loath to go against the word of a medical expert.

Sex and the Vagina

83. Will my vagina feel the same to my partner after a vaginal birth? Will sex feel the same for me?

After a vaginal birth, your vagina might be a bit wider, which both you and your partner might notice in the first few months after birth. But as you continue to do those Kegels and your vagina settles into its new normal, the changes will be less and less noticeable. In addition, some women experience vaginal dryness as their hormones shift, but this will work itself out after a few months.

Beyond the physical components of sex, you, your partner, or both of you might experience some mental blocks. One of the big ones is feeling comfortable connecting to your sexual side when so much of your identity has suddenly shifted into parent mode. It can be tricky to reconcile these two pieces of yourself. Because of this, it's normal for your sex life to go through a dry patch in the early months of parenthood. Just take it easy on yourselves, commit to continuing to have sex every now and then — even when it's awkward — and know that you can find your way back to a steamy sexual connection.

What to do

Go to a vagina spa. I'm kidding. But doesn't that sound like something that could actually exist in Los Angeles? Until we discover a vagina spa, try these ideas:

- **Do Kegels.** This exercise is a sexual game changer as it strengthens the pelvic floor muscles that surround the vagina, making it tighter. It also increases circulation to the vagina and pelvic floor, which can enhance arousal and lubrication — Kegels are a great way to get you going before sex. To do them...
  - Identify your pelvic floor muscles by stopping your stream of urine midflow. Release after a few seconds.
  - Focus on pulling the pelvic floor muscles in and up, hold for the count of ten, and then fully release to the count of ten.

- ◆ Maintain smooth and easy breathing during reps, slowly inhaling with the intake of muscles, and exhaling with the release.
- ◆ Do ten sets, three times a day.
- **Use lube, if needed.** Because nothing kills the mood quicker than a dry vagina, purchase an organic lube to utilize until your hormones start providing natural lubrication again.
- **Get creative with positions.** The temporary changes in your vagina could make positions that used to be lovely feel painful; and positions you haven't tried, the bee's knees. Go into sex with curiosity, trying out different positions until you find the one (or many) that do the trick. It's also important to let your partner know you're going to lead the way with this, as you're the one who will know when something is working for, or against, your pleasure.
- **Consider amping up foreplay.** If you've tried all the positions and none are doing the trick, return to the tried-and-true techniques of oral sex and fondling. Sex will eventually feel good again, but there's no need to forgo pleasure in the meantime.
- **Love yourself.** A transformed vagina, leaking boobs, a shift in identity, fatigue, seriously limited time to get frisky…it can all lead to some bummer thoughts about yourself. Common thoughts I had in the fourth trimester were, "I'm no longer a sexual being, but a bloated baby bottle. I can't possibly seem sexy to Eric. I feel so gross. Why am I so sticky? My vagina is probably disgusting, but I'm too scared to look." I was so mean to myself. And needless to say, this meanness didn't enhance my connection with myself or Eric.

  Do as I didn't, and tell yourself that the mean voice is full of lies. Instead of allowing yourself to fall down the rabbit hole of those damaging thoughts, be gentle with yourself, continually coming back to the knowing that things will settle down, you'll reclaim your sense of self and sexiness, and your sex life will get back on track. It won't happen all at once, and that's okay. Instead of focusing on what's not working, pay attention to what is — like the fact that you can create, birth, and nurture a new human. And that stretchy pants exist.

84. I've been avoiding sex because I now associate my vagina and breasts with my baby, and I can't reconcile motherhood with

arousal. Is there a way to shift my mind and body out of mom mode so I can enjoy sex again?

When I was a few months into motherhood, my husband and I had a big fight about sex — and not for the first time. Not surprisingly, he wanted more of it, and I couldn't get into it. I associated my breasts with breastfeeding, and when I thought of my vagina I could think only of our baby coming out of me. My erogenous zones had turned into mommy zones. This severe shift in perspective suddenly made an act I had always enjoyed feel dirty, and not in the fun way.

To make myself feel better, I started rage journaling (obviously!). During this journaling session I drew what I called my sexuality spectrum. On one end of the spectrum was "using my body to care for a baby" (acts I perceived as requiring 0.01 percent of my sexuality), and on the other end was "using my body to feel sexual pleasure" (acts I thought required 100 percent of my sexuality). I wholly believed the dichotomy of that spectrum was accurate, and it screwed up my sex life for the first year of motherhood. Living by that model meant I had to push through intense mental, physical, and emotional shifts anytime my husband wanted sex, because I'd have to get all the way from one side of the spectrum to the other.

What I failed to realize when I created that spectrum was that the act of breastfeeding and vaginally birthing a baby is a lot more sexual than I realized. After all, my sexuality is what led to me becoming pregnant, birthing consists of the same uterine contractions that happen during orgasms (hence the phenomenon of orgasmic birth, see question 56), and breastfeeding causes nipple stimulation that releases oxytocin, or "the love hormone." Some women even have orgasms while breastfeeding.

Sex and motherhood mingle a lot more than we realize. But I think that also puts a lot of women off postpartum sex. For example, I have a client who felt aroused when breastfeeding and experienced a lot of shame around that. She then developed negative connotations about anything that caused arousal because it reminded her of what she called the "wrong feeling" when she fed her baby. This caused issues when it came to sex. She used the techniques in the "What to do" section to restructure her beliefs around motherhood and sexual arousal, and eventually found her way back to enjoying sex.

Something else that can turn a new mom off is the shift in identity that she and her partner experience. Our society often paints "good parents" as virtuous, wholesome, married citizens who never curse and have sex only to procreate. Little room is left for arousal, eroticism, and orgasm. I think that's a shame. Sexual pleasure is an innate, healthy desire — something to be explored and celebrated instead of suppressed and shamed. But that takes work, because many of us have to reprogram our beliefs on having sex as a parent before we can enjoy having sex as a parent. So how do we start that reprogramming and get to the place where we want and enjoy carnal pleasures as much as our partner does?

What to do

Don't give up on your sex life. Just because it feels awkward now doesn't mean you can't transition into a passionate, deeply pleasing sexual relationship with your partner. These tips can help you start that transition:

- **Look at where your beliefs about sex and parenthood come from.**
  Many times, our blocks around postpartum sex were implanted long before we became mothers. To remove these blocks, take some time to examine where they came from. You could ask yourself…
  - What messages did my parents share about sex?
  - How did my parents navigate their own sexuality?
  - What messages have I received about what it means to be a good parent?
  - What societal messages about sex and parenthood have impacted me?
  - Do I associate aspects of sex with traits I've been made to feel are inappropriate for a parent to have? (For example, do you think dirty talk, oral sex, or masturbation aren't appropriate for a mother?)

  Continue asking these questions until you have a solid idea of the forces that impacted your perception of postpartum sex. From there, you can decide what can be thrown out — for example, outdated ideas passed to you from your parents, the media, or society at large. And then, determine how you would like to perceive postpartum sex. Because that's the thing, you have the right to create your own definition of what sex after birth looks like, and you don't need anyone's permission to live by that new definition. Here's an example of a new definition: "I perceive postpartum sex as a beautiful dance between me and my partner that allows us to bond and to enjoy pleasure. Being a good parent means honoring my need for pleasure." Here's to a shift in perspective that fosters unfettered arousal, rolling orgasms, and a shame-free afterglow!

- **Tell your partner how you feel.** I can almost guarantee you that unless you tell your partner what's actually going on, you not wanting sex will make them feel rejected, like there's something about them that's causing you to not want sex. Fill them in on the blocks you're having, why they're coming up, and how you want to navigate them. If you don't yet know how you want to navigate them, ask your partner if they're interested in helping you in this process. If so, you can read through these suggestions together or come up with other possible solutions that suit your unique relationship. This communication can foster connection and prevent rifts or resentment that might be caused by changes to your sex life. An added bonus is your partner will probably put less pressure on you to have sex when you're not feeling it.

- **Ask to lead the way during sex.** When you're first finding your bearing as a mother who is also a sexual being, ensure that sex moves at your pace by asking to set the pace. Move as fast or slow as you want. Tell your partner how you want to be touched. Let them know when you're ready to be penetrated or intimately touched on the vagina — or if you're not ready for that. Teach them what kind of touch on your breasts does and does not feel good. While this instruction might seem strange at first, it can help you feel empowered in your sexuality, and support you and your partner in understanding how to please this new version of you.

- **Take solo "warm-up" time before sex.** For many women, the mind needs to be aroused before the body can get on board. So before you and your partner get frisky, slip away to the bathroom or another private space, and start thinking about things that turn you on. You can also pleasure yourself. Take your time, giving your mind and body time to warm up. Then, when your freshly aroused self is ready, go to your partner.

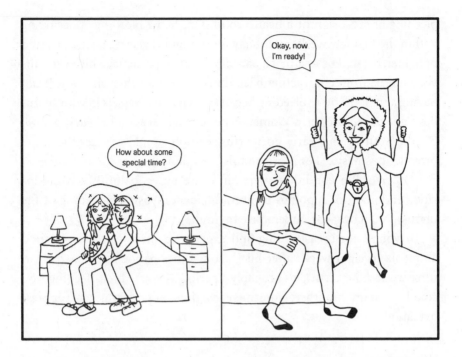

- **Flip to question 89, about feeling pleasure when breastfeeding.** The "What to do" section for that question has additional tips on navigating postpartum sex.

85. I've been having the heaviest, most insanely painful periods since having my baby. Is this normal?

Can I start with a rant? Okay, thanks! I think it's so unfair that after having monthly periods for many years, then growing a baby for nine months, then birthing said baby, we may have to deal with wildly painful periods — sometimes while our vagina or abdominal scar is still healing. Unfair. And all dudes have to deal with is a slightly lowered testosterone level when they become a dad. Pshh.

Okay, rant over! Thanks for listening.

So what to do about your heavy, painful periods? First off, let's look at why it's happening. For many women, a larger postpregnancy uterine cavity is to blame for heavier periods, as it produces more mucus lining that has to be shed each cycle. But we also want to make sure the pain and bleeding aren't a sign of a health condition. If the bleeding is occurring within the first few weeks after baby is born and is getting heavier instead of lighter, it could be a sign of a partially retained placenta, which prevents your uterus from contracting back down to size. In this case, you're not having a period, you're bleeding because open blood vessels in your uterus have not closed properly. Women experiencing excessively heavy, painful bleeding during this early postpartum period should contact their care provider posthaste. (For more on this, see question 65.)

Other health conditions that can cause heavy, painful bleeding include endometriosis, polyps or fibroids, adenomyosis (thickening of the uterus), or an over- or underactive thyroid.

If you're not breastfeeding and experience what feels like a period about six to eight weeks after birth (sometimes periods start as early as three weeks after birth), it's probably a period. If you're breastfeeding, you could go many months before menstruating, as prolactin can suppress ovulation.

What to do

Don't suffer in silence. Look into the following to find relief:

- **Have your iron levels checked.** Because heavy periods can screw with your iron levels, and low iron levels can lead to exhaustion and other unpleasant symptoms, have your care provider check for an iron deficiency. If you do have a deficiency, they might recommend iron supplements, IV iron therapy, or diet shifts.
- **Rule out underlying health issues.** In addition to having your iron levels checked, ask your care provider to help you confirm your heavy periods are not being caused by conditions like fibroids or endometriosis. If your care provider is not a specialist in women's health, ask for a referral.
- **Consider birth control.** As many types of birth control reduce uncomfortable period symptoms or can completely stop periods, you might want to talk to your care provider about getting a prescription for one that's right for your unique needs. However, make sure birth control doesn't mask the symptoms of an underlying issue by first having an OB-GYN confirm your reproductive health.

- **Get some exercise.** Exercise is a whiz at helping the body manage hormone imbalances, potentially reducing the heaviness of your next flow. Even going on a thirty-minute walk a few times a week can be helpful.
- **Know that time may alleviate uncomfortable period symptoms.** As your intense periods may be caused by your uterus getting used to life after pregnancy, you can likely expect the heavy flow and pain to somewhat subside after a few months, as your uterus and hormones adapt to their new normal.

Breastfeeding

86. I feel like I should want to breastfeed, but I'm totally freaked out by the idea. Why do I feel like this? What should I do?

It's normal to be nervous about breastfeeding, although this feeling is rarely talked about. Most women hear only about how breastfeeding is the most natural thing in the world, and so great for our babies. While the latter is definitely true, it doesn't always feel natural.

If you try breastfeeding and find it's not a fit for your family, you can of course stop. But for many women, there are a slew of "breastfeeding fear sources" that can be unraveled, and often healed, helping them move from fear to gratitude and excitement about breastfeeding. Here are the main concerns:

- **Shift in the relationship with your breasts:** It can be startling when a part of your body that's probably been sexualized most of your life suddenly becomes a source of food. Some women organically make this shift, while others find it strange to have a little human sucking on a part of their body society has labeled sexual. If you're in the latter camp, take heart that every woman I've worked with who had this block found that once she started, the act felt more natural every day until it finally became second nature. There's nothing wrong with you if breastfeeding initially feels bizarre. (I dive deep into this topic in the next question.)
- **Possibility of not producing enough milk:** There's a chance your breasts won't produce enough milk, because of circumstances like excessive blood loss during birth, limited milk ducts, hormonal imbalances, various medications and herbs, and other factors. While this can be incredibly frustrating and disheartening, a lactation consultant can help you determine why you're not producing enough milk, and provide effective solutions.

  It's also good to know that the only way to confirm you're not producing enough milk is baby's weight. Not being able to get much out while pumping or feeling like baby is not eating enough does not mean your supply is low. Your baby's pediatrician can help you determine if you need to get your supply up.

- **Pain from cracked nipples:** The first two weeks of Hudson's life were unreasonable torture for my nipples. I didn't know he had a shallow latch (because I didn't call a lactation consultant), so I suffered through bloody, mind-bending pain until my nipples finally toughened up and everything was fine — or maybe he figured out a better latch.

  The suffering didn't need to happen. If I had only asked for support, a lactation consultant could have provided tips to eliminate, or at least lessen, the discomfort. But I didn't ask because I naively thought it was supposed to be like that — that I had to martyr myself to breastfeed. Don't follow my lead. Speak up if breastfeeding is confusing or painful.

- **The newborn being entirely dependent on you for food:** It can feel overwhelming to have a tiny, defenseless human dependent on you for protection, booty cleaning, connection, language acquisition, bathing, entertainment, and, well, pretty much everything. But these are all tasks others can help you with. The exception is sustenance — if you choose to breastfeed. This form of feeding is all you. Even if you plan on your partner giving baby bottles of breastmilk, you still have to produce that breast milk. It feels like a big responsibility because it is.

  I felt buried by this responsibility until I realized it forced me to foster a powerful bond with Hudson. We were together *all the time* (he was a cluster feeder), which led to us quickly finding a rhythm for our relationship. And because oxytocin was released each time I fed him, I was blissed out at the end of each feeding. A study published in the *International Journal of Psychiatry in Medicine* even found that breastfeeding can decrease a woman's chances of developing postpartum depression during the first four months of the baby's life. But of course, it's not a panacea. Some women will still develop postpartum depression no matter how much they breastfeed.

  The gist: While I totally get the concern of being the sole source of food for your infant, it's been my experience that the early demands of breastfeeding could provide innumerable benefits for your transition into motherhood.

- **Others seeing your breasts:** I *never* thought I'd be okay with my brothers, father, father-in-law, and pretty much everyone I encountered in the first few years of my child's life seeing my boobs — or at least some side- or underboob. And yet, I quickly stopped caring. There's an assortment of breastfeeding covers that allow women to get out the milk jugs without anyone seeing, but I couldn't be bothered. I just got the fullest boob out, my voracious child latched on, and people looked away. However, I would sometimes breastfeed when Hudson was in the Ergobaby, my all-time favorite baby carrier, which provided ample coverage.

Luckily, I never encountered comments from breastfeeding-in-public shamers, but even if I had, I'm pretty sure I would have just rolled my eyes. Feeding my baby when he was hungry felt like the most innocent, natural act, and I felt no shame.

With that said, you have every right to want breastfeeding to be a more private experience, and there are ways to achieve that. You can utilize one of the aforementioned covers, pop into one of the pumping stations that are showing up in more public spaces, or do anything else that makes you more comfortable breastfeeding.

- **Becoming nutritionally depleted:** As breastmilk is made from your body, it can deplete you if you don't stay on top of your food and water intake. Typically, a breastfeeding mother needs an additional five hundred calories a day, ideally from nutrient-rich sources.

  Much like in pregnancy, during breastfeeding the body takes what it needs to provide baby with the ideal ingredients for health. If you have a surplus of nutrients and are consistently adding to the supply, you and baby will be fine. But if you're lacking, you could experience postnatal depletion, which could cause exhaustion, poor concentration and memory, and big emotional shifts.

  Maintain your vitality by drinking lots of water and eating breastfeeding superfoods like salmon, eggs, avocado, green leafy veggies, sweet potatoes, legumes, whole-fat yogurt, whole grains, nuts and seeds (especially chia and flaxseeds), fenugreek, ashwagandha, and turmeric. If possible, buy organic.

As you can see, many factors can understandably make you hesitant about breastfeeding. But with the right support and techniques, you can get past these blocks and have a successful journey through this amazing aspect of motherhood.

What to do

Know that breastfeeding is initially a struggle for many women. Needing help with this dynamic undertaking is so normal, and it's often made much easier with the right support.

- **Hire a lactation consultant.** A great lactation consultant helps you solve logistical issues with breastfeeding, figure out the best ways to make the experience more physically comfortable, and resolve any mental blocks. Because not every lactation consultant will be a good match for you, interview various candidates before your baby is born. This allows you to pick someone you're comfortable with and have go-to breastfeeding support when baby arrives.
- **Join a support group.** Connecting with women who have similar concerns and struggles can normalize your breastfeeding experience and provide a safe space to share your thoughts and receive supportive feedback.
- **Soothe pain by expressing milk onto topless breasts.** Beyond ensuring that baby has a good latch, one of the best ways to pacify painful nipples is to push a bit of milk out of your breasts and dab it on each nipple, as breastmilk has amazing healing properties. Then, go topless for a while, allowing the milk to soak into the cracked skin.
- **Make healthy snacks and a big metal water bottle easily accessible.** Prevent breastfeeding from draining your vitality by regularly restocking it with nutritious food and lots of water. I would get hungry and thirsty almost the moment I started breastfeeding. If I didn't have water and food within arm's reach, I felt trapped. Make sure you're equipped for the multiple daily feeding sessions by having a bag filled with healthy goodies (that no one but you is allowed to pull from) and an always-filled reusable water bottle (metal is the safest).
- **Remind yourself how good breastfeeding is for you and baby.** When you're feeling overwhelmed by your breasts and babe, remind yourself that breastfeeding can do the following:
  - Lower your baby's risk of SIDS (sudden infant death syndrome), childhood leukemia, stomach viruses, lower respiratory illnesses, ear infections, and meningitis
  - Decrease their chances of developing allergies or becoming obese

- Provide regular helpings of vitamins, nutrients, and other disease-fighting substances that serve as natural immunizations for your baby the first few months of life
- Improve cognitive development
- Save your baby in the case of an emergency, as it protects them from the effects of a contaminated water supply, helps prevent hypothermia, and requires zero supplies
- Reduce your chance of developing ovarian and breast cancer

Making breastmilk even more amazing is the fact that it's custom made for your baby. Your milk ducts contain sensors that pick up signals in your baby's saliva, telling your body what your baby's unique body requires; your body then responds by creating customized milk. Your body also responds to pathogens you're exposed to by producing customized milk that helps protect your baby from the pathogens' potentially harmful effects.

- **Know that there's no shame in stopping.** If after trying all these sources of support, breastfeeding is still causing more stress than solace in your life, you have every right to stop. While I'm all about the benefits of breastfeeding, I'm more about women doing what is best in their unique situation. If the thought of switching to formula fills you with relief, follow that instinct.

87. I feel self-conscious about my massive leaking boobs. How do I make them stop leaking? And how do I stop feeling ashamed of my body? Especially when I'm in public.

My boobs were so leaky the first six months of Hudson's life that I once dripped onto a woman who was pushing a baby out. Yup. I was her doula and had been away from Hudson for about twelve hours. My boobs were bursting. As I held her leg while she pushed, I wasn't paying attention to what was happening under my shirt. And then I saw something wet drop onto her arm. It was raining, and the old hospital we were in had some leakage issues, so I looked up. But it wasn't the ceiling, it was my mammaries. I. Was. Horrified. Thank the birthing gods I was wearing a black shirt; no one seemed to notice, and I flew to the bathroom to change and squeeze milk into the sink. Oy vey.

That's a long way of saying, I get it. I was constantly embarrassed by my leaky jugs, instead of being thrilled they were producing so much milk. This is something many women experience in early motherhood. I'll get to how to physically deal with the seepage, but I want to start with the shame you might feel when this happens. As I noted in the previous question, it takes a while to stop sexualizing our breasts, meaning we still think of them in "that way" when they start drawing attention, especially when they're leaking. I have a friend who had DD-size breasts before pregnancy. They were a G after baby was born. She once said, "I can't go into public. It's bad enough that these puppies are so massive, but they start leaking unexpectedly. Obviously, I'm not doing it on purpose, but I feel like people are going to think I'm trying to draw attention to them or something. Leaking from anywhere is embarrassing, but this is next level." Her words hit on many important points.

First, many women I've worked with also think people will judge them for having leaky breasts in public. And maybe some people do, but those aren't the people we should care about. The people we should care about are the little humans relying on those glorious boobs for sustenance, and your glorious self, who has every right to get out of the house when your body is still trying to figure out the whole milk supply thing. You're doing nothing wrong when you're out and all of a sudden you have wetness spreading across your shirt.

While it's easy for me to write that, I understand it can be tricky to turn off the shame tap we've been taught to open at the slightest provocation. I turned off the shame by forcing myself to laugh at the situation. Whenever I was in public and my milk volcanoes erupted, I would shrug my shoulders, laugh, and in my own time, change into the extra shirt I always kept in my bag. I was totally faking this lighthearted attitude in the beginning, but the more I did it, the more I felt genuine humor instead of shame. It also seemed to give others permission to brush it off as no big deal, instead of something to uncomfortably ignore.

The second excellent point my aforementioned buddy made is that we are deeply conditioned to associate a leaking body part with serious humiliation. Peed your pants? Thought you needed to fart, but turned out it was something more? Got boogies coming out your nose? All are situations our society has said should produce mortification. Most people are ashamed even to cry in public. I think that's all whack. Our bodies don't stop doing body stuff just because we're outside the privacy of our home. Leaks happen — to every body. Every single person. I encourage you to remember this when you're met with seeping boobs in public. Remind yourself that what's happening is the most natural thing in the world, and if you're able to give yourself the grace to handle it with amusement instead of humiliation, you're helping us all take a small step toward being more accepting of our bodies. Hey girl, you can be a leaky boob trailblazer!

What to do

And now for the logistics of that soaked bosom — because while we've canceled the Shame Game, it's still not a fun feeling to have a sticky, wet chest.

- **Know the leaking triggers.** Often hearing a crying baby, seeing a baby, or just thinking about your baby can induce a letdown. Knowing these triggers and any others you notice can give you a heads-up about a milky surge that's on the way.
- **Press on your nipples when you feel tingling in your breasts.** This preemptive measure can dam the milk flow. If you want to be incognito with this motion, just stretch an arm across your boobs and press it into your chest with your other hand.
- **Feed baby or pump before you go out.** Emptying your breasts before you leave the house can minimize the chance of a leak.
- **Use breast pads.** These absorbent boob buddies can soak up milk before it reaches your shirt. Keep a supply in your car, diaper bag, and purse so you always have replacements on hand. Be sure to change them when they're wet, as your nipples being in a moist, enclosed space for long periods could lead to a yeast infection. (Aren't we lucky — we can get yeast infections in the vagina *and* on our boobs!)
- **Keep tissues and organic wet wipes handy.** I was the worst at remembering breast pads, but I almost always had tissues on hand. I would stuff them in my bra when I sensed an impending leak. And because the stickiness of breastmilk was irritating, I would try to have wet wipes on hand. I recommend organic wipes, as the alternative could leave chemical residue on your breasts.

- **Keep an extra shirt in your purse and diaper bag.** Despite all the pads and tissues, you'll still have moments where the milk reaches the shirt. So keep a patterned or dark-colored (with the exception of gray) shirt in your going-out bags. Avoid silk. I also recommend a cover-up you can throw on until you're able to change.

- **Sleep on a waterproof pad that's covered by a pillowcase.** I had to wash my sheets *every single day* for the first week of Hudson's life because I soaked the bed in milk nightly. I then wised up and bought a few waterproof changing pad liners. I would cover the liner with a pillowcase to make it less scratchy, and bam, I only had to change out a small liner and pillowcase instead of all the sheets. If it was chilly, I would sleep in a zip-up sweater so I wouldn't have to pull the covers over my drippy boobs.

- **Wear a milk saver while breastfeeding.** Many women leak out of one breast while feeding baby from the other. Save those precious drops by popping a "milk saver" onto the boob not being used. These are boob-shaped pieces of plastic and rubber, with a hole in the middle for your nipple and a catchment area below it. Once you've finished that side, you can pour the collected milk into a container. It can add up to a lot of extra milk!

88. Why are my milk-producing boobs constantly changing size? Why have my nipples changed color? And what can I do to ensure they don't look defeated when I'm done breastfeeding?

Solidarity, sister. This largely selfless act takes previously perky boobs and puts them through multiple, daily metamorphoses. During my breast-feeding days, my B-cup tatas would suddenly inflate to DDs in the morning, and after thirty minutes of baby-feeding, they looked like deflated water balloons. Then a couple hours later, they were back in Pamela Anderson territory. As you likely suspect, these size shifts are thanks to the boob-filling and draining that takes place multiple times a day. The constant change does a number on your breasts' skin and tissue — so when a woman weans her baby, she's often left with a flatter, saggier version of her former chest. But not always! Women with smaller breasts and those with more elastic skin sometimes don't notice a big change when they're done breastfeeding. (I get into ways to nurture your bosom buddies in the "What to do" section.)

Now for your nipples. The darkening, which is normal, is caused by pregnancy hormones stimulating pigment-producing cells. The nipples often appear bigger because they're being drawn out each time baby feeds. These darker, larger nipples can be helpful, as they serve as bull's-eye "Eat Here" signs for baby. Nipples usually return to their pre-pregnancy size and color (or something close to it) after you wean.

You might also notice those little bumps on your areolas (aka Montgomery glands) plumping up. These bumps secrete sebum, a light yellow, oily substance that keeps your nipples moisturized and clean and emits an odor that attracts baby.

Another thing you can expect from your nipples — for now and forever more — is that they'll pretty much always be at attention. Months of being sucked train them to stay alert. I enjoy this change, as it gives the illusion that my boobs are perkier than they are.

What to do

While there's no way to avoid the boob restyling that comes with breastfeeding, there are ways to support your skin and emotional health during the changes:

- **Become one with organic oil and shea butter.** Regularly massaging your breasts with organic oil or shea butter increases suppleness and blood flow. This can minimize stretch marks and help skin bounce back after weaning.
- **Drink plenty of water.** Hydration has a big impact on your skin's elasticity, which is why you want to drink a minimum of eight glasses of water a day — preferably more.
- **Eat vitamin-rich foods.** The vitamins in healthy foods have a big impact on what's going on in and under your skin. Here are the vitamins you want to get more of:
  - **Vitamin A** stimulates the growth of new skin cells, which can prevent dryness. It can also curb cell damage and premature skin aging. Foods rich in vitamin A include salmon, eggs, carrots, tomatoes, sweet potatoes, and leafy greens.

- **Vitamin C** helps your skin bounce back from stretching, promotes collagen production, heals damaged skin, reduces the appearance of wrinkles, and hydrates skin. As an added bonus, it has cancer-fighting properties. Get your vitamin C on by noshing on citrus fruits, strawberries, broccoli, and spinach.
- **Vitamin D** helps skin stretch, grow, and repair. Get your vitamin D with about ten minutes of sun each day and eating foods like salmon, cod, tuna, and mushrooms. It's also present in fortified foods like milk, yogurt, cereal, and orange juice.
- **Vitamin E** is a powerful antioxidant that can reduce wrinkles, inflammation, and dryness, and it might minimize the appearance of scars (aka stretch marks). You can get it from sunflower seeds, almonds, hazelnuts, spinach, mangoes, avocados, and butternut squash.

- **Exfoliate.** Once a week, gently rub your breasts with a dry brush or use a sugar scrub in the shower, as exfoliation can promote new skin growth and increase blood circulation, which can regenerate skin and enhance elasticity. Make a homemade sugar scrub by mixing one-half cup of brown sugar with three tablespoons coconut or olive oil and two tablespoons raw honey.
- **Talk with your partner about your insecurities.** If the changes in your breasts make you insecure, tell your partner, as these feelings might impact your willingness to be naked in front of them. It's also important for them to know so they can be sensitive about how you're feeling and can maybe even pump up your confidence with compliments about your amazing lactating breasts.

  It's natural to develop insecurities when experiencing rapid changes in various parts of the body, but you don't have to navigate the emotions these changes trigger alone.
- **Honor the shifts as a reminder of the gift you're giving your child.** If you get bummed because breastfeeding is almost constantly remodeling your boobs, shift your focus from what they look like to what they can do. They make milk that's custom designed for your baby! That's so cool — and something not all boobs can do. Some women would happily give up their breasts' constant perkiness for the ability

to make enough milk for their baby. While you have every right to feel all the feels about your breasts, I encourage you to bring yourself back to gratitude as often as possible.

89. I feel pleasurable sensations when I breastfeed, and it's messing with my head. I can't reconcile having what I can only describe as a sexual feeling while doing something that's far from sexual. It's making me resist breastfeeding. What should I do?

One of the causes of those pleasurable sensations is oxytocin. Your body pumps it out when breastfeeding to encourage you to keep doing it and bond with baby. It's the most natural thing in the world. And the reason it's messing with your head is likely that our culture oversexualizes breasts. You've probably been programmed your entire life to associate breasts with sex. Because of this, breastfeeding can turn you on and even cause sexual fantasies. And there's nothing wrong with that. You're not fantasizing about your baby; you're fantasizing about a tryst with your partner, or Thor, or whomever. And more women than you realize experience this; you just don't hear about it because society has made the topic super taboo.

Speaking of taboo, some women even report orgasming while breastfeeding. In most of these cases, the woman has her legs crossed, which causes clitoral stimulation. That stimulation, coupled with uterine contractions from the oxytocin and nipple stimulation from the breastfeeding, pushes them over the edge. While many of these women say they're horrified by this reaction, they don't need to be. They suddenly had a baby sucking on a part of their body that's always been an erogenous zone, while other parts of their body that play a part in arousal (the clitoris and uterus) were also being stimulated. They weren't making a conscious choice to be aroused — biology was doing it for them. It's understandable to feel resistance to this type of situation, but know that the emotional discomfort will pass. Here's how it happens…

As you continue breastfeeding, your perspective on your breasts will shift from "sexy-time trigger" to "feeder of child." In addition, the prolactin your body is pumping out to produce milk will induce maternal behavior, like a desire to cuddle your baby, fostering the shift in your relationship with your breasts. While you wait for this change, keep reminding yourself that you're not a pervert for enjoying the sensations of breastfeeding — that's just biology rewarding you for giving your baby the gift of mega-nutrients.

In addition to feeling pleasure when breastfeeding, it's common for your nipples to get hard. This is another phenomenon we usually associate with being turned on (or being cold), and it makes some women uncomfortable. But the nipples are hardening just to meet breastfeeding's anatomical requirements, as your nipples have to be somewhat erect for baby to latch on. It's normal for your nipples to harden when stimulated, whether that stimulation is your baby's mouth, your shirt rubbing against them, or a fondle from your partner. The hardening is sexual only when you give it that label.

It's also helpful (and maybe a little frustrating) to know that lactating will shift your sexual encounters in a few ways. According to an article published in the *Journal of Perinatal Education*, during lactation you experience little to no vaginal lubrication when you're turned on (Oh hi there, lube!), and milk can potentially eject from the breasts during orgasm. In addition, the longer you breastfeed, the more your perspective on your breasts gets embedded in "mom zone," to the point where you may have little sexual response when they're touched sexually. The researchers go on to explain that the mix of prolactin and oxytocin that's released during breastfeeding can also satisfy your need for connection and affection in such a complete way that you don't seek it as much from your partner. Being aware of all this can help ensure you don't unintentionally neglect your bond with your honey.

What to do

Here are a few ways to avoid shaming yourself for feeling pleasure when breastfeeding and to maintain a connection with your partner.

- **Shift your perception of physical pleasure.** Many of us associate pleasure in the more sensual areas of our body (e.g., breasts and vagina), and definitely orgasm, with sexual encounters. This is understandable, as sexual encounters (with yourself or someone else) are the primary reason you experience these sensations…until you have a baby. But the "sexual" label we put on these sensations is all in our head. Our body doesn't care why it's feeling good; it just likes to feel good. The mind is what gets in the way when we have those warm, tingly feelings while breastfeeding. So give yourself permission to take sexual meaning away from those sensations — at least when breastfeeding. You can start thinking of them as a lovely by-product of feeding your baby — a present for all the hard work you're putting in. And just like that, you can wipe away shame and guilt.

- **Find ways to stay connected to your partner.** Because breastfeeding can satisfy your need for physical connection, you might find your desire to be affectionate with your partner is weakening. While there's nothing wrong with this in the short term, it could negatively impact your relationship if it goes on for too long. To fortify that connection, find ways to be intimate with your partner without sacrificing your needs. For example, if you can't stand being touched after a marathon round of breastfeeding, ask your partner to keep their hands off for at least an hour. When you feel your resistance to touch wearing off, ask them if they want to cuddle while you both play with the baby or watch a movie.

  This might feel contrived in the beginning, but the more you commit to re-establishing that physical bond, the more you'll enjoy it. The key is that the connection be on your terms as you find your way back to intimacy. Feeling forced to be intimate could make you resent your partner, which isn't good for anyone. Take it slow and steady, and eventually you'll relish a long hug, or a roll in the sheets.

- **Create new rules for breast fondling.** Once I started breastfeeding, nothing turned me off more than having my boobs touched by my husband. I never told him how I was feeling, and understandably, he took it personally when I swatted him away. Be wiser than me, and talk to your special person if you notice yourself cringing when they go for your milk jugs. Explain that it has nothing to do with them, and everything to do with your new relationship with your breasts. You can also reassure them that when baby eventually weans, you'll probably become more comfortable with boob play.

  With that said, you might be cool with certain types of breast touch, but not all. For example, I have a friend who enjoyed her husband gently cupping her breasts, but couldn't stand him touching her nipples with his hands or mouth. She let him know how she felt, and he honored her guidelines. If you're not quite sure what you are and aren't comfortable with, have your partner test out various types of fondling and let them know what feels good.

90. My baby bit my nipple while breastfeeding, and I yelled at them. They're now scared of me, and I'm scared of them biting me again. It's breaking my heart. How can we move through this?

Dang those little nipple biters. I remember the first time it happened to me. An ungodly pain ripped through my chest, I arched my back, unintentionally chomped the side of my tongue, and held my breath, unable to look down. I was sure my nipple had been beheaded. When I finally peeked, I expected to see a wicked grin on my six-month-old's face. Instead I saw his perfect, soft, squishy, innocent sleep face. "How can something so adorable do something so evil?" I thought. Thus began the one-month nightmare of living in breastfeeding purgatory.

Hudson had inexplicably developed the habit of chomping on my nipple while falling asleep. As the nipple would start sliding out of his mouth, he would clamp down. It felt personal, and it pissed me off. "How dare you bite me when I'm feeding you my milk." Sometimes I would actually say that. One time I flicked him so hard on the cheek he started to cry. Then I started to cry. During the few biting encounters when I could hold it together, I'd slide my finger between his gums, break the latch, and refuse to nurse him until the memory of the trauma faded. No one was happy. But after a month, it just stopped and we started liking each other again.

My story is not unique. I've had countless women call me, crying that they'd screamed at their baby after being bit. Many said the reaction made their baby hesitant to nurse. And, not surprisingly, the mothers were hesitant to hand over the nipple.

I'll start to break down the cruel phenomenon of nipple biting by first stating the obvious: your baby is not biting you because they secretly hate you. Here are a few reasons why this oh-so-unfortunate scenario might be occurring:

- The biting is a reflex. Just like the reflex to root, suck, swallow, and gag, babies sometimes have the instinct to bite.
- You baby is teething and wants to chew on everything. *Everything.*
- Their brain is curious about cause and effect, so they chomp the nip to see what happens.
- They have a cold or an ear infection. If baby has a hard time swallowing because of a stuffy nose or pain in the ear, they might be inclined to bite when nursing. Luckily, that should cease when the cold or infection clears up. In the meantime, get them in a sitting position while nursing and use a humidifier as often as possible. If they're tugging on their ear, take them to the pediatrician for treatment for a potential ear infection.

What to do

Kindly ask your baby not to bite, as they're very responsive to logical requests. What's that you say? Your baby doesn't acquiesce when you request they sleep through the night, stop puking on your favorite shirt, and not pee on you while you change their diaper? Well in that case, here are a few ideas for surviving the biting phase. Solidarity, my sore-nippled sister.

- **Be vigilant about positioning.** Baby will be less likely to bite when their head is angled back, their tummy is pressed against your upper abdomen, and they have a deep latch. When they have this good latch and are actively nursing, they can't bite, as their tongue will be covering their lower teeth or gums.
- **Learn the pre-biting signs.** Start paying attention to what your baby is doing right before they bite, as this can help you remove the nipple before it turns into a teething tool. For example, Hudson would bite when he was really drowsy. Some babies bite when they've emptied the breast but are still sucking for comfort. Other babies are prone to biting when they're teething, so if they seem to be extra fussy and are cutting teeth, be wary. I've also heard of babies biting when they get distracted and turn their head away from mama's body. Another big sign of a potential, impending bite is baby pulling their tongue back.
- **Make sure baby is on a "loaded" breast.** As I mentioned before, babies

don't bite when they're swallowing. So pay attention to how full the breast they're feeding off is, and switch to the other side when it seems nearly drained. This helps prevent the lull in swallowing that can lead to a bite.

- **Unlatch baby with your finger.** While your first instinct may be to yank baby away from your breast when they bite, this could further damage the offended nipple. Instead, slip your finger between their gums to break the latch. When you feel the release — you might also hear a little pop — remove the nipple *tout de suite*.

- **Stop nursing, but not forever.** After baby bites, stop nursing to inform them that nursing can't continue after a bite. However, when the bite's no longer fresh in everyone's mind (I'm talkin' around fifteen minutes, not many days), you're probably safe to recommence nursing.

- **Offer something else for them to chew on.** If you suspect baby is using your nipple as a teether, give them something else to gnaw on. When Hudson went through this, I kept a few teethers by my prime breastfeeding locations and swapped my nipple for a teether as soon as he stopped consistently swallowing.

- **Don't beat yourself up for a loud reaction.** While we obviously don't want to respond to a bit nip with a physical action that could hurt the baby, it's only natural that you yelp, or curse, or let out some other loud noise. I can almost guarantee you didn't stop to think, "Hmm, what kind of noise can I make that will scare my baby?" No, I'll bet it just happened, because that's what happens when a private part (or any part) is bit out of nowhere. Your baby might cry or look offended at your noise-of-not-choice, but you did nothing wrong and don't need to feel guilty.

- **Apologize.** Not feeling guilty is easier said than done. So if that guilt is sparked after you've screamed bloody nipple, just apologize — it's a classic way to make amends. While baby can't fully understand your apology, they will be soothed by your calm voice and loving facial expression. And they get over slights shockingly fast.

- **Don't wean, unless you were wanting to wean before the biting started.** If you love breastfeeding, don't let the biting scare you away, as it will likely be a short-lived phase.

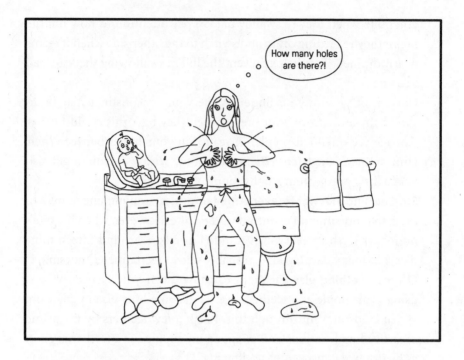

91. Sometimes my breastmilk starts squirting in all directions. Is that normal? How many holes do my nipples have?

A woman typically has four to twenty milk duct orifices (aka tiny holes) in each nipple. So if you have engorged or just really full, bare breasts, and they're triggered to let down by something like your baby crying, thinking about your baby, or having an orgasm, milk might start shooting out in all directions. This can also happen if baby is breastfeeding and suddenly turns their head away, leaving the nipple exposed. Hudson received a face-ful of milk many times because of this. So, my fellow milk-maker, your squirting boobs are completely normal and something to celebrate. Some women can barely get their breasts to eke out an ounce of milk, and you have so much it's spraying across the room! Yay!

What to do

Know your letdown triggers, and be prepared for blastoff if they occur. For example, if you know you often have a letdown when you hear your baby cry or you're turned on, throw on a bra or simply hold tissues against your breasts to prevent a spray when those circumstances crop up. If the spraying doesn't stop on its own, you can self-express some milk, pump, or breastfeed. Beyond that, enjoy your milk fountains!

92. I'm tempted to drink my extra breastmilk. Is it safe? Is it worth it? Should I just donate it?

It's safe, so long as you're drinking only your own breastmilk. Because when you're drinking milk from your body, you're not exposed to anything you haven't already been exposed to. That safety does not extend to the strange trend among bodybuilders of purchasing untested breastmilk at high prices on the internet. I even had an ex-boyfriend text me after I gave birth, brazenly asking if I would give him my leftover milk. My response: "Uh, *no*. I don't have milk to spare, and if I did, I would donate it to a milk bank, not your vanity." Many milk banks create a safe environment for the exchange of breastmilk, as they ensure that the mother donating milk is free of health conditions, medications, and other substances that could contaminate breastmilk. Milk sold through shady sources online could contain anything from germs found in human waste to *Staphylococcus* and *Streptococcus* bacteria (not dinosaurs). Yummy.

Back to your milk. While you can definitely benefit from the proteins and vitamins in it, it's not nearly as amazing for you as it is for baby. It's custom made for them, helping ensure they get the exact nutrients and immune-boosting goodies they need during early development. Much of what you get from breastmilk is akin to what you'd get from eating a healthy diet. But if you have enough to spare and are motivated to make your breastmilk part of your diet, *anecdotal* evidence has shown it could...

- Increase energy
- Boost immunity
- Clear up acne when applied to the face
- Soothe Crohn's disease and rheumatoid arthritis symptoms
- Build muscle
- Help erectile dysfunction (No wonder steroid-filled bodybuilders are all about breastmilk.)

So swigging breastmilk could have some perks, but it might be put to better use by a baby whose mama can't produce enough. But that's 100 percent your call — no judgment either way! I have a friend who can't consume dairy but also can't stand plant-based milk. She tried her breastmilk in her cereal and coffee and loved it. She now has a massive frozen supply of her milk to use for breakfast.

What to do

You might as well…

- **Give it a try.** If you're curious about sipping your special sauce, go for it. If you're primarily interested in it for potential health benefits, try it for a week and notice whether you experience any positive changes. Or if you just like the taste and prefer using it over cow or plant milk, keep on drinkin'.
- **Consider donating the milk.** If you're not fully committed to drinking your milk but want something to do with your surplus, contact local hospitals to see if they accept donations. You can also reach out to legit milk banks at the following websites:
    - hmbana.org
    - medolac.com
    - prolacta.com
    - lactalogics.com

93. Is any amount of marijuana safe to consume while breastfeeding? Is it bad that I'm craving it?

Sister, you've just spent nine months abstaining from all the relaxing vices and are now in the thick of motherhood. I don't blame you for wanting to indulge in some Mary Jane. And now that it's decriminalized in many states and legalized in others, it's even more tempting. But like any responsible breastfeeding mama, you want to make sure what you put in your body doesn't screw with your baby's body.

The tricky thing with marijuana is that it sticks around in your body longer than something like alcohol, so you can't "pump and dump." Various studies have detected small quantities of THC (the psychoactive component of cannabis) in breastmilk from six days to more than six weeks after use. And a study published in *Pediatrics* found that more than four hundred chemicals in marijuana can transfer into breastmilk. The researchers also reported that typically less THC was detected when the mother used edibles or topicals, instead of smoking. As an added bonus, edibles and topicals don't expose baby to secondhand smoke. However, all delivery methods expose the baby to THC.

Shedding a less damaging light on marijuana use and breastfeeding is a 2018 study published in *Obstetrics & Gynecology* that reported the concentration of THC in breastmilk was about 2.5 percent of what the mother received, and of that, only around 1 to 5 percent is absorbed by the baby. So the dose is pretty minimal. In addition, they found that levels of THC in breastmilk were undetectable twenty-four hours after a mother who only occasionally used marijuana ceased use. But because it's hard to go twenty-four hours without breastfeeding (at least with an infant), it's assumed a baby would consume some THC before it was metabolized out of the milk. In the case of chronic marijuana users, the study discovered that it took much longer than twenty-four hours for THC levels to become undetectable — it could potentially take up to four days. This study suggests that risks might be minimal if a mother uses marijuana infrequently and waits twenty-four hours between use and breastfeeding. However, they still urge caution.

Regarding the effects of marijuana — specifically, THC — on the baby, limited research has found that occasional maternal use of marijuana during breastfeeding didn't have noticeable effects on the infant — but this research did not rule out long-term risks. It's also believed that THC could alter baby's brain and motor development, slow weight gain, reduce milk production, and diminish the baby's ability to suckle.

The bottom line: I don't have a straight answer for you. Limited research has indicated marijuana can have negative impacts on baby. Continued research might discover a safe amount for a breastfeeding mother to consume, but unfortunately, we don't currently have that information. So in many ways, the choice of whether to use marijuana when breastfeeding comes down to the level of uncertainty and risk you're comfortable with.

What to do

Make informed decisions by trying the following:

- **Check with your care provider:** With something as little understood as consuming marijuana when breastfeeding, it's best to check with your care provider before proceeding. While they'll likely tell you to "just say no," if you push you may be able to get some information about the amount they think would probably, maybe, possibly be safe. And if you're hoping to use marijuana for a condition like anxiety and you'd be using it in place of a pharmaceutical, your care provider might determine that the risks of marijuana for the baby are less than the risks of a certain pill. You can also get a second or third opinion to gain a more well-rounded perspective.
- **Purchase from a dispensary:** If you choose to occasionally partake in ganja, know that it's not all created equal, which is why it's best to purchase it from a dispensary instead of getting it from a friend. Dispensaries typically have staff trained in the various strains and delivery methods and can help you choose an option best suited to your unique needs. But again, I wouldn't take this route until you get the go-ahead from your care provider.
- **Don't bed-share.** If you use marijuana, hold off on bed-sharing the same day, as you might experience heavier sleep.

C-sections and VBACs

94. I elected to have a C-section, but my community of moms is super crunchy. I'm afraid I'll be judged if I talk honestly about my child's birth. Should I lie?

I'm in a similar community. (Hi, Ojai!) Many moms here have home births, and those who need a C-section, or even an epidural, are often embarrassed to talk about it. But what I've discovered is that almost every time someone is brave enough to talk honestly about their birth experience, they're met with understanding, regardless of the type of birth they had. Often the source of judgment about our birth that we face comes more from within, than from our community. In essence: you don't need to lie.

I was at a baby shower once where moms sat in a circle sharing their birth stories. Woman after woman told tales of empowering home births (some orgasmic!), until it came to a woman who would not look away from her hands, clenched in her lap. The host asked if she wanted to pass, but she took a deep breath and said no. Then she told us about her C-section. It wasn't an emergency situation that led her to the C-section, but a series of events that made her feel that a C-section was the best option. "I feel weird saying this," she said, "but it was actually a pretty positive birth. I had a great doctor who didn't pressure me into anything, and a surgeon who talked to me in a really encouraging way through the operation." As she spoke, I scanned the faces of the other women. No one was looking judgy — everyone was smiling and nodding. The woman sharing looked so relieved when she was done. And then, something really cool happened. One of the women who had already told us about her home birth said that her second birth experience had been a C-section, but she had been nervous to talk about it. Then another woman shared a similar story. That one woman having the courage to talk about her C-section in the land of home births made other women feel safe to do the same. I think more often than not this is what happens. Women are afraid they'll be judged for their cesarean birth story, but instead they're met with compassion and even relief that someone else is openly talking about it.

But what about that rare person who does pass judgment? Even if the judgment is as subtle as a slight lift of the eyebrows when you tell them about your C-section? Well, that person can go to h-e-double-hockey-sticks. Just kidding. But really, it's so lame when people are critical about someone else's very personal journey. If you get stuck in this type of unfortunate encounter, remind yourself that their reaction has so much more to do with them than with you. They likely have a mental catalog of stories, information, and personal experiences that have formed their biased opinion of C-sections. That's where their reaction is coming from — it's not an indication that your choice was wrong or that you're a "bad mom." Let them feel how they feel about C-sections, and make a mental note to not discuss your birth with them again.

What to do

Here are some ideas to help you not take judgments about your C-section personally and hopefully avoid those condemnatory conversations entirely:

- **Come to terms with your birth experience before you talk to your community about it.** If you're still processing your C-section, you'll understandably be much more sensitive to reactions to your birth story. For example, if you're still trying to decide if the C-section was something you wanted, and you talk to a person who believes pretty much all C-sections are just a money-making scheme, their feedback will likely color how you see your own experience.

  To help ensure that your feelings about your birth are built by *your* beliefs and experiences instead of those of others, spend time reviewing the events that led up to your C-section. How did you feel before, during, and after the surgery? What elements do you feel good about? What do you not feel good about? Do you have questions about the birth? After considering these questions, discuss your findings with the people who were with you during the birth.

  Sit with your birth story until you have a solid understanding of what happened, and how you feel about it. Getting to this place before you give the story up for interpretation can make you less vulnerable to judgment, and more capable of sharing the story only with people you believe will be supportive.

- **Be selective about who you share your story with.** First of all, you're under no obligation to share your story with anyone. If someone asks how your birth went, you can be super general. For example, "It went great. Baby and I are both healthy." But it can feel good to share your story with certain people, especially if you're disappointed by the birth and need to vent or mourn. Set yourself up for positive, cathartic encounters by sharing your story only with people you trust, people who won't pass judgment.

- **Have a go-to response for the rare time when someone is judgmental.** If you unexpectedly find yourself in a conversation with a Fault Finder, have a script ready to get you out of it. For example, if someone starts going on about the dangers of C-sections, how much risk you put yourself in, how you let yourself be manipulated, how difficult it will be to have a vaginal birth now, or one of the other common objections some people have about C-sections, you can simply say, "You know, I'm still trying to figure out how I feel about the experience and would love to press pause on this conversation until I have time to do that." You're not required to get sucked into their vortex of opinions.

- **Be sure you're not the one passing judgment.** As it's often easier to spot someone else's judgments than our own, stay aware of your own responses to the birthing decisions of others. Because even when we know how hurtful it is to be on the receiving end of judgment, we can still give in to the impulse to throw around criticism, especially toward the person throwing it at us. But we're better than that. And while passing judgment can provide initial satisfaction, it often leaves a yucky emotional residue. So let's make our kindergarten teachers proud and practice that Golden Rule: treat others the way we want to be treated.

- **Remember that you don't need to justify your choice.** You have every right to choose whatever type of birth feels best to you, regardless of the circumstances. No one has to agree with your choice for that to be true. While it's obviously fine to justify your decision, you don't have to. If someone seems judgmental of your C-section, it's not your job to change their mind — it's their job to examine their biases and figure out how to be accepting of other people's choices.

Skin and Appearance

95. I have so many hemorrhoids I can barely sit down. Will they go away? And how do I make them stop itching?

Oh, hemorrhoids. Those little demons were my constant companions from month six of pregnancy to six months postpartum. And they still like to come for unwelcome visits every now and then. Their specialties are soreness, itchiness, and embarrassment, and they take great pride in being the ultimate pain in the.... They range in size from chickpea to grape.

So first off, what are they? They are swollen veins in the lowest area of your rectum, or anus. Internal hemorrhoids often go unnoticed, while external hemorrhoids — swollen lumps poking out of the anus — are constantly saying hi. If a blood clot forms in the hemorrhoid (thrombosis), it will likely turn blue or purple. Often, a bit of blood on your poop is caused by hemorrhoids. These beauties can be caused by the following:

- The weight of the baby pressing on the rectum
- Progesterone during pregnancy relaxing the walls of the veins, making them more prone to swelling
- Heavy-duty pushing when pooping (often a result of constipation) or pushing a baby out
- Serious exertion when doing something like lifting a heavy object
- Excess weight

While hemorrhoids usually go away after a few weeks, there will likely be "skin bags" poking out of the anus forevermore. (But they shouldn't hurt or itch.) And now for some pictures! Just kidding.

What to do

Here's how to soothe the fury of the hemorrhoid:

- **Sit on soft surfaces.** Soften the impact of sitting by swapping hard surfaces for soft. You can also make a pillow your constant companion.
- **Ice 'em.** Sit on the toilet and hold a piece of ice, or an ice pack, on the hemorrhoids to reduce swelling.

- **Swap toilet paper for witch hazel wipes.** Standard TP usually doesn't do the trick when trying to wipe away all the poop particles stuck in the crevices of hemorrhoids. So use witch hazel wipes instead. The moisture of these wipes does a better cleanup job, and the witch hazel helps relieve itchiness, pain, and swelling.
- **Become one with hemorrhoid cream.** Many hemorrhoid creams contain lidocaine (hello, numbness!) as well as healing ingredients like hydrocortisone, vitamin E, and aloe vera.
- **Drown them in a warm bath.** Soaking in a regular tub or a sitz bath minimizes itchiness, pain, and swelling. You can add Epsom salt or a splash of apple cider vinegar to the water to promote healing.
- **Load up on fiber, and drink more water.** As hemorrhoids can be caused and agitated by constipation, eat fiber-rich foods like avocados, lentils, chickpeas, oats, chia seeds, almonds, pears, raspberries, and of course, prunes. In addition, drink plenty of water, as it helps soften fecal matter and keeps it moving.
- **Use a footstool when pooping.** Propping your feet up on a stool when using the bathroom helps you get into a squatting position, which stimulates the bowels, making it easier to get it all out without too much force.
- **See your care provider if they're really bugging you.** If the external hemorrhoids seem excessively uncomfortable or are regularly causing rectal bleeding, check in with your care provider.

General

96. I'm disappointed by my birth experience. People keep telling me I should just be happy I have a healthy baby, but I feel like a failure. How can I reconcile with my child's birth story and move past these emotions?

Don't you hate it when people discount your feelings with the "at least you have a healthy baby" line? I mean, sure, they don't mean to discount your feelings and are (probably) trying to cheer you up, but they're missing the point. You don't *want* to be cheered up, at least in the beginning. You want someone to make you feel like your disappointment is okay and normal. That you have every right to be bummed about a labor and delivery that didn't go as you'd hoped. You likely put in significant preparation to have a certain type of birth experience, and it's a real loss when aspects of it (or all of it) don't go as planned.

Speaking of that preparation, it's irritating and hurtful when people make us feel foolish for having hopes for birth beyond getting the baby out, and having the audacity to write out these hopes in the form of birth preferences. But we have every right to infuse our birth experience with hope and intention. And often, that positive forethought and preparation does enhance the birth experience, even if it doesn't unfold in the exact way we wanted it to. When it doesn't happen as we'd hoped — even if there are only a few pieces we're upset with — we should be free to feel mad, upset, or whatever else is coming up.

As you feel those emotions and work through the process described below, I want you to hold on to the truth that you did everything you could with the tools at your disposal to have the best possible birth experience. Even if you're kicking yourself for making a decision that you feel derailed your experience, like saying yes to an intervention that went awry, know that you don't deserve the blame or shame you're probably dumping on yourself. What you do deserve is to take the birth story and emotions you have and put in the time and care to work through them, instead of masking them.

What to do

Feel the feelings. Before you give up your story and emotions for interpretation, allow it to all flow through you. This unobstructed feeling can help you figure out what you're actually upset about. Start this process by taking these steps:

- **Seek privacy.** Have someone watch baby for a set period of time and go to a private space to cry, rage, write — do whatever you need to begin the process of exploration and release.

- **Talk to someone who was present at your birth.** It's common for women to forget many of the details of their birth experience, which can make it difficult to figure out why we're upset. By gathering all the facts from someone who was there, you can gain clarity about the circumstances your feelings are stemming from.

- **Hold your birth story and emotions close.** Now that you're understanding the root of your emotions and have given yourself permission to feel them, choose the people you talk to wisely. If your intuition tells you that your mother-in-law or sister, for example, might brush off your feelings, you'll want to choose someone else to confide in. If you want a sure bet, find a therapist you trust, as they're almost guaranteed to be an active listener and abstain from "at least you have a healthy baby" comments.

- **Stand tall in your emotions.** When you're met with an unsympathetic response to your reaction to your birth experience, resist the urge to agree with it. Many of us are so wary of disagreement that we agree with someone even when we don't actually agree. Although smiling, nodding, and saying, "Yeah, I guess you're right" when someone says, "At least you have a healthy baby" sounds harmless enough, it's actually giving your mind the message that your feelings aren't valid. So instead of agreeing, just change the subject. Realize that this person isn't the right recipient for your birth concerns, and commit to finding someone else to talk to.

If you're feeling guilty about prioritizing the acknowledgment and processing of your feelings, remember that it's not frivolous or ungrateful. It's the best way to fully integrate with the intense journey you went through, extract the insights that live within that journey, and move forward with a clear emotional canvas.

97. What's the deal with cosleeping (aka bed-sharing)? Is it as dangerous as many imply?

Before I get into this question — a gray area for many — I need to make it clear that I'm not advocating cosleeping. As you'll soon discover, I coslept with Hudson, as it made sense to me in our circumstances. But as someone who offers guidance to women, I cannot give an official thumbs-up to cosleeping. What I can do is share studies and anecdotes about this practice, and leave it up to you to make the decision that feels best for your family.

I coslept with Hudson, and he's still in our bed many nights. The literature told me repeatedly not to do it, but my instincts overpowered it all on his second night home. The moment I placed him in the crib a few feet from our bed, I felt off. Each time I couldn't hear him breathing I would get up and stare at his chest until I saw it rise and fall — that happened about every fifteen minutes. I wasn't getting any sleep. I was relieved when he finally cried for milk, as I could bring him into the bed. But then, staying true to the recommendations I had received, I carried him back to the crib and laid him down. He immediately woke up and started crying. We repeated the nurse, crib, cry, nurse again routine until the sun came up. I hadn't fallen asleep once. The next day, I reread the studies, or at least their conclusions.

Here's how I interpreted the information: cosleeping is most dangerous in a bed with parents who drink, smoke, take drugs, or are extremely heavy sleepers. Eric and I were none of those. "They" also advised against cosleeping in a soft bed. We had a super firm mattress. Regarding bedding, we didn't sleep with a top sheet, and I knew I could keep the blanket away from Hudson by tucking it around my waist.

So I defied the expert advice and we coslept the following night — and it felt right. My blanket strategy worked, and I naturally slept with my arm arched around the top of his head (preventing the pillow from getting near his face), and my legs tucked up under his feet. He was in a mama cocoon, and I was immediately aware of anything that tried to invade it. I also stirred at his every movement — there was no heavy sleeping happening. But overall, we both got more sleep, as minimal shuffling and waking were needed when he was ready to nurse. He never rolled out of the supine position (lying on his back), and he would simply turn his head to the side when he wanted milk. For me, this practice transformed early motherhood by allowing me to get decent sleep, almost entirely dissolving my fear of SIDS, and solidifying my bond with Hudson.

I don't say any of that to convince you to do as I did. Because as I've learned from working with hundreds of mothers and babies, every pair has a unique experience with just about everything. I tell you that story because I want you to understand the thought process that led me to the decision to cosleep. Do with it what you will.

Now, let's hear from science.

Cosleeping: What the Experts Say

Medical Experts

Here are key findings about bed-sharing from the medical community:

- A report published by the American Academy of Pediatrics states that regardless of parental smoking or breastfeeding status, there is an increased risk of SIDS when bed-sharing if the baby is younger than four months.
- A study in *Morbidity and Mortality Weekly Report* found that 61 percent of respondents from a 2015 Pregnancy Risk Assessment Monitoring System (PRAMS) survey reported bed-sharing with their infant, at least some of the time.
- According to a study published in *Pediatrics*, breastfeeding infants who routinely shared a bed with their mother breast-fed approximately three times longer during the night than infants who slept separately. The study also suggested that because bed-sharing could increase breastfeeding, it might protect against SIDS "in some contexts."
- Showing how much care providers can impact our choices, a study published in *JAMA Pediatrics* stated that out of the 54 percent of 18,986 participants who talked with a doctor

about bed-sharing, 73 percent reported receiving negative advice; 21 percent, neutral advice; and 6 percent, positive advice. Not surprisingly, those who received negative advice were less likely to bed-share, and those who received neutral or positive advice were more likely to bed-share.

- A study in *Pediatrics* analyzed 239 cases of SIDS, finding that bed-sharing was reported in 39 percent. In addition, 43 percent noted maternal smoking and 72 percent did not breastfeed. Researchers found that the bed-sharing cases had increased bedding risks and more babies in the prone (facedown) position. They also reported that bed-sharing was especially risky when the mother smoked, the mother slept with the baby on a sofa, the infant was younger than eleven weeks, or there was someone in the bed that wasn't one of the baby's parents, like a sibling.

- A study published in the *British Medical Journal* suggested that the risk of bed-sharing seems to be more connected to the infant being exposed to secondhand smoke than to the possibility of a parent rolling on the baby, or to overheating.

- Another study in the *British Medical Journal* found that cosleeping on a sofa significantly increased the risk of SIDS. The study also found that when parents do not smoke and the infant is older than fourteen weeks, cosleeping did not increase the risk of SIDS. In addition, the study stated that the SIDS risk for younger infants seems to be associated with recent parental consumption of alcohol, overcrowded housing conditions, extreme parental tiredness, and the infant being under a duvet.

- And to exhibit just how unlikely SIDS is while bed-sharing with a healthy baby: a person is more likely to be hit by lightning during their lifetime in the United States (1 in 15,300) than a low-risk baby is to die of SIDS while bed-sharing (1 in 16,400).

The takeaway from medical experts is that the risk of cosleeping is not the same across the board. It largely depends on the health of the baby and the risk factors in the sleeping environment, such as parents who smoke and drink.

Anthropologists

While I think it's important to honor the research performed by medical professionals, I believe it's equally valuable to consider the findings of experts in the field of human behavior and cultures.

- Anthropologist James McKenna at the University of Notre Dame performed a comprehensive cosleeping study that found that mothers create a type of "shield" around the baby as they sleep. Being in this shield helps the baby regulate their heart rate, and carbon dioxide from the mother collects around the baby's face, prompting them to take a breath. They also observed that the baby rarely moved around during sleep, instead staying next to the mother, with their face pointed toward the breast. It's like the mother's body creates a microenvironment that helps the baby's body learn how to stay alive.
- McKenna has also found that safe bed-sharing can be an important mechanism in regulating an infant's sleep development, and that mothers in many other cultures, and in species like nonhuman primates, understand this connection and have thus practiced bed-sharing from the beginning.

  He also comments on how US culture strongly values independence and fails to honor the fact that infants are inherently dependent, especially on the mother. In addition, countries that commonly practice bed-sharing, like Japan, have children who gain a sense of safety and comfort from this close contact with the parents, which then gives them confidence to flex their autonomy. Instead of fostering dependence, the bed-sharing is promoting independence.
- Bed-sharing is a common practice in Japan, where it is referred to as *kawa no ji*. This term is represented by the character for *river*, which looks like this: 川. According to a study

published in *Pediatrics*, Japan has one of the lowest rates of SIDS in the world, and the United States has one of the highest. Cross-cultural data also shows that cultures where co-sleeping and breastfeeding are the norm have either no cases of SIDS or incredibly low rates.

- Studies have shown that bed-sharing causes mother and infant to spend more time in light sleep than deep sleep, and that they often arouse around the same times. This is especially supportive of bed-sharing with infants who have difficulty waking themselves when experiencing something like apnea (temporary cessation of breathing), which is a risk factor for SIDS.

- Historians have documented the origin of the practice of having infants sleep alone; it likely began in the last five hundred years, when poor, starving women in areas of Europe smothered the infant during sleep because they didn't have the means to provide for them. After hearing women confess this, Catholic priests began banning parents from having their infants sleep in the parental bed.

- It's common practice in Bali to hold a baby until it falls asleep, then have the baby sleep in its parent's bed, as the Balinese believe the child is "vulnerable to spirit risks" during sleep.

- Research has shown that early mother-infant separation can impact a child's long-term mental health. A study of 2,080 families showed that regular mother-child separation was related to higher levels of negativity and aggression in the child. The researchers found that it was essential that the child believe their mother would respond if they called, or cried in the case of an infant. They found that children who were securely attached to their mother were better able to tolerate physical distance as they aged. Essentially, more close contact with the mother in early life equaled more independence as the child grew up.

- A study done by anthropologist Helen Ball found that parents who bed-shared with their breastfed babies had safer sleeping conditions than parents who bed-shared with formula-fed babies. The formula-fed babies typically slept with their head level with the mother's head, either on a pillow or between the parents' pillows, did not arouse as much as their breast-fed counterparts, and had mothers who slept in a variety of positions. In contrast, the mothers who breastfed their babies slept the entire night with their baby level with the breast (far away from pillows), formed a protective arch around the baby, and aroused more often, usually at the same time as their infant.

What to do

Make the decision that feels safest to you. If you try cosleeping and you're panicked the entire night, switch to a bassinet, bedside sleeper, or whatever your baby-bed of choice is. But if your instincts are screaming at you to try cosleeping, make sure you do the following first:

- **Confirm there aren't obvious risks.** I want to reiterate that although the American Academy of Pediatrics does not recommend cosleeping under any circumstance, they note that it's especially dangerous if you or your partner drink, smoke, take drugs (even if they're prescribed drugs — as they can make you drowsy), or are heavy sleepers. If you fall under any of those categories, cosleeping is ill advised. In addition, a baby under twelve months should not sleep in a bed with another child.
- **Create a safe bed.** Before cosleeping, make sure you have a firm mattress, without a cushy topper. In addition, move out any nonessential bedding. For example, you could move all pillows out of the bed with the exception of one pillow for yourself and one for your partner, ditch the top sheet, and tuck the blanket under your hips to make sure the blanket won't bunch up around baby's face.
- **Consider baby's health.** Because a baby who was born prematurely, is underweight, or has health issues has a higher risk of SIDS, you might want to hold off on cosleeping until any health risks have passed. Your

baby's pediatrician can help you develop a thorough understanding of your child's current health status.

- **Evaluate how the cosleeping trial went.** After your first night of co-sleeping, consider how safe it felt. Did it transform your sleep and baby's? Did feeling their warm breath on your chest the entire night make you feel secure? Or did it keep you awake and anxious? Did anything happen that could have threatened their safety? Does it feel like the most natural thing in the world? Or something you're forcing? Listen to your instincts.

- **Continually reassess.** Evaluate your decision as things change. For example, because respiratory infections are believed to increase the risk for SIDS, you might consider reassessing your cosleeping arrangement if baby develops this type of illness. Or if you or your partner drink one night, smoke a cigarette (or are even just around smoke), or take a medication that can cause drowsiness, carefully consider whether it's safe for baby to sleep in your bed. The main point: always be considering what the safest sleeping arrangements are for your baby.

How's that for a murky answer to this question?! This was one of the hardest questions for me to answer, as my feelings around cosleeping are such a mixed bag. As I recommend with all the information I provide, take it with a grain of salt, seek information from various sources, and make decisions that feel best to you. You are so much wiser than you likely give yourself credit for.

98. Sometimes, I'm so painfully tired I'm tempted to let my baby cry while I try to sleep. What should I do?

When Hudson was three weeks old, he fell asleep in his infant-carrier-baby-chair-thing, and I passed out facedown on the couch. He woke up first. His crying was loud and urgent and pierced through my sleep...but not enough to cause me to pull myself out of my pool of drool. I was so tired, and my limbs felt so heavy, I just lay there, willing myself to go to him but not actually going to him. After what felt like an excessive amount of time I rolled off the couch, crawled to him, pulled him out of the chair thing, laid us both on the carpet, pulled up my shirt, and fell back asleep on the floor as he nursed. It got better, but whoa, man, those first few weeks were brutal. I would get so tired I hallucinated. I fell asleep on the toilet twice.

So yup, super-duper extreme fatigue is a natural by-product of being a new mom. You know what's also a by-product of new mamahood? Feeling guilty about feeling like you'd rather slip into a three-month coma than go to your baby. I've had so many moms tell me with guilt-ridden faces that they sometimes hated their babies for messing with their sleep. I would have fleeting moments of thinking I loved my pregnancy pillow more than Hudson.

Even though exhaustion comes with the territory, certain levels of it could be a sign of bigger issues. For example, I later discovered that the postpartum blues I experienced the first two weeks of Hudson's life likely contributed to my falling-asleep-on-the-floor-and-the-toilet situation. For some moms, the fatigue is a symptom of postpartum depression or various physical ailments. But the thing is, regardless of why you're bone-tired, you want to find a solution like yesterday. Fortunately, there are ways to temper that tired.

What to do

Drink more coffee! Just kidding. (Although a little coffee doesn't hurt.) But really, the main thing we want to do is figure out how to get you more sleep, help you feel more energized when you have to be awake, and discover if there's a deeper reason you're so pooped. Here's how:

- **Reconsider your sleeping arrangement.** One of the biggest reasons new mamas are so tired during the day is because they get so little sleep at night. Part of this is that baby's body does not yet know that humans are supposed to sleep when it's dark and be awake when it's light. Another part is that baby's stomach is so small they need some nosh in the wee hours. But the last part, the part you can actually do something about, is *your* sleeping situation. For example, if you're spending half your night dragging yourself down the hall to baby's room, rocking them until they fall asleep, then dragging yourself back to your bed, you might want to talk to baby's pediatrician about how to create a safe environment for bed-sharing. Or, if you're bed-sharing and constantly waking up because you're afraid you've rolled on your baby, consider having them sleep in a bedside sleeper, or a bassinet by your bed. To sum it up, toy around with sleeping arrangements until you find one that safely allows you to get more sleep.

- **Embrace the "nap when they nap" cliché.** I rarely listened to this advice and instead did unimportant stuff while Hudson partook in day sleeping. I probably would have been a less scary human if I had just put down the vacuum and napped when he napped. Be smarter than me, and give in to your fatigue when baby gives in to theirs. It will make almost every part of life easier.
- **Get some help.** If the "nap when they nap" thing is laughable to you because you have so dang much to do, get your partner to kick it up a notch with their support. If you don't have a partner, reach out to friends or family members. If you don't know anyone in your area, contact a local parent support center that can point you in the direction of a postpartum doula or a program that pairs new moms with a volunteer, in-home helper.
- **Take all the shortcuts.** I'm pretty sure exhausted moms invented things like grocery delivery services, frozen meals, cleaning services, those robot vacuums, and dry shampoo. Let yourself off the hook for making home-cooked meals, maintaining a pristine house, and doing all the other nonessential tasks society has told us are essential. All you need to do right now is sleep as often as you can, prioritize your other basic needs, and care for your baby — which doesn't need to include a daily bath and chic outfits. A wet wipe, fresh diaper, and clean-enough onesie will do just fine.
- **Take a walk, or just step outside...or at least open a window.** The body has to work harder for oxygen when it's indoors, as it's mainly working with recirculated air. This can exaggerate fatigue. By simply stepping outside or opening some windows, you're making oxygen more readily available and minimizing your body's workload. This equals more energy.

    If you're up for a walk, even better, as you'll get a dose of vitamin D, exercise, and a change of scenery; at least the first two are proven to increase energy. When Hudson was a newborn, my husband Eric suggested a walk around the block *every day* when he got home from work. I would roll my eyes and resist. "I'm too tired," I would moan. "I don't wanna." But he was persistent, and we'd go. I always felt happier, more energized, and less hostile when we were done. It worked so well, I started taking Hudson on a walk every morning.

- **Drink more water.** Water makes up 55 to 75 percent of our body, and 90 percent of our blood, and it's essential for cellular homeostasis. As the most essential nutrient, water plays a huge role in how tired we feel. When we're well hydrated, pressure is relieved on organs like the kidneys, bodily functions don't have to work as hard, and our blood has more oxygen to carry through the body. This leaves us with enhanced energy for baby tickles, smiling, and general life enjoyment.

  My go-to method for drinking enough water is to always have a forty-ounce metal water bottle by my side. I shoot for drinking three of these a day, but even if I just get through it twice I'm still feeling pretty good.

- **Avoid bottomless coffee.** One or two cups of coffee in the morning can work wonders for energy levels. But it's usually downhill from there. For many, having more than two cups of coffee daily leaves them susceptible to anxiety, which can be really exhausting. This occurs because too much caffeine can prompt your body to pump you full of adrenaline and cortisol. I'm always pretty certain catastrophe is around every corner if I drink more than 1.5 cups a day.

  And then there's *when* you drink it. Sipping on caffeine after two in the afternoon can make it harder to fall asleep during those precious blips of time when baby allows you to sleep.

- **Stash healthy snacks everywhere.** Food and fatigue are interesting bedfellows. Eat too many heavy, processed foods, and you're more fatigued. Don't eat enough food, and you feel fatigued. Eat fresh, nutrient-rich fare, and your fatigue lifts (at least a bit). Help food help you feel less wiped out by keeping healthy snacks in the prime baby-feeding areas. I kept a bag with mixed nuts, dried mangoes, carrot sticks, and some other goodies by my glider chair, bed, and couch.

- **Explore your emotions.** Is your fatigue accompanied by sadness or anxiety? Do you feel incapable of summoning joy? Do you feel like motherhood is just an awful chore? If you answered yes to one or all of these questions, you should not lock yourself in a closet of shame. Some of your fatigue might be caused by postpartum blues or depression (something I covered more thoroughly in question 72). If you suspect that might be what's up, start the process of seeking support ASAP by scheduling an appointment with your care provider.

- **Get a physical.** While fatigue is a normal (albeit unfortunate) by-product of early motherhood for most women, you might also have a condition that enhances drowsiness, like anemia, certain allergies, fibromyalgia, or hypothyroidism. Let your doctor know how you're feeling, and request a physical that includes blood work.

99. I don't want another baby but am met with shocked looks and judgmental questions when I share this information. Is it selfish to not want another child?

Well…you're not a good American unless you have 2.5 children.…Just joshin'. Throw those white-picket-fence, June Cleaver expectations out the window when deciding how many children you want to have. Every human has different circumstances that influence the number of humans they want to raise, and none are wrong. The people who don't want to have any children should get to have no children without judgment. The one-and-done folks should get to have one child without judgment. The folks that want to raise a soccer team should get to have that soccer team without judgment. Dreams, careers, finances, emotional landscapes, relationships, childhood memories, past birth experiences, and a slew of other factors influence how many children we want to have. And because those factors are unique for each person, everyone will have varying ideas on what the right number of children is for them.

The unfortunate thing is, some people mistakenly assume that the number of children that's right for *them* is also "right" for everyone else. Some people don't want kids and are perplexed by anyone who does want them. Some people think that people who want only one child are selfish, and those who don't want any are insane. I don't think any of these people have a right to pass judgment on anyone's family planning. It's one of the most personal decisions you'll ever make, and a decision that needs to be made by you.

I even think that the decision to have more children is ultimately up to the partner who would be carrying the pregnancy. And sure, if both partners are on the fence, it's a decision you'll want to make together. But if you're certain you don't want more children, I don't think anyone, not even your partner, should make you feel shame for that decision. Because as you know, navigating pregnancy, childbirth, and early motherhood is an intense experience for women, and one that they should be on board with. They shouldn't be shoved on board.

That's my long way of saying that no, you aren't selfish for not wanting another child. If you're making this decision because you've tuned in to your inner knowing and it's saying, "No way! One and done, lady. *One and done!*" you get to listen to that knowing. And sure, if your inner knowing really wants another child, but you're afraid for a variety of reasons, you may want to explore that, determining whether it's worth it to you to work past that fear in favor of expanding your family. But if that's not the case for you, stand tall in your decision to only have one child.

Regarding where people are coming from when they judge you for your decision, it often stems from three places:

1. **Resistance to that which is different from what they believe in.** If someone feels strongly that having a large family is an important part of life, they might want you to feel the same. When they discover you don't, their judgment and defensiveness could be triggered. They might see your differing choice as a sign that you don't think their life decisions are "right." While your choice to have only one child likely has nothing to do with anyone but your nuclear family, some people won't be able to see that.

2. **The belief that you're robbing your child of the opportunity to have a sibling.** Here's the thing with this argument: there's no guarantee a sibling will enhance someone's life. There are plenty of only children who have rich lives and fulfilling relationships. There are plenty of people with siblings who have fractured relationships with those siblings and have instead fostered deep bonds with friends. While a sibling can be a beautiful thing in some circumstances, it's not a golden ticket to happiness.

3. **Buying into the myth that the only child is destined to be self-centered, lonely, and spoiled.** While we don't need studies to know this stereotype is hogwash, there are still plenty of studies showing that only children have the same chance of being happy and whole as those with siblings, and that they aren't more likely to be egocentric brats. For example, a study published in *Social Psychological and*

Personality Science found that only children are not more likely to be narcissistic than those with siblings. Research has also found that only children typically have the same number and quality of friendships as their peers with siblings.

Now let's look at some examples of people who chose to have one child. My friend Amy and her wife June stopped procreating after their daughter was born because they had limited finances and the dream of traveling full-time. They felt a second child would hinder that dream. So they followed the path that felt right to them and spent ten years home-schooling their daughter in forty-seven countries. Their daughter is now in her late teens and says she feels like she has siblings all over the world.

Another friend, we'll call her Celeste, had extreme postpartum depression and OCD for a year after her son was born. "It almost broke me," she said. "There were days I couldn't be around my baby and was bombarded by suicidal thoughts. I eventually got past it, but I can't imagine exposing myself to that emotional trauma again, even with the meds and therapy." Her husband didn't push her to change her mind, and they're four years into enjoying their happy family of three.

The last woman I'll mention, Caitlyn, didn't have any dreams a second child would thwart or crippling postpartum depression; she simply felt complete after her son was born. "I had always assumed I'd have two, but after Henry was born I just didn't feel a need for more. Our family feels whole."

So there you have it. Having one child is not a situation reserved for those who experience secondary infertility or have another medical circumstance that makes it impossible for them to become pregnant again. It's also a perfectly fine decision for any reason that feels right to you. No one knows the inner workings of your body, emotions, and family like you do, which is why you get to make the decision without allowing anyone to make you feel shameful or selfish.

What to do

Hold true to what feels right for your family, and try the following to fortify that right-feeling:

- **Listen to your inner knowing.** Your inner knowing (aka gut instinct) knows. Regardless of the decision you're trying to make, if you drift within and really listen, you'll receive an answer. And usually, this answer — an answer that comes from your truest self — will lead you down the path you're meant to follow.

  So if external opinions are making you feel shame for or doubt about your decision to not have another child, tap into that inner knowing and trust its feedback. It knows more than all those people sticking their nose where it doesn't belong.

- **Reserve the right to change your mind.** If you're currently set on having one child and change your mind years down the line, that's obviously fine! You get to make that choice without anyone having the right to say, "I told you so." As life circumstances change, our preferences for what we want in life can also change. If that happens to you, don't let your early assertions about having one child stop you from following this new dream.

- **Decide what you want to say when people ask about baby number 2.** It's a foregone conclusion that someone will eventually ask you about another baby. Avoid being sucked into a conversation you don't want to have by planning what you'll say. For example, you could say, "We're still deciding." Or "We've decided we're just going to have one. That's what feels best for us." If the person pushes, asking why you made that decision, you can just reiterate, "It feels like the best choice for our family right now." You don't owe anyone an explanation and can keep your answers short and vague. Then you can change the subject or make an excuse to slip away.

- **Consider egg freezing if you need to buy time.** If you don't currently want more children but think you could want more in the future, you might feel pressured by your biological clock to speed up your timeline. If the idea of speeding things up is stressful, consider freezing your eggs.

  Of course, this is not a light or cheap decision, as it costs thousands of dollars and requires you to take fertility injections, then undergo an egg retrieval. From there, you have to pay an annual fee for egg storage and utilize IVF when you're ready to use your eggs. However, this option can provide peace of mind and the gift of time if it's financially and physically feasible for you.

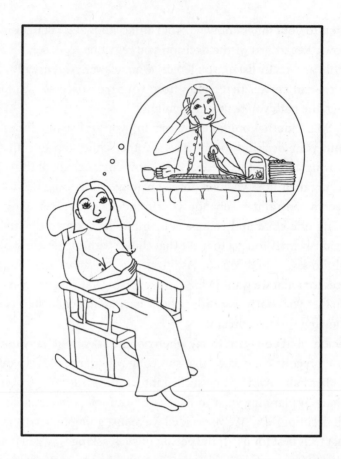

100. I really want to get back to work and am considering finding full-time childcare or asking my partner to stay home with the baby. Am I not bonding properly? How do I broach the subject with my partner?

In the early days of Hudson's life, I felt rudderless. The home organizing business I had before he was born couldn't continue without me driving to Los Angeles every day, and I couldn't afford regular childcare. And because my husband was a teacher, it wasn't an option for him to stay home. I suddenly found myself without a job or a passion outside motherhood. I felt like life was a VHS that rewound as I slept and replayed every day. Then one day, driving home from a RIE (Resources for Infant Educarers) class, I had an idea for a book. Suddenly pumped, I sat in my driveway for an hour breastfeeding Hudson and making notes on my phone. From that point, I wrote every time Hudson fed. This new project pulled me out of the postpartum blues I'm pretty sure was on its way to becoming depression. Ideally, I would have had numerous uninterrupted hours to work each day, but I took what I could get.

So I get it. I get the pull to return to work, whether that's retreating to your home office five hours a day or heading back to your job outside the home. Some women feel relieved when they can become a stay-at-home mom, others are bummed when they have to return to work, and a few of us are yearning to dive back into our career. There's nothing wrong with any of these feelings — it just shows we're all different in our needs. It's okay if your cup doesn't runneth over from motherhood alone — this in no way indicates you're not bonding properly or aren't meant to be a mother. It means you're a dynamic human who requires an array of activities and passions to be fulfilled. And it doesn't hurt to feel financially independent.

However, I get why you're wary about this desire. An ongoing issue in the United States is the severe lack of maternity leave available to most women. This leads many mothers to dread the return to work, and the rest of us to assume there must be something wrong with us if we're looking forward to that return. Some of us might even think we're not as maternal or selfless as the women wanting to extend their leave. But the best path for each mother-baby pair is unique. There will be some who crave constant togetherness for the early phase of baby's life, and others perfectly happy seeing one another in the morning and evening. There's not one right way. You get to miss your job and figure out how to go back early. You get to love your job without feeling like that means you love your baby less.

Making a plan with your partner about how to get you back to work may be simple, or really tricky. If you have the money for childcare and your partner understands your need to get back to career mode, you should have relatively smooth sailing. But if that's not the case, things might be more challenging. For example, if your partner would need to stay home, or at least share more childcare duties, to enable you to go back to work, you may get pushback — especially if your partner is male.

While our culture is slowly shifting, a deeply embedded societal norm still gives the woman responsibility for things at home, with the man working outside the home. This is of course rubbish, but it might, consciously or subconsciously, impact how your male partner responds to your request, and how firm you are in that request. You and your partner might be required to really examine your views on gender roles and determine if they're coloring your decision making. This isn't a quick fix, but starting the process of acknowledging how social expectations impact your thinking can help you both make more objective decisions.

What to do

As much as possible, let excitement replace any guilt and shame you may feel about wanting to go back to work. If you love your job, it will likely be joyful to incorporate this important aspect of yourself back into your life. It might even make you a more present, happy mother. Essentially, keep reminding yourself that there's nothing wrong with your desire as you work through the following suggestions:

- **Determine if there's an underlying issue behind your desire.** While it's completely normal to want to return to work, I encourage you to analyze whether you're using it as a Band-Aid. For example, I had a client who was desperate to go back to work but couldn't figure out why. She enjoyed her job but had never been crazy about it. When she got honest with herself, she realized she was trying to escape the anxiety she felt when caring for her baby. She was always worried she was going to screw something up and felt calmer when the baby was in someone else's care. While spending more time at work would have masked the problem, it wouldn't have helped her work through it. Once she realized this, she sought therapy, which eventually dissolved her anxiety. When she returned to work, she was happy to do so but was also happy to return home every afternoon.

  It's natural to want to escape some aspects of motherhood, like rarely talking to adults, changing nappies all day, and not having reasons to dress up, but if you're trying to escape deep-seated emotional challenges, make sure returning to work isn't your only solution.
- **Remember your right to love your career.** As you become vocal about your desire to return to work, you could face resistance. Some people might be perplexed by your desire and offer opinions that could

make you question your decision. I urge you to remember that this pushback has little to do with you and likely everything to do with those aforementioned gender roles. Too many people are trained to believe a woman's primary desire should be staying home with her baby. Hold tight to your right to love your career, and make moves to return to it. Ultimately, this decision won't really impact anyone but your baby, your partner, and yourself, so consider only those people when determining what to do. No one else gets a vote.

- **Advocate for your needs.** If your partner is the one pushing back on your desire to return to work, you might need to do some major advocacy on your behalf. You might need to help them understand where you're coming from, explaining how your career makes you feel, how you think it will benefit your homelife, and what your ideas on childcare look like. And this issue shouldn't be about you asking for permission, but instead, you informing your partner of a need and letting them know they must work with you to find a solution that works for all involved. You are partners — they're not your gatekeeper. You have just as much right to nurture your career as they do. Advocate for that right.

- **Get creative with childcare and work hours.** If you can't afford daily childcare, you might need to brainstorm with your partner about how you can make your return work. For example, maybe you both shift to working part-time on-site and part-time at home, staggering your schedules so someone is always with baby. Or you could do some kind of trade with friends or family members willing and able to offer childcare. Even if at first it seems like nothing can work, you might be surprised by an enlightened idea as you continue to explore options. Don't give up!

101. I have a baby with special needs, and while I feel intense love for them, I'm devastated they won't have the life I imagined. I also resent how much my life will change. How can I work through my emotions and find acceptance for our situation?

The minute I found out I was pregnant, I began building expectations for my child's life. I think most parents do. And as pregnancy progresses, these expectations expand and become embedded in our psyche. So when baby's special needs are discovered, whether it's during pregnancy or after birth, many of those expectations are shattered — and not just expectations about the child's life, but your life as well. In an instant, everything changes.

After the discovery of special needs, many parents move through the seven stages of grief but try to suppress the process because they feel guilty for feeling anything but gratitude for their child's survival. Some feel they should have immediately accepted the situation. But I don't think that's fair. I think it's the most natural thing in the world to move through shock, denial, anger, bargaining, depression, and reconciliation (finding solutions) before reaching acceptance — and people much smarter than me would agree. In some ways, the discovery of special needs is like a death. You have to grieve the child and life you thought you were going to have, to create emotional space for the child and life you do have. It can be a painful, expansive, uncertain, and unexpectedly beautiful journey.

What to do

Try the following ideas, all the while holding on to hope that one day your situation won't feel so shocking or foreign. You will get through this initial grief, even if it's the hardest thing you ever do.

- **Surrender to the seven stages of grief.** Repressing the stages of grief only prolongs the process. Those emotions are coming up one way or another. So instead of pushing them away, I encourage you to accept them. And because it's hard to fully immerse yourself in emotions when you're caring for a newborn, you can make a plan with your partner or a friend or family member to watch the baby for one hour every day while you go to a private space and fully surrender to whatever stage of grief you're in. Let yourself really go there. Journal about your dashed dreams. Cry. Rage. Feel with abandon. This concentrated release can create the emotional space for you to care for your baby and self without being constantly distracted by grief. It might even help you reach acceptance faster than if you tried to force acceptance by denying your feelings.
- **Find a community that understands what you're going through.** I

once worked with a woman whose baby had Down syndrome. "I can't stand being around people who have the children they expected," she once told me. "I know it's not logical, but I try to figure out if they're somehow morally superior, or did some special health thing I didn't do during pregnancy, or, I don't know, are just somehow better or luckier than I am. I get so jealous. It drives me crazy."

This frustration persisted until her pediatrician referred her to a support group for parents of children with special needs. She met caregivers for children of all ages who had a range of needs. They supported her through grief, provided hope, and helped her realize that what happened wasn't some cosmic punishment. They also supported her in finding specialized care for her child and herself, and they eventually became like a family. "In a lot of ways, I feel more connected to them than my actual family because they really get what we're going through. I couldn't do this without them," she said.

- **Communicate with your partner.** Some partners are inclined to hide their grief from one another in an effort to be strong for the other. But consider that it might be more helpful for you and your partner if you're both honest about what you're thinking and feeling, as this could normalize what you're experiencing. For example, hearing that your partner is also feeling devastated and resentful about the dashed expectations they had for your child could be a huge relief. Be raw and vulnerable with each other, instead of putting on a mask of strength.

- **Know that acceptance will come and go.** Many of us believe (or want to believe) that finding acceptance is a linear process — that once we find it we'll never regress. But that's rarely true, especially when navigating life with a child with special needs. For example, after you've settled into acceptance of life with a baby with special needs, that acceptance might fade when they reach school age because you'll be faced with a new set of decisions and challenges. It's normal to lose your grip on acceptance and be pulled back into grief. But this time, you'll likely have an effective tool kit for navigating the grief and can find your way back to acceptance quicker. The point is, you're not failing if you don't always feel acceptance. Life is like a maze: it will stop you in your tracks, force you to retrace your steps, and set you on a new path.

- **Don't punish yourself for feeling resentment.** Although your child's special needs are no one's fault, it's normal to feel resentment for the situation, or even resentment toward the child. While many parents report feeling horrible when they view their child in this way, it's not a sign you're a selfish or cruel parent. You're a human who has their own dreams and desires — dreams and desires that are likely thwarted (at least initially) by your family's new circumstances. While the natural inclination is to push away the resentment, this only causes it to fester.

  If possible, slip away to the bathroom or another private space when the resentment is ignited. Let it move through you. Get angry. Curse the Universe. Then, literally shake your body, envisioning the resentment breaking away from you, leaving you emotionally renewed and ready to commence caregiving.

- **Seek support so you can nurture yourself.** Not surprisingly, many children with special needs require more time and attention than children without these needs. This can be taxing. Avoid surrendering to martyrdom by doing the hard task of asking for help. Ensure you and your partner are sharing childcare tasks as evenly as possible, and seek out people qualified to care for your child's needs, like "respite providers," or teach willing friends or family members how to provide this care. And as much as possible, use the free time this creates to do something for yourself — something that recharges you and makes you feel like a whole, separate being.

- **Learn as much as you can about your baby's unique needs.** Immersing yourself in learning about your child's mental, physical, and emotional needs can help you transition into your new reality. And as you build your base of knowledge, you'll likely feel a sense of empowerment regarding your ability to support your child and family through the changes you'll experience.

- **Create new dreams for your family.** Once you've reached acceptance, you get to begin the exciting process of crafting new dreams for your child, and yourself. Because you now know more about what to expect from your child's needs, you can dream up fresh ideas for how you can both lead fulfilling, joyful lives.

- **Prepare yourself for unsolicited advice and platitudes.** People who care for you but do not fully understand what you're going through might offer words of comfort that are anything but comforting. Or, in an attempt to be helpful, they might share misguided advice. Ready yourself for these awkward encounters by reading the unsolicited-advice suggestions from question 73.

There are resources for parents of children with special needs in the "Recommended Resources" section.

Farewell, My Friend

Welp, we've done it! We've come to the end of our journey into motherhood taboos, and I don't know about you, but I feel free. Free of the fear of judgment. Free to speak up when I have a question or concern that's typically "discussed behind closed doors," or not at all. And free to live a life of truth and openness. I'm all in for those candid conversations. I hope you feel similarly. I hope you realize there's nothing shameful about expressing and exploring your true self. I hope you know that you're a whole, dynamic woman who has permission to craft your transition into motherhood, and life in general, any way you see fit. You no longer have to shackle yourself to societal norms or shy away from taboo topics. You get to step into your full, unique glory. It was an honor sharing this ride with you.

xo
Bailey

Join the Sisterhood

If you'd like further information about topics covered in this book, have new questions, or would like to connect with other women navigating this wild journey, join the private *Asking for a Pregnant Friend* group on Facebook. I'm the sole admin and respond to all questions within twenty-four hours. I also keep a close eye on the activity of the group, ensuring it is 100 percent free of shame and judgment. This is a safe space to feel heard and supported.

Blatant Plugs: To receive well-rounded support, I recommend checking out my first book, *Feng Shui Mommy: Creating Balance and Harmony for Blissful Pregnancy, Childbirth, and Motherhood*, which is a comprehensive, holistic guide to this wild journey you're on. In addition, my bestselling online course Childbirth Preparation: A Complete Guide for Pregnant Women is an excellent complement — you can find it here: udemy.com /course/childbirth-preparation-a-complete-guide-for-pregnant-women/. You can also receive a free download of "The Ultimate Birth Prep Workbook" at baileygaddis.com.

Acknowledgments

To all the women brave enough to share their intimate questions and stories with me, thank you. You made this book possible and inspired me to open up about my own raw experiences. Together, we can dissolve taboos by continuing to get real and refusing to let our true, messy, powerful selves be censored. I'm honored to be on this journey with you.

And then there's my child and husband, Hudson and Eric. Thank you for being integral parts of my wild path into motherhood and allowing me to air our complicated laundry.

To my mom, Anna Lee. Thank you for forging a mother-daughter relationship where taboos don't exist. I've felt safe talking to you since I first remember having taboo thoughts. And I'm sorry that you know way more about my sex life than you ever wanted to.

Thank you to my amazing editor, Georgia Hughes, who planted the seed of this book and gave me the honor of fostering its growth. Seeing *New World Library* on the spine of my books is such a thrill. You all are changing the world.

My deepest gratitude to Meghan Rudd Van Alstine. You were not only a steadfast friend through the birthing of this book (and always), but you also provided invaluable expert insights into the psychology of many of the taboos tackled in the book.

Amanda Sandoval, my goddess of graphic design — thank you for taking my strange ideas and turning them into comics that far surpass my initial vision. You are a badass.

Mel Lubey, many of the questions in this book wouldn't be nearly as juicy if it weren't for you. Thank you for your support with this book and all that you do for the birth community.

And finally, the women of Ojai. What a kaleidoscope of creators, visionaries, and powerhouses we have in this magical valley. My time with each of you (you know who you are!) is filled with expansion, joy, and a refreshing audacity to talk about all the things.

Essential Tips for the Journey

This section includes suggestions that support various aspects of the journey into motherhood.

Rest

To ensure you're not constantly in the "trying to keep my head above water" mode, allow yourself to rest as often as possible. When you're feeling depleted, scared, or overwhelmed, and you just want to curl up in your bed — do that. Let yourself escape into sleep, or a book, or whatever your instincts are telling you to do.

If you feel like to-dos pile up every time you rest, determine what can be handed off, at least for the time being. Ask your partner, family member, or friend to help out with housework, ask a colleague to temporarily take some of your workload, remind yourself that missing a workout in favor of rest is not going to derail your fitness. Give yourself permission to pause.

Move

Moving your body is one of the best ways to reduce stress and anxiety and keep your body healthy. Regular movement can also strengthen your birthing muscles, potentially making birth easier. But my favorite thing about movement is that it causes endorphins to release. Endorphins are your body's natural pain relievers and can be up to two hundred times more powerful than morphine. This hormone blocks your brain's ability to receive messages of pain from the sensory nerves, improves your mood, and can be passed through the placenta to baby. The more you move, the more skilled your body becomes at producing and releasing endorphins, which could cause more of these pain relievers to help you out during birth.

If you don't currently have an exercise routine, talk with your care provider about safe options. Walking, swimming, and prenatal yoga are typically safe and effective choices.

Eat

In addition to movement, what you eat has a significant impact on how you feel during pregnancy and beyond. Your care provider can help you determine if you're lacking in certain nutrients and need to eat more of a particular type of food or take a supplement. And because heartburn is an unsavory bedfellow of pregnancy, aim for eating six small meals a day, instead of three big ones.

Following are general guidelines for what types of food, and how much, you'll want to consume each day during pregnancy. It's also important to supplement your diet with prenatal vitamins.

- **Protein:** 2 to 3 servings (1 serving = 3 ounces, or the size of a deck of cards)
- **Green veggies:** 2 servings (1 serving = 1 cup)
- **Orange and yellow veggies:** 3 servings (1 serving = ½ cup)
- **Fruits and berries:** 2 to 3 servings (1 serving = ½ cup)
- **Fiber-rich foods (legumes, nuts, etc.):** 2 to 3 servings (1 serving = ½ cup), or enough to get the recommended 25 to 35 grams of fiber per day
- **Whole grains:** 3 servings (1 serving = ½ cup or 1 slice)
- **Calcium:** 1,000 milligrams per day; found in dairy, poultry, beans, nuts, salmon, turnip greens, and more
- **Water:** about 100 ounces each day, or 12 to 13 eight-ounce cups
- **Omega-3 fish oil:** Daily, take a high-quality fish oil supplement that has at least 300 mg of DHA (docosahexaenoic acid). Or, each week, have at least two servings of an omega-3-rich fish that has low levels of mercury, like salmon (1 serving = 3 ounces, or the size of a deck of cards).
- **Pink Himalayan sea salt:** To taste

Breathe

When stress, anxiety, or fear start taking over, dissolve them by focusing your attention on your breath. Envision peace, clarity, and courage flowing in with each inhalation, while fear, tension, and stress flow out with every exhalation. You emit a brightening glow with each breath, until you find yourself enveloped in healing energy. Let this energy enter every nerve and cell of your being — grounding you and filling you with a deep sense of calm.

Prepare Your Home

As you'll likely be spending a lot of time in your home once your baby arrives, you want it to feel like an oasis. One of the first steps to crafting this oasis is evicting all clutter. If you don't love it or regularly use it, donate or recycle it.

From there, fill your space with fresh air by opening windows when the weather allows, and placing air-purifying plants in your room (in a location baby can't reach when they become mobile). NASA found that the peace lily, spider plant, florist's chrysanthemum, red-edged dracaena, and English ivy all do wonders at removing toxins from the air.

As good lighting is also crucial, let in natural light during the day and use lamps in the evening, as they create a more soothing energy than overhead lighting. Placing three lamps at three different levels is ideal.

Finally, go through each room in your home and ask yourself, "How do I feel in this space?" If the answer isn't "amazing," brainstorm how you can enhance the space. Do you need to rearrange the furniture? Invest in attractive storage solutions? Paint the walls? Get rid of some focal points you hate looking at? Investing time in this project will help ensure you feel calm and clear when stuck at home (at least most of the time).

Find a Care Provider Who Believes in Patient Autonomy

Patient autonomy refers to a person's right to make a decision about their health care without their care provider trying to control that decision. Having a care provider who believes in patient autonomy will go far in ensuring your rights are honored during birth. Your care provider can (and should) share information with you about the state of your health, and baby's, and provide options if it looks like intervention is needed. However, they'll ideally share this information with as little bias as possible, encouraging you to make the decision that feels best to you and then honoring that decision.

Practicing patient autonomy — and being urged to do so — does wonders for self-governance, helping you have a more satisfying birth experience and fostering trust in yourself to make decisions without intervention from an authority figure. And this can seriously enhance your parenting experience.

Turn Your Birth Environment into a Sanctuary

Any location you birth in can be transformed into an environment filled with a sense of safety, calm, and joy by nurturing your five senses in that space. You can do this by making a list of your five senses — sight, sound, smell, taste, and touch — and then listing ideas on how you can support each during birth. For example, you could collect a few soothing prints to hang in your birthing room, in addition to some battery-powered candles; create a playlist with your favorite sleepy-time music and guided meditations; purchase an essential oil diffuser and a few of your favorite scents; pack a bag with coconut water, honey sticks, and breath mints; and find a cozy robe to wear during birth. I also recommend creating a sign to hang on the door of your birthing room that says, "Please knock gently, and enter only when invited in." This helps ensure you have control over who comes in and out of your space.

Maintain a Strong Voice during Birth

You can stay empowered during birth by making it clear to your care provider, during a prenatal appointment close to your due date, that much of your comfort during childbirth will depend on their ability to listen rather than pressuring you into anything. In the absence of a true emergency, they should honor your birth preferences, give you ample information about any interventions they recommend and what the alternatives are, and provide time and space for you to make your final decision in privacy. In addition, be super clear about not wanting to hear any fear-based language or tactics.

EFT (Emotional Freedom Technique) Instructions

This effective exercise can replace any fearful, chaotic energy running through the body with calm and clarity. I recommend using the EFT technique, also called *tapping*, before moving into any activity that may trigger negative emotions or physical responses.

Setup

Move through the following steps to begin experiencing emotional freedom. With practice, this technique can become a quick and easy tool to release negative emotions and physical reactions on the fly.

Pinpointing the Concern

Before you begin resetting your energy around a particular issue, you need to decide what issue you would like to work with. For example, the first time I tried EFT I chose to focus on my panic-attack-inducing fear of ultrasounds — specifically, the fear that there would be no heartbeat. (The EFT dissolved my fear.) Once you clear the energy for one issue, you can move on to others. So pick a specific issue that you'd like to start with. Because the fear of vaginal bleeding is common during pregnancy, we'll use that as our example; just insert your fear where appropriate.

Distress Assessment

We now need to determine how much distress this issue is causing. Close your eyes and focus on your fear of vaginal bleeding. On a scale of 0 to 10 — 0 being no pain or anxiety around this issue, and 10 being extreme pain or anxiety around it — decide what your current level of distress is.

Affirmation

Next, you'll tune your energy system in to the issue you're working on. To do this, locate two tender spots about two or three inches below your collarbone on each side of your chest. Rub those spots in a circular motion while saying the following affirmation three times out loud (or in your head):

"Although I have [insert issue here], I still profoundly and wholly love and honor myself."

So in our example the affirmation would be, "Although I have a fear of vaginal bleeding, I still profoundly and wholly love and honor myself" (again, said three times while rubbing your upper chest, not your boobs).

Tapping Points

Your fear (of vaginal bleeding, or childbirth, or spiders, or *The Real Housewives*, or fill in the blank) is now ripe for the resetting. Using the diagrams below, you're going to tap each point from 1 to 10, on both sides

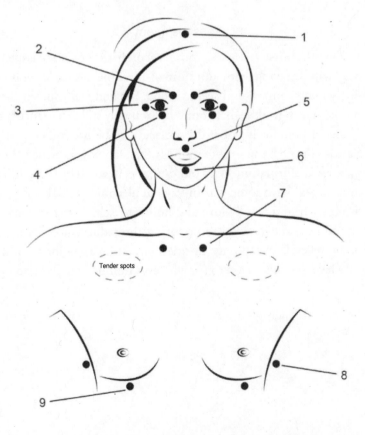

of the body, and repeat your affirmation with each number. Use your pointer and middle finger on each hand, so you can cover each side of your body with each round of counting. For a demonstration, go here: yourserenelife.wordpress.com/eft/.

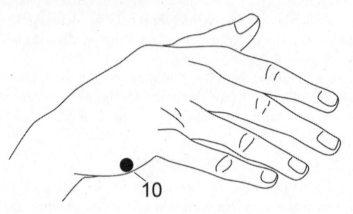

Repeat the sequence a few times, then close your eyes for a moment.

Reassessment

As you sit with yourself, reassess your level of distress over the issue you're working with. Staying with our fear-of-bleeding example, you might imagine wiping yourself and seeing blood. See and feel yourself there, in that moment, and notice what comes up. You may still experience hints of fear or anxiety, but likely not at the same level as before you tapped.

Now, go through a few more rounds of the tapping sequence, this time using a revised affirmation. With our example, it would be something like, "Although I still have some fear of vaginal bleeding, it's subsiding, and I still profoundly and wholly love and honor myself." We're still acknowledging the fear, and now we're honoring the reduction of its intensity. Continue the cycle of tapping, affirmations, and reassessment until your intensity level is down to a zero (or whatever number you feel good with).

APPENDIX 3

Fear Release Exercise

S uppressing fear-induced emotions infuses life into them, often causing a manifestation of depression or unpleasant physical symptoms. Here is a plan to liberate the emotions surrounding your fears so they can have their moment and then go bother someone else.

1. Meditate on the various elements of your life (e.g., friends, family, career, body, home, upcoming childbirth, etc.) and any fears that may be attached to them.

2. Write down the fears. If you've made it this far, tremendous progress has already been made. Fears hold the greatest power when they exist without you recognizing them.

3. Choose the fear that's causing you the greatest struggle and move through steps 4 and 5. There's no need to move through your entire list of fears in one day; be gentle with yourself, creating time for rest in between fear release sessions.

4. Set a timer for ninety seconds. Now close your eyes, visualize the fear, and allow the emotions attached to it to be expressed. Let yourself notice and experience the emotions and any accompanying physical sensations moving through you — let go of resistance and judgment toward the fear. Hold the intention that the emotions attached to the fear will be flushed out of you by the time your alarm chimes.

   (The fear you're working with may still be triggered after this exercise — that's normal, just give yourself the ninety seconds again to rerelease any attached emotions.)

5. Now that you've released the emotions attached to the fear, examine the fear objectively and decide whether it is:

   • **Completely outside your control, and able to be fully released by doing the ninety-second-release work anytime it comes up:** There is no benefit in stewing over a potential outcome you have no control over. For example, I was really nervous I'd

309

go into labor when stuck in traffic. As I had little control over when labor would begin, and I couldn't just stop driving, I did the fear release every time this concern popped up.

- **An issue you need to educate yourself on:** Knowledge gained pushes away uncertainty and invites in confidence. For example, I was so fearful of testing positive for group B strep (an infection caused by a common bacterium — often found in pregnancy) that I educated myself on what it actually is (not as scary as I thought), and what my options would be if I tested positive. When I did test positive, I felt calm and prepared.

- **A fear you need to talk through with another person:** Honest communication fosters peace, harmony, and connection. For example, if you're fearful of how your romantic relationship will shift after birth, share these concerns with your partner.

6. Do the work, mama. Just do it. When you release the emotions that hold up your fears, and you release the fear of them poking their heads up again (which they may do), you live from a space of love and trust, versus suffering and doubt.

Do It Daily

Every morning before you get out of bed, clear any negativity that may have made itself known as you slept by closing your eyes and envisioning any and all fears, doubts, or stressors being pulled from your mind, body, and spirit and collecting in a bubble floating in front of you. Then, deeply inhale, and as you exhale imagine the bubble being blown away from you and picked up by the wind. Imagine it being pulled so far out on the horizon it becomes a minuscule dot that pops and dissolves everything the bubble carried. Now smile, open your eyes, and claim your fresh day.

APPENDIX 4

List of the 101 Questions in This Book

Pregnancy

Mothering

Glossary

active labor: The phase of labor when your cervix dilates from six to eight or nine centimeters. This is when the intensity of labor really picks up and you're rarely able to talk during contractions.

afterbirth: The placenta and membranes that exit the uterus after the birth of baby. You will continue having contractions as the afterbirth comes out, but you'll be so distracted by baby you'll barely notice them. It can take thirty to sixty minutes for the afterbirth to emerge.

amniotic fluid: The protective fluid in the amniotic sac baby is floating in, made of water, nutrients, hormones, and antibodies. Near the end of gestation, the fluid is composed primarily of baby's urine. Beyond offering protection, the amniotic fluid supports the development of baby's lungs and gastrointestinal tract when it's breathed in and swallowed, helps to prevent the umbilical cord from being compressed, provides lubrication so webbing doesn't occur in areas of the body like the fingers and toes, and facilitates baby's muscle and bone development, as it gives them space to move.

birth preferences: A list of preferences the mom has for her birth experience. It's often organized by phases of birth: onset of labor, active labor, baby's descent, and preferences for mom and baby after birth. It's best to present this document to your care provider around week thirty-six of gestation to ensure they understand your desires.

Braxton Hicks contractions: These are like practice contractions. They can start as early as six weeks' gestation but usually aren't felt until the third trimester. They often consist of tightening and pulling sensations in the abdomen, sometimes accompanied by light cramping. To tell the difference between a Braxton Hicks contraction and one that indicates you're going into labor, drink a cup of water and walk around. This hydration and movement often causes a Braxton Hicks to dissolve, but will do little to stop a real contraction.

breech baby: The fetal position wherein baby's feet or butt are facing down toward the cervix. Many babies are breech throughout various phases of gestation but turn into the cephalic (head-down) position by around week thirty-six. However, it is possible for baby to turn into the head-down position after week thirty-six. In some cases of a breech position, an ECV (explained on page 143) will be recommended. While some care providers will deliver a baby in the breech position, many won't, as they're not comfortable with the challenges a breech delivery can present. To access a guided meditation for encouraging a breech baby to turn, go here: yourserenelife.wordpress .com/breech-baby/.

cervix: The narrow passageway that connects the vagina and uterus. It's primarily made of fibromuscular tissue and must open to ten centimeters before baby can be born.

cesarean birth: A surgical birth consisting of an incision through the mother's abdomen and uterus, also called a C-section. A care provider then removes the baby through the incision. The mother usually receives a regional anesthetic so she's numb from the waist down. In rare cases, general anesthesia is used.

colic: The phenomenon of a healthy infant frequently crying or being fussy for prolonged periods. Colic typically begins at around six weeks of age and usually resolves around three or four months. While the exact cause of colic is unknown, some believe digestive issues, food allergies, migraine, or stress triggers it.

contraction: The motion of uterine muscle tissue wherein the outer, longitudinal muscles in the uterus pull up, out, then push down. As they do this, the innermost, circular muscles of the uterus are pulled up and out, which is what causes the cervix to dilate and efface. Contractions usually intensify and become longer as labor progresses. They also typically occur in steady intervals. Often, the more relaxed you are during contractions, the more effective (and less painful!) they'll be.

crowning: When your baby's head remains visible and does not retract back into the vagina after pushing, it is crowning! Some women experience numbness during this phase, because of the pressure of baby's head on the nerves, while others might experience burning or stinging.

dilation: How open the cervix is. When the cervix is at ten centimeters (about the same diameter as a softball! Or a baby's head...), you're fully dilated.

early labor: The phase of labor from the onset of labor until the cervix is three centimeters dilated. Some women barely feel early labor, while others experience contractions strong enough to require deep breathing and other pain-relieving techniques.

engorgement: When your milk comes in and you get giant, rock-hard boobies! It's great. Oh wait, it's not. They'll also occasionally harden up as you and baby find your rhythm with feedings. To soften the breasts, place a warm compress on them, then self-express until they're soft enough for baby to nurse.

epidural: A local anesthetic that blocks nerve impulses from the lower spinal segments, creating numbness from the waist down; the most common type of pharmaceutical pain relief during birth. After the woman is given one to two liters of IV fluids, an anesthesiologist numbs the injection site in the lower portion of the spinal cord, then administers a small catheter attached to a needle. After application, the needle is removed, while the catheter remains to deliver medications administered by pump or occasional injection — these medications are usually a combination of numbing agents and opioids. After the epidural is placed, women typically feel only pressure during contractions. While many women don't feel the "let me tell you all my secrets" loopiness these types of meds are often associated with, some might feel a little drowsy or loose-lipped.

episiotomy: A surgical cut made in the perineum (tissue between the vaginal opening and anus) to make it easier for baby to emerge. While they used to be commonplace, episiotomies are now typically performed only in emergency situations.

fourth trimester: The first three months after baby's birth. Many have nicknamed this period the "fourth trimester" because the baby is still completely dependent on the mother, and they're both going through a time of profound change and integration.

gestational diabetes: Diabetes (high blood sugar) that develops in a pregnant woman who didn't have diabetes before conception. It is often managed through healthy eating and exercise. In some cases, insulin injections are needed.

glucose tolerance test: The test given to women between weeks twenty-four and twenty-eight of gestation to check for gestational diabetes. It consists of going to a lab (after fasting for at least eight hours) and having your blood drawn. You then drink a delightful beverage that tastes like the offspring of a sports drink and cough syrup. An hour later you're given another blood test, which evaluates how your blood reacted to the sugar blast. Because some women feel like poo after drinking the sugar drink, ask your care provider about other, more natural, foods or drinks you can use for the test — for example, apple juice or bananas.

high-risk pregnancy: Many care providers consider a pregnancy "high risk" if a woman has pre-existing conditions like high blood pressure or diabetes, is obese, is carrying more than one baby, or is over the age of thirty-five.

jaundice: A yellow discoloration in a newborn's skin and eyes, caused by a yellow pigment, called bilirubin, that's a by-product of the breakdown of red blood cells in the liver. While jaundice is usually harmless, it's best to alert your baby's pediatrician if you suspect they have it. To check, lightly press your finger against their forehead — if the skin turns yellow, they may have jaundice. It's often treated by placing the baby in the light of a window for around ten minutes twice a day.

lactation consultant: A professional breastfeeding specialist trained to support mothers with breastfeeding issues like latch, positioning, and milk production. Some hospitals employ lactation consultants who check your breastfeeding progress soon after baby's arrival. There are also lactation consultants who make house calls. I recommend hiring a board-certified lactation consultant (with *IBCLC* after their name).

linea nigra: The sexy, dark pregnancy line from the belly button to the pubic hair. It's actually always there but is often so faint at other times that you can't see it — that good ole shift in hormones causes the line to darken during pregnancy. It often fades after baby is born.

meconium: Baby's first poops, which often look like greenish-black tar, have no scent, and are sterile. They're composed of everything baby swallowed in the womb, like skin cells, lanugo, mucus, amniotic fluid, bile, and water. Sometimes, baby has a bowel movement in the womb, which would present as discoloration in the amniotic fluid. If this occurs and you're having a hospital birth, the NICU team will be present when baby is delivered in case they've aspirated any of the meconium.

mucus plug: The thick, jelly-like cervical mucus lodged between your cervix and uterus. It keeps bacteria and viruses from entering your uterus, and it comes out when your body is preparing for labor. You'll never be so excited to see a heap of discharge come out your vagina! It's typically clear, but it's normal to see a bit of a pink, red, yellow, or brown tinge in it. If a significant amount of bright red blood comes out with it, call your care provider.

NICU: The neonatal intensive care unit. It's the area of the hospital where baby will go if they need specialized care.

oxytocin: A hormone produced by the hypothalamus and secreted by the pituitary gland; also called *the love hormone.* It supports sexual reproduction, childbirth, and bonding, and it causes contractions. It's also released when baby breastfeeds, a phenomenon that's especially helpful right after birth, as it causes contractions that help the uterus shrink back to pre-pregnancy size and slows bleeding.

pelvic floor: A group of muscles in the floor of the pelvic area that stretch like a trampoline from the tailbone to the pubic bone. The pelvic floor muscles support the bladder, uterus, and colon, and the urine tube, vagina, and bowels pass through them. Keeping these muscles strong helps prevent lovely circumstances like wetting your pants when laughing, sneezing, and walking with a bounce in your step; and being surprised by flatulence. Because no one wants a saggy trampoline, it's important to strengthen these muscles with Kegel exercises, but it's equally important for pregnant women to practice relaxing the pelvic floor, as this relaxation is a crucial component of allowing the pelvic area to soften and widen as baby passes through at birth.

perineal tissue massage: A stretching technique to prepare your perineum for expansion during birth. This massage that feels nothing like a massage consists of coating your pointer and middle finger, or thumb, with an unscented, organic oil, inserting the fingers two inches into the vaginal opening, and moving the fingers in a U-shape along the edge of the perineum. I recommend applying more pressure when you reach the tautest skin (area between the vagina and anus), as this is the skin most likely to tear during birth. Push to the point of discomfort, utilizing pain-relieving techniques like deep breathing and facial relaxation. This makes the perineum become more elastic and helps mentally prepare you for the vaginal stretching during crowning. I recommend doing this nightly for about ten minutes, starting at around week thirty-five of gestation. If you want to test your partner's devotion, have them do the massage for you.

perineum: The area between the vulva and the anus.

Pitocin: A synthetic version of oxytocin, sometimes given to induce contractions. Pitocin is administered through an IV, and the dosage is gradually increased until the woman is having regular contractions, typically every two to three minutes. Pitocin can make contractions unnaturally strong, which can sometimes lead to the need for an epidural. However, it can be turned off at any time.

placenta: The organ that grows in your uterus during pregnancy and provides nutrients and oxygen to the baby and removes waste from baby's blood through the umbilical cord. Ideally, it attaches itself to the top or side of the uterus. It's made of tissue from the mother and the embryo, and is birthed about thirty minutes after baby. Question 64 covers the pros and cons of ingesting the placenta.

posterior or "sunny-side up" baby: The fetal position wherein baby is head down, but their face is pointed toward the front of your body, instead of toward your spine (called the anterior position, which is optimal). Laboring with a baby in this position can increase discomfort — especially in the back — and lengthen the time it takes to get little one out. In the "Recommended Resources" section, there's a link to a video with tips on how to turn a posterior baby into the anterior position.

postpartum: The period following childbirth.

postterm pregnancy: A pregnancy that has lasted longer than forty-two weeks' gestation.

pregnancy mask: A type of hyperpigmentation that causes tan or brown patches on the face; also called *melasma*. You can minimize it by wearing organic zinc oxide sunscreen and staying out of the sun as much as possible. It will often go away after birth.

preterm labor: Labor that occurs between twenty and thirty-seven weeks' gestation.

relaxin: A hormone that is secreted by the ovaries even when a woman isn't pregnant but is also produced by the placenta when she is pregnant. Higher levels of relaxin during pregnancy relax the walls of the uterus, minimizing the chance of contractions early in the pregnancy. It also relaxes ligaments in the pelvis and softens and widens the cervix in preparation for birth.

ring of fire: Comforting term used to describe the burning sensation some women feel as baby's head is crowning during delivery, causing the labia and perineum to stretch to capacity. If you have an epidural, you likely won't feel much more than pressure. Women having an unmedicated childbirth might not feel this burning either, as the endorphins that build up throughout labor and the pressure of the baby's head on nerves can cause a numbing sensation. While the pushing phase was the most exhausting for me, it was strangely the most comfortable because all I felt was intense pressure and fullness.

rupturing of membranes: Another term for the water breaking, which happens when the amniotic sac ruptures and the fluid drains out. While movies often depict this as a surprise gush that occurs when a woman is standing in public (often at a fancy restaurant), it usually doesn't happen until labor is well underway. It can happen naturally, or the care provider can break the sac to potentially speed up labor. Contractions usually become more intense after the water has released because there's no longer a "cushion" between baby and the uterus.

transition: The last, and often most intense, part of active labor, when you dilate to ten centimeters. Transition is usually a short phase consisting of incredibly strong contractions that typically last sixty to ninety seconds. If your water hasn't already broken, it might release during transition. You could also experience nausea and spotting. However, the most common indication you're moving through transition is a feeling like you can no longer do it — that you would like to pause labor and come back another time after you've had a full night's rest and gone to the spa. For women having an unmedicated birth, this is usually when they ask for an epidural. But no. By this point, you've come so far that all there is to do is remind yourself you're *so* close to meeting your baby *and* that you got to ten centimeters! That's a big deal. You're a big deal.

umbilical cord: The cord that goes from the placenta to baby's belly button and transports blood, oxygen, nutrients, and hormones.

VBAC: Stands for "vaginal birth after cesarean," meaning you've had at least one baby via cesarean but are having a subsequent baby vaginally. Question 50 in this book is devoted to VBACs.

walking epidural: A type of epidural that allows for more movement than the standard epidural, as it consists of a lower dose of medications; also called a *combined spinal-epidural*. While a woman can't actually walk with a "walking epidural," she can usually get into a variety of positions that facilitate birth. Many hospitals don't offer walking epidurals, so speak with your care provider if this is something you're interested in.

water birth: Laboring in warm water, which can promote relaxation, more effective contractions, enhanced flexibility in the perineum, and lower blood pressure. While some women choose to stay submerged for delivery and are often allowed to do so during a home or birth center birth, most hospitals require women to get out of the water before they deliver. Typically, baby won't take their first breath until exposed to air and continues receiving oxygen from the umbilical cord.

Endnotes

Pregnancy

p. 9   *a fetus's exposure to these hormones could potentially cause*: Sherri Lee Jones, Romane Dufoix, David Laplante, et al., "Larger Amygdala Volume Mediates the Association between Prenatal Maternal Stress and Higher Levels of Externalizing Behaviors: Sex Specific Effects in Project Ice Storm," *Frontiers in Human Neuroscience* 13, no. 144 (2019), https://doi.org/10.3389/fnhum.2019.00144.

p. 9   *maternal stress could increase the risk for preterm birth*: Aleksandra Staneva, Fiona Bogossian, Margo Pritchard, and Anja Wittkowski, "The Effects of Maternal Depression, Anxiety, and Perceived Stress during Pregnancy on Preterm Birth: A Systematic Review," *Women & Birth* 28, no. 3 (2015): 179, https://doi.org/10.1016/j.wombi.2015.02.003.

p. 9   *prenatal stress could result in low birth weight*: Mary Coussons-Read, "Effects of Prenatal Stress on Pregnancy and Human Development: Mechanisms and Pathways," *Obstetric Medicine* 6, no. 2 (2013): 52–57, https://doi.org/10.1177/1753495X12473751.

p. 12   *The bad news is that 10 percent of males cheat*: Robert Garrett Rodriguez, *What's Your Pregnant Man Thinking? A Roadmap for Expectant & New Mothers* (AuthorHouse, 2005), 71.

p. 25   *pregnant women with chronic high levels of anger*: Tiffany Field, M. Diego, Maria Hernandez-Reif, et al., "Prenatal Anger Effects on the Fetus and Neonate," *Journal of Obstetrics and Gynaecology* 22, no. 3 (2002): 260–66, https://doi.org/10.1080/01443610220130526. '

p. 31   *there were 2,457,118 reported cases of STDs*: CDC, "Reported STDs in the United States, 2018," n.d., https://www.cdc.gov/nchhstp/newsroom/docs/factsheets/STD-Trends-508.pdf.

p. 36   *only about 2 percent of women will have a repeat miscarriage*: Yadava Jeve and William Davies, "Evidence-Based Management of Recurrent Miscarriages," *Journal of Human Reproductive Sciences* 7, no. 3 (2014): 159–69, https://doi.org/10.4103/0974-1208.142475.

p. 36   *while women who have had a stillbirth have*: Kathleen Lamont, Neil Scott, Gareth Jones, and Sohinee Bhattacharya, "Risk of Recurrent Stillbirth: Systematic Review and Meta-analysis," *BMJ* 350, no. 3 (2015), https://doi.org/10.1136/bmj.h3080.

p. 37   *various factors that could potentially help you avoid*: Jeve and Davies, "Evidence-Based Management of Recurrent Miscarriages."

p. 37   *50 percent of miscarriages are unexplained*: Hayden Anthony Homer, "Modern Management of Recurrent Miscarriage," *Australian and New Zealand Journal of Obstetrics and Gynaecology* 59, no. 1 (2018): 1, https://doi.org/10.1111/ajo.12920.

p. 40   *I was ten weeks along, so according to a study*: Anne-Marie Nybo Andersen, Jan Wohlfahrt, Peter Christens, Jørn Olsen, and Mads Melbye, "Maternal Age and Fetal Loss: Population Based Register Linkage Study," *BMJ* 320, no. 7251 (2000): 1708, https://doi.org/10.1136/bmj.320.7251.1708.

p. 40   *To assure you even more that bleeding is pretty normal*: Juan Yang, David Savitz, Nancy Dole, et al., "Predictors of Vaginal Bleeding during the First Two Trimesters of Pregnancy," *Pediatric and Perinatal Epidemiology* 19, no. 4 (2006): 276, https://doi.org/10.1111/j.1365-3016.2005.00655.x.

p. 77   *pregnant women who ate oily fish*: Juliana dos Santos Vaz, Gilberto Kac, Pauline Emmett, John Davis, Jean Golding, and Joseph R. Hibbeln, "Dietary Patterns, n-3 Fatty Acids Intake from Seafood and High Levels of Anxiety Symptoms during Pregnancy: Findings from the Avon Longitudinal Study of Parents and Children," *PLOS One* 8, no. 7 (2013): e67671, https://doi.org/10.1371/journal.pone.0067671.

p. 77   *"sushi that was prepared in a clean and reputable establishment"*: Nathan Fox, "Dos and Don'ts in Pregnancy," *Obstetrics & Gynecology* 131, no. 4 (2018): 713–21, https://doi.org/10.1097/aog.0000000000002517.

p. 78   *most seafood-related illnesses are caused by shellfish*: Martha Iwamoto, Tracy Ayers, Barbara Mahon, and David Swerdlow, "Epidemiology of Seafood-Associated Infections in the United States," *Clinical Microbiology Reviews* 23, no. 2 (2010): 399–411, https://doi.org/10.1128/CMR.00059-09.

p. 79   *pregnant women over the age of thirty-four had only a slightly increased risk*: Dan Shan, Pei-Yuan Qiu, Yu-Xia Wu, et al., "Pregnancy Outcomes in Women of Advanced Maternal Age: A Retrospective Cohort Study from China," *Scientific Reports* 8, no. 1 (2018): 12239, https://doi.org/10.1038/s41598-018-29889-3.

p. 80   *women aged eighteen to thirty-four had a stillbirth rate*: M. Jolly, N. Sebire, J. Harris, S. Robinson, and L. Regan, "The Risks Associated with Pregnancy in Women Aged 35 Years or Older," *Human Reproduction* 15, no. 11 (2000): 2433–37, https://doi.org/10.1093/humrep/15.11.2433.

p. 85   *The use of misoprostol is controversial*: Madeline Oden and Doula Certificate, "The Freedom to Birth — The Use of Cytotec to Induce Labor: A Non-Evidence-Based Intervention," *Journal of Perinatal Education* 18, no. 2 (2009): 48–51, https://doi.org/10.1624/105812409X426332.

p. 86   *10 to 29 percent of fetuses experience nuchal cord*: Morarji Peesay, "Nuchal Cord and Its Implications," *Maternal Health, Neonatology and Perinatology* 3 (2017): 28, https://doi.org/10.1186/s40748-017-0068-7.

Birthing

p. 102   *a woman's positive and negative perceptions of her birth experience*: Katie Cook and Colleen Loomis, "The Impact of Choice and Control on Women's Childbirth

Experiences," *Journal of Perinatal Education* 21, no. 3 (2012): 158–68, https://doi.org /10.1891/1058-1243.21.3.158.

p. 112 *tokophobia — a morbid, pathological fear of childbirth*: Manjeet Singh Bhatia and Anurag Jhanjee, "Tokophobia: A Dread of Pregnancy," *Industrial Psychiatry Journal* 21, no. 2 (2012): 158, https://doi.org/10.4103/0972-6748.119649.

p. 114 *there was a 50 percent reduction in elective C-sections*: Bhatia and Jhanjee, "Tokophobia," 158.

p. 116 *planned home births for low-risk women result in*: Melissa Cheyney, Marit Bovbjerg, Courtney Everson, Wendy Gordon, Darcy Hannibal, and Saraswathi Vedam, "Outcomes of Care for 16,924 Planned Home Births in the United States: The Midwives Alliance of North America Statistics Project, 2004 to 2009," *Journal of Midwifery & Women's Health* 59, no. 1 (2014): 17–27, https://doi.org/10.1111 /jmwh.12172.

p. 120 *The importance of speaking up throughout childbirth*: Elsa Montgomery, Catherine Pope, and Jane Rogers, "The Re-enactment of Childhood Sexual Abuse in Ma-ternity Care: A Qualitative Study," *BMC Pregnancy and Childbirth* 15 (2015): 194, https://doi.org/10.1186/s12884-015-0626-9.

p. 121 *Read Penny Simkin's book* When Survivors Give Birth: Penny Simkin and Phyllis Klaus, *When Survivors Give Birth: Understanding and Healing the Effects of Early Sexual Abuse on Childbearing Women* (Seattle, WA: Classic Day Publishing, 2011).

p. 131 *To learn more, check out the article*: Amali Lokugamage and S. Pathberiya, "The Microbiome Seeding Debate — Let's Frame It around Women-Centred Care," *Reproductive Health* 16, no. 1 (2019): 91, https://doi.org/10.1186/s12978-019-0747-0.

p. 133 *this book helps you nurture your postpartum self*: Heng Ou, Amely Greeven, and Marisa Belger, *The First Forty Days: The Essential Art of Nourishing the New Mother* (New York: Harry N. Abrams, 2016).

p. 134 *a VBAC often decreases the risk of maternal mortality*: F. G. Cunningham, S. Bangdiwala, S. S. Brown, et al. for the National Institutes of Health Consensus Development Conference Panel, "National Institutes of Health Consensus Development Conference Statement: Vaginal Birth after Cesarean: New In-sights," *Obstetrics & Gynecology* 115, no. 6 (2010): 1293, https://doi.org/10.1097 /AOG.0b013e3181e459e5.

p. 134 *if you had a previous cesarean with a low transverse incision*: Cunningham, Bangdiwala, Brown, et al., "National Institutes of Health Consensus Develop-ment Conference Statement," 1296.

p. 134 *A survey done by the American College of Obstetricians and Gynecologists*: Cunningham, Bangdiwala, Brown, et al., "National Institutes of Health Consen-sus Development Conference Statement."

p. 139 *90 percent of women who have had a cesarean birth are candidates for a VBAC*: "Vaginal Birth after Cesarean: VBAC," American Pregnancy Association, April 25, 2019, https://americanpregnancy.org/labor-and-birth/vbac/.

p. 143   *reported that 33 percent of first-time mothers*: E. K. Hutton, J. C. Simioni, and
L. Thabane, "Predictors of Success of External Cephalic Version and Cephalic
Presentation at Birth among 1,253 Women With Noncephalic Presentation Using
Logistic Regression and Classification Tree Analyses," *Obstetric Anesthesia Digest*
38, no. 2 (2018): 105–6, https://doi.org/10.1097/01.aoa.0000532303.98988.72.

p. 143   *the following treatments may improve the outcome of an ECV*: Catherine Cluver,
Gillian Gyte, Marlene Sinclair, Therese Dowswell, and G. Justus Hofmeyr,
"Interventions for Helping to Turn Term Breech Babies to Head First Presenta-
tion When Using External Cephalic Version," *Cochrane Database of Systematic*
Reviews, 2012, https://doi.org/10.1002/14651858.cd000184.pub4.

p. 149   *women with epidurals typically have to push*: Yvonne Cheng, Brian Shaffer, James
Nicholson, and Aaron Caughey, "Second Stage of Labor and Epidural Use: A
Larger Effect than Previously Suggested," *Obstetric Anesthesia Digest* 35, no. 1
(2015): 49–50, https://doi.org/10.1097/01.aoa.0000460423.58316.20.

p. 149   *women who receive an epidural are more likely to develop a fever*: Scott Segal,
"Labor Epidural Analgesia and Maternal Fever," *Anesthesia & Analgesia* 111, no. 6
(2010): 1467–75, https://doi.org/10.1213/ane.0b013e3181f713d4.

p. 150   *only 1.2 in 10,000 women experience this*: Muhammad Atif Ameer, Thomas Knorr,
and Fassil Mesfin, "Spinal Epidural Abscess," *StatPearls* (StatPearls Publishing,
2020), https://www.ncbi.nlm.nih.gov/books/NBK441890/.

p. 150   *Limited research has found that babies of women who had Pitocin*: Melissa Small-
wood, Ashley Sareen, Emma Baker, Rachel Hannusch, Eddy Kwessi, and Tyisha
Williams, "Increased Risk of Autism Development in Children Whose Mothers
Experienced Birth Complications or Received Labor and Delivery Drugs," *ASN*
Neuro 8, no. 4 (2016): 1759091416659742, https://doi.org/10.1177/1759091416659742.

p. 150   *babies exposed to Pitocin during birth had 2.4 times increased odds*: David
Freedman, Alan Brown, Ling Shen, and Catherine Schaefer, "Perinatal Oxytocin Increases the Risk of Offspring Bipolar Disorder and Childhood Cognitive
Impairment," *Journal of Affective Disorders* 173 (2015): 65–72, https://doi.org
/10.1016/j.jad.2014.10.052.

p. 151   *when these two questions are asked, the rate of unnecessary intervention*: Tamara
Kaufman, "Evolution of the Birth Plan," *Journal of Perinatal Education* 16, no. 3
(2007): 47–52, https://doi.org/10.1624/105812407X217985.

p. 152   *the estimated risk of permanent harm following a spinal anesthetic*: T. M. Cook, D.
Counsell, and J. A. W. Wildsmith for the Royal College of Anaesthetists, "Major
Complications of Central Neuraxial Block: Report on the Third National Audit
Project of the Royal College of Anaesthetists," *British Journal of Anaesthesia* 102,
no. 2 (2009): 179–90, https://doi.org/10.1093/bja/aen360.

p. 154   *genes account for 34 to 45 percent of a woman's ability to climax*: Kate Dunn, Lynn
Cherkas, and Tim Spector, "Genetic Influences on Variation in Female Orgasmic

Function: A Twin Study," *Biology Letters* 1, no. 3 (2005): 260–63, https://doi.org/10.1098/rsbl.2005.0308.

p. 155   *Most women who have orgasmic births prepare thoroughly*: Elizabeth Davis and Debra Pascali-Bonaro, *Orgasmic Birth: Your Guide to a Safe, Satisfying, and Pleasurable Birth Experience* (Emmaus, PA: Rodale, 2016); *Orgasmic Birth: The Best Kept Secret*, directed by Debra Pascali-Bonaro and available at www.orgasmicbirth.com.

p. 178   *a retained placenta occurs in only 1 to 3 percent of deliveries*: Nicola Perlman and Daniela Carusi, "Retained Placenta after Vaginal Delivery: Risk Factors and Management," *International Journal of Women's Health* 11 (2019): 527–34, https://doi.org/10.2147/ijwh.s218933.

p. 179   *prolonged use of Pitocin could increase the risk of a retained placenta*: Perlman and Carusi, "Retained Placenta after Vaginal Delivery."

Mothering

p. 200   *one in nine women experience symptoms of postpartum depression*: Jean Ko, Karilynn Rockhill, Van Tong, Brian Morrow, and Sherry Farr, "Trends in Postpartum Depressive Symptoms — 27 States, 2004, 2008, and 2012," *Morbidity and Mortality Weekly Report (MMWR)* 66, no. 6 (2017): 153–58, https://doi.org/10.15585/mmwr.mm6606a1.

p. 201   *Sadly, about 60 percent of women with symptoms of depression*: Ko, Rockhill, Tong, Morrow, and Farr, "Trends in Postpartum Depressive Symptoms."

p. 201   *As added incentive to seek support, consider this*: Emma Robertson, Sherry Grace, Tamara Wallington, and Donna E. Stewart, "Antenatal Risk Factors for Postpartum Depression: A Synthesis of Recent Literature," *General Hospital Psychiatry* 26, no. 4 (2004): 289–95, https://doi.org/10.1016/j.genhosppsych.2004.02.006.

p. 213   *74 percent of mothers and 70 percent of fathers reported preferential treatment*: Barbara Shebloski, Katherine Conger, and Keith Widaman, "Reciprocal Links among Differential Parenting, Perceived Partiality, and Self-Worth: A Three-Wave Longitudinal Study," *Journal of Family Psychology* 19, no. 4 (2005): 633–42, https://doi.org/10.1037/0893-3200.19.4.633.

p. 219   *Read* Good Dog, Happy Baby: Michael Wombacher, *Good Dog, Happy Baby* (Novato, CA: New World Library, 2015).

p. 221   *when serotonin-producing neurons are inhibited*: Ryan Dosumu-Johnson, Andrea Cocoran, YoonJeung Chang, Eugene Nattie, and Susan M Dymecki, "Acute Perturbation of *Pet1*-Neuron Activity in Neonatal Mice Impairs Cardiorespiratory Homeostatic Recovery," *ELife* 7 (2018), https://doi.org/10.7554/elife.37857.

p. 221   *the prone (facedown) position has been found*: Jhodie Duncan and Roger Byard, eds., *SIDS Sudden Infant and Early Childhood Death: The Past, the Present, and the Future* (Adelaide, Australia: University of Adelaide Press, 2018).

p. 222   *a mild degree of respiratory viral infection was observed*: E. Athanasakis, S. Karavasiliadou, and I. Styliadis, "The Factors Contributing to the Risk of Sudden Infant Death Syndrome," *Hippokratia* 15, no. 2 (2011): 127–11, PMID: 22110293.

p. 222   *common bacterial toxins found in the respiratory tract*: Jane Blood-Siegfried, "The Role of Infection and Inflammation in Sudden Infant Death Syndrome," *Immunopharmacology and Immunotoxicology* 31, no. 4 (2009): 516–23, https://doi .org/10.3109/08923970902814137.

p. 222   *smoking during pregnancy is considered one of the*: Duncan and Byard, *SIDS Sudden Infant and Early Childhood Death.*

p. 222   *And exposure to secondhand smoke after birth*: Blood-Siegfried, "The Role of Infection and Inflammation in Sudden Infant Death Syndrome."

p. 223   *many premature babies have impaired blood pressure control*: Nicole B. Witcombe, Stephanie R. Yiallourou, Scott A. Sands, Adrian M. Walker, and Rosemary S. Horne, "Preterm Birth Alters the Maturation of Baroreflex Sensitivity in Sleeping Infants," *Pediatrics* 129, no. 1 (2011), https://doi.org/10.1542/peds.2011-1504.

p. 223   *long QT syndrome accounts for 12 percent of SIDS cases*: Nikolaos Ioakeimidis, Theodora Papamitsou, Soultana Meditskou, and Zafiroula Iakovidou-Kritsi, "Sudden Infant Death Syndrome Due to Long QT Syndrome: A Brief Review of the Genetic Substrate and Prevalence," *Journal of Biological Research-Thessaloniki* 24, no. 1 (2017): 6, https://doi.org/10.1186/s40709-017-0063-1.

p. 223   *A New Zealand scientist and chemist, Dr. James Sprott*: David Tappin, Hazel Brooke, Russell Ecob, and Angus Gibson, "Used Infant Mattresses and Sudden Infant Death Syndrome in Scotland: Case-Control Study," *BMJ* 325, no. 7371 (2002): 1007, https://doi.org/10.1136/bmj.325.7371.1007.

p. 224   *babies of women who obtain regular prenatal care*: Rachel Moon for the Task Force on Sudden Infant Death Syndrome, "SIDS and Other Sleep-Related Infant Deaths: Updated 2016 Recommendations for a Safe Infant Sleeping Environment," *Pediatrics* 138, no. 5 (2016): e20162938, https://doi.org/10.1542/peds.2016 -2938.

p. 224   *babies who are exclusively breastfed have a 50 percent lower*: Moon, "SIDS and Other Sleep-Related Infant Deaths."

p. 225   *swaddling might increase the risk for SIDS*: Anna Pease, Peter Fleming, Fern Hauck, et al., "Swaddling and the Risk of Sudden Infant Death Syndrome: A Meta-Analysis," *Pediatrics* 137, no. 6 (2016): e20153275, https://doi.org/10.1542 /peds.2015-3275.

p. 225   *babies sleep in their parents' room for the first twelve months*: Moon, "SIDS and Other Sleep-Related Infant Deaths."

p. 227   *new mothers report unwanted intrusive thoughts of infant-related harm*: Fanie Collardeau, Bryony Corbyn, John Abramowitz, Patricia Janssen, Sheila Woody, and Nichole Fairbrother, "Maternal Unwanted and Intrusive Thoughts of Infant-Related Harm, Obsessive-Compulsive Disorder and Depression in the

Perinatal Period: Study Protocol," *BMC Psychiatry* 19, no. 94 (2019), https://doi
.org/10.1186/s12888-019-2067-x.

p. 249　*breastfeeding can decrease a woman's chances of developing postpartum depression*: Aisha Hamdan and Hani Tamim, "The Relationship between Postpartum
Depression and Breastfeeding," *International Journal of Psychiatry in Medicine* 43,
no. 3 (2012): 243–59, https://doi.org/10.2190/pm.43.3.d.

p. 258　*In addition, the prolactin your body is pumping out*: Viola Polomeno, "An Independent Study Continuing Education Program — Sex and Breastfeeding: An
Educational Perspective," *Journal of Perinatal Education* 8, no. 1 (1999): 29–42,
https://doi.org/10.1624/105812499x86962.

p. 259　*during lactation you experience little to no vaginal lubrication*: Polomeno, "An
Independent Study Continuing Education Program."

p. 266　*Various studies have detected small quantities of THC*: "Cannabis," Drugs and
Lactation Database (LactMed) [Internet], US National Library of Medicine,
February 7, 2019, https://www.ncbi.nlm.nih.gov/books/NBK501587/.

p. 267　*more than four hundred chemicals in marijuana*: Kerri Bertrand, Nathan Hanan,
Gordon Honerkamp-Smith, Brookie Best, and Christina Chambers, "Marijuana
Use by Breastfeeding Mothers and Cannabinoid Concentrations in Breast Milk,"
Pediatrics 2, no. 3 (2018): e20181076, https://doi.org/10.1542/peds.2018-1076.

p. 267　*Shedding a less damaging light on marijuana use*: Teresa Baker, Palika Datta,
Kathleen Rewers-Felkins, Heather Thompson, Raja Kallem, and Thomas Hale,
"Transfer of Inhaled Cannabis into Human Breast Milk," *Obstetrics & Gynecology*
131, no. 5 (2018): 783–88, https://doi.org/10.1097/aog.0000000000002575.

p. 267　*Regarding the effects of marijuana*: "Cannabis," Drugs and Lactation Database
(LactMed).

p. 277　*regardless of parental smoking or breastfeeding status*: Moon, "SIDS and Other
Sleep-Related Infant Deaths."

p. 277　*found that 61 percent of respondents from a 2015*: Jennifer Bombard, Katherine
Kortsmit, Lee Warner, et al., "Vital Signs: Trends and Disparities in Infant Safe
Sleep Practices — United States, 2009–2015," *Morbidity and Mortality Weekly Re-
port (MMWR)* 67, no. 1 (2018): 39–46, https://doi.org/10.15585/mmwr.mm6701e1.

p. 277　*breastfeeding infants who routinely shared a bed*: James J. McKenna, Sarah S.
Mosko, and Christopher A. Richard, "Bedsharing Promotes Breastfeeding,"
Pediatrics 100, no. 2 (1997): 214–19, https://doi.org/10.1542/peds.100.2.214.

p. 277　*out of the 54 percent of 18,986 participants*: Eve Colson, Marian Willinger, Denis
Rybin, et al., "Trends and Factors Associated with Infant Bed Sharing, 1993-2010,"
JAMA Pediatrics 167, no. 11 (2013): 1032, https://doi.org/10.1001/jamapediatrics
.2013.2560.

p. 278　*bed-sharing was reported in 39 percent*: Barbara M. Ostfeld, Harold Perl, Linda
Esposito, et al., "Sleep Environment, Positional, Lifestyle, and Demographic

Characteristics Associated with Bed Sharing in Sudden Infant Death Syndrome Cases: A Population-Based Study," *Pediatrics* 118, no. 5 (January 2006): 2051–59, https://doi.org/10.1542/peds.2006-0176.

p. 278   *the risk of bed-sharing seems to be more connected*: R. Scragg, E. Mitchell, B. Taylor, et al., "Bed Sharing, Smoking, and Alcohol in the Sudden Infant Death Syndrome. New Zealand Cot Death Study Group," *BMJ* 307, no. 6915 (1993): 1312–18, https://doi.org/10.1136/bmj.307.6915.1312.

p. 278   *cosleeping on a sofa significantly increased the risk*: Peter Blair, Peter Fleming, Iain Smith, et al., The CESDI SUDI Research Group and E. Mitchell, "Babies Sleeping with Parents: Case-Control Study of Factors Influencing the Risk of the Sudden Infant Death Syndrome," *BMJ* 319 (7223): 1457–62, https://doi.org/10.1136/bmj.319.7223.1457.

p. 278   *a person is more likely to be hit by lightning*: National Weather Service, "How Dangerous Is Lightning?" 2019, https://www.weather.gov/safety/lightning-odds.

p. 278   *than a low-risk baby is to die of SIDS*: Robert Carpenter, Cliona McGarvey, Edwin Mitchell, et al., "Bed Sharing When Parents Do Not Smoke: Is There a Risk of SIDS? An Individual Level Analysis of Five Major Case-Control Studies," *BMJ Open* 3, no. 5 (2013), https://bmjopen.bmj.com/content/3/5/e002299.

p. 279   *mothers create a type of "shield" around the baby*: James McKenna, Helen Ball, and Lee Gettler, "Mother–Infant Cosleeping, Breastfeeding and Sudden Infant Death Syndrome: What Biological Anthropology Has Discovered about Normal Infant Sleep and Pediatric Sleep Medicine," *American Journal of Physical Anthropology* 134, S45 (2007): 133–61, https://doi.org/10.1002/ajpa.20736.

p. 279   *McKenna has also found that safely bed-sharing*: McKenna, Ball, and Gettler, "Mother–Infant Cosleeping, Breastfeeding and Sudden Infant Death Syndrome."

p. 280   *Japan has one of the lowest rates of SIDS*: Fern Hauck and Kawai Tanabe, "International Trends in Sudden Infant Death Syndrome: Stabilization of Rates Requires Further Action," *Pediatrics* 122, no. 3 (2008): 660–66, https://doi.org/10.1542/peds.2007-0135.

p. 280   *Cross-cultural data also shows that cultures where cosleeping*: McKenna, Ball, and Gettler, "Mother–Infant Cosleeping, Breastfeeding and Sudden Infant Death Syndrome."

p. 280   *bed-sharing causes mother and infant to spend more time*: McKenna, Ball, and Gettler, "Mother–Infant Cosleeping, Breastfeeding and Sudden Infant Death Syndrome."

p. 280   *Historians have documented the origin of the practice*: McKenna, Ball, and Gettler, "Mother–Infant Cosleeping, Breastfeeding and Sudden Infant Death Syndrome."

p. 280   *It's common practice in Bali*: McKenna, Ball, and Gettler, "Mother–Infant Cosleeping, Breastfeeding and Sudden Infant Death Syndrome."

p. 280   *A study of 2,080 families showed that regular*: Kimberly Howard, Anne Martin, Lisa Berlin, and Jeanne Brooks-Gunn, "Early Mother–Child Separation,

Parenting, and Child Well-Being in Early Head Start Families," *Attachment & Human Development* 13, no. 1 (2011): 5–26, https://doi.org/10.1080/14616734.2010. 488119.

p. 280   *parents who bed-shared with their breastfed babies*: Helen Ball, "Parent-Infant Bedsharing Behavior," *Human Nature* 17, no. 3 (2006): 301–18, https://doi.org /10.1007/s12110-006-1011-1.

p. 285   *Water makes up 55 to 75 percent*: Barry Popkin, Kristen D'Anci, and Irwin Rosenberg, "Water, Hydration, and Health," *Nutrition Reviews* 68, no. 8 (2010): 439–58, https://doi.org/10.1111/j.1753-4887.2010.00304.x.

p. 288   *only children are not more likely to be narcissistic*: Michael Dufner, Mitja Back, Franz Oehme, and Stefan Schmukle, "The End of a Stereotype: Only Children Are Not More Narcissistic than People with Siblings," *Social Psychological and Personality Science* 11, no. 3 (2019): 416–24, https://doi.org/10.1177/19485506198 70785.

p. 288   *only children typically have the same number*: Katherine Kitzmann, Robert Cohen, and Rebecca Lockwood, "Are Only Children Missing Out? Comparison of the Peer-Related Social Competence of Only Children and Siblings," *Journal of Social and Personal Relationships* 19, no. 3 (2002): 299–316, https://doi.org/10.1177 /0265407502193001.

Recommended Resources

Affordable Doula Care

Birth Options Alliance (Washington, DC): birthoptionsalliance.org/free
-and-low-cost-birth-doulas-and-postpartum-doulas.html

Doula Medicaid Project: healthlaw.org/doulamedicaidproject/

The Doula Project (New York City): doulaproject.net

List of volunteer doula programs across the United States: radicaldoula
.com/becoming-a-doula/volunteer-programs/

Joy In Birthing Foundation (Los Angeles County):
joyinbirthingfoundation.org

Breech Babies

Breech-Baby-Turn Hypnosis Recording: yourserenelife.wordpress.com
/breech-baby/

Dr. Stuart Fischbein: birthinginstincts.com

Spinning Babies: spinningbabies.com

Childbirth Preparation

Childbirth Preparation: A Complete Guide for Pregnant Women
(Bailey's online course): udemy.com/course/childbirth-preparation
-a-complete-guide-for-pregnant-women/

Birthing from Within: birthingfromwithin.com

The Bradley Method: bradleybirth.com

The Complete Guide to the Alexander Technique: alexandertechnique.com

HypnoBirthing: us.hypnobirthing.com

Lamaze International: lamaze.org

Cosleeping

Safe Cosleeping Guidelines: cosleeping.nd.edu/safe-co-sleeping-guidelines/

Counseling Resources

Psychology Today: psychologytoday.com/us

Doula Resources

American Pregnancy Association — What Is a Doula?:
    americanpregnancy.org/labor-and-birth/having-a-doula/
Birth Doula Services: yourserenelife.wordpress.com/birth-doula-services/
DONA International: dona.org/what-is-a-doula/find-a-doula/
DoulaMatch.net

Guided Meditation Downloads

Awaken the Courage to Advocate for Your Birthing Rights:
    yourserenelife.wordpress.com/birthing-rights/
Discovering the Ideal Environment for Birth:
    yourserenelife.wordpress.com/ideal-birth-space/
Enhancing Your Confidence for Childbirth:
    yourserenelife.wordpress.com/enhancing-birth-confidence/
Enjoying Your Rainbow Baby Pregnancy:
    yourserenelife.wordpress.com/rainbow-baby/
Feeling Calm as an Epidural Is Placed:
    yourserenelife.wordpress.com/epidural-meditation/
Journey through a Gentle C-section:
    yourserenelife.wordpress.com/gentle-csection/
Journey through a Peaceful VBAC: yourserenelife.wordpress.com/vbac/
Making Peace with the Unknowns of Childbirth:
    yourserenelife.wordpress.com/unknowns-of-childbirth/
Preparing for an Orgasmic Birth:
    yourserenelife.wordpress.com/orgasmic-birth/
Releasing Disappointment about Your Baby's Gender:
    yourserenelife.wordpress.com/babys-gender/
Releasing Shame during Pregnancy:
    yourserenelife.wordpress.com/releasing-shame/
Releasing the Fear of Dying during Childbirth:
    yourserenelife.wordpress.com/fear-of-dying/

Releasing the Fear of Tearing during Childbirth:
   yourserenelife.wordpress.com/fear-of-tearing/
Turning a Breech Baby: yourserenelife.wordpress.com/breech-baby/

Midwife Associations

American College of Nurse-Midwives: midwife.org
Midwives Alliance of North America: mana.org
National Association of Certified Professional Midwives: nacpm.org
North American Registry of Midwives: narm.org

Parenting Classes and Books

*How to Talk So Little Kids Will Listen: A Survival Guide to Life with
   Children Ages 2–7* by Joanna Faber and Julie King (Scribner, 2017).
No Bad Kids: Toddler Discipline without Shame by Janet Lansbury
   (CreateSpace, 2014).
*Parenting with Presence: Practices for Raising Conscious, Confident, Caring
   Kids* by Susan Stiffelman (New World Library, 2015).
Respectful Parenting Sessions with Janet Lansbury:
   sites.fastspring.com/jlmlpress/product/sessions
RIE Parenting Classes: rie.org
*The Whole-Brain Child: 12 Revolutionary Strategies to Nurture Your
   Child's Developing Mind* by Daniel Siegel and Tina Payne Bryson
   (Bantam, 2012).

Parenting Children with Special Needs

ARCH National Respite Network: archrespite.org
Caregiver Action Network: caregiveraction.org
Center for Parent Information & Resources, Find Your Parent Center:
   parentcenterhub.org/find-your-center/
Complex Child E-Magazine: complexchild.org
Different Dream Living: differentdream.com
Mommies of Miracles: facebook.com/MommiesofMiracles
Nancy's House (Mid-Atlantic region): nancys-house.org

National Down Syndrome Society, "Welcome to Holland":
ndss.org/lifespan/a-parents-perspective/
Parent to Parent: p2pusa.org

Your Rights during Childbirth

American College of Obstetricians and Gynecologists' Committee
Opinion on Refusal of Medically Recommended Treatment during
Pregnancy: acog.org/clinical/clinical-guidance/committee-opinion
/articles/2016/06/refusal-of-medically-recommended-treatment
-during-pregnancy
Childbirth Connection — Making Informed Decisions:
childbirthconnection.org/maternity-care/making-informed-decisions/
Human Rights in Childbirth: humanrightsinchildbirth.org
Improving Birth: improvingbirth.org

SIDS (Sudden Infant Death Syndrome)

American SIDS Institute: Sids.org
International Society for the Study and Prevention of Perinatal and
Infant Death: ispid.org
Pregnancy after Loss Support: pregnancyafterlosssupport.org
SleepFoundation.org

VBAC (Vaginal Birth after Caesarian) Support

International Cesarean Awareness Network (ICAN): ican-online.org
ICAN's hotline: 1-800-686-4226

Videos

Gaddis, Bailey. "How to Reposition a Posterior, or 'Sunny Side Up,' Baby."
March 7, 2019. YouTube video, 0:5:57, youtu.be/wgN41r5i7gQ.

Index

abscesses, epidural, 150, 152

abdominal pain, 76

abdominal surgery, 134

abortion, xiii, 44–45

abuse, 10, 118–23

acceptance, 295, 296

acne, 65–66, 265

acupuncture, 12, 38, 57, 109, 141

addictions, 64

adenomyosis, 246

adrenaline, 25, 285

advanced maternal age (AMA), 79–80

advice, unsolicited, 202–5, 296–97

affection, 202, 234

affirmations, 136–37

afterbirth, 318

age issues, 78–81

air fresheners, 75

air purifiers, 225, 304

air quality, 284, 304

alcohol: cosleeping and, 276, 278, 281, 282;
pregnancy and safe amounts of, 77,
78; pregnancy loss prevention and, 38;
SIDS risk and, 224

Alexander Technique, 335

allergies, 251, 286

alone time, 25, 231, 275

American Academy of Pediatrics, 224, 225,
277

American College of Nurse-Midwives, 337

American College of Obstetricians and
Gynecologists, 134; Committee on
Refusal of Medically Recommended
Treatment during Pregnancy, 338;
Resource Center, 100

American Pregnancy Association, 139, 336

American SIDS Institute, 338

amniocentesis, 82

amniotic fluid, 50; amniocentesis test and,
82; defined, 318; discoloration of, 321;
levels of, 70, 143, 147; "pruning" effects
of, 88

amniotic sac, 324

anchors, 124–25

androgens, 65, 67

androstenedione, 67

anemia, 176, 286

anesthesia, 127–28, 319, 320. *See also* epidurals

anesthetic spray, 160

anger, 296

anterior cingulated cortex, 154

antibacterial products, 72–73

antibiotics, 58, 179

antibodies, 237

anti-itch products, 69

antioxidants, 63, 257

anxiety: birthing environment and, 118,
156; desire to return to work and, 285;
diet and, 63, 77, 285; due dates and,
108; exercise and, 302; fatigue and, 285;
fetus and, 9; intrusive thoughts and,
229; marijuana use and, 268; mother/
baby relationship and, 200; of pets
toward babies, 218; postpartum, 230;
prenatal testing and, 113; rainbow
baby pregnancies and, 36; release tools
for, 41, 153, 303, 306–8; sexual trauma
history and, 118–23; over SIDS risk,
220; social, 25; STDs and, 33; stress
and, 9–10; therapy and, 285; women of
AMA and minimization of, 80–81

About the Author

Bailey Gaddis is the author of *Feng Shui Mommy: Creating Balance and Harmony for Blissful Pregnancy, Childbirth, and Motherhood* (New World Library, 2017). She is also a certified hypnotherapist, certified birthing doula, HypnoBirthing® practitioner, HypnoMothering® practitioner, founding member of the Ojai Valley Birth Collective, and past IVF coordinator. She's contributed to *Working Mother, Fit Pregnancy, Pregnancy, Newborn*, Disney's parenting site *Babble, Elephant Journal, Cosmopolitan, Redbook, Woman's Day, Good Housekeeping, Scary Mommy, Natural Solutions, Natural Mother, YourTango, American Baby, Green Child, Huffington Post*, and more.

Bailey also supports families navigating cancer by volunteering her hypnotherapy services at the cancer resource center OjaiCARES. In addition, Bailey volunteers for the ParentCare Program at Secure Beginnings, where she offers in-home support to parents of newborn babies. She lives in Ojai, California, with her husband and son.

For a list of Bailey's online courses and to download "The Ultimate Birth Prep Workbook," visit baileygaddis.com.